MALABSORPTION IN COELIAC SPRUE

MALABSORPTION IN COELIAC SPRUE

O. J. J. CLUYSENAER M.D.
and
J. H. M. VAN TONGEREN M.D.

Department of Medicine, Division of Gastroenterology, Sint Radboud Hospital,
University of Nijmegen, The Netherlands.

with a foreword by
C. C. BOOTH M.D., F.R.C.P.
Professor of Medicine, Royal Postgraduate Medical School, London

Springer-Science+Business Media, B.V. 1977

ISBN 978-90-247-2000-2   ISBN 978-94-010-1093-1 (eBook)
DOI 10.1007/ 978-94-010-1093-1

© *Springer Science+Business Media Dordrecht 1977*
Originally published by Martinus Nijhoff The Hague in 1977

Cover illustration from Andreas Vesalius
(De humani corporis fabrica V, 1543).

FOREWORD

For at least three centuries, Holland has been at the centre of research on intestinal malabsorption. In the 17th and 18th centuries, early descriptions of coeliac disease and tropical sprue were published by physicians trained in Holland, and it was in 1950 that Dicke published his painstaking and vital observations that coeliac disease in children was caused by the ingestion of wheat flour. Subsequent careful work with van de Kamer and Weijers showed that the harmful agent was gluten.

Since these discoveries were made, research in intestinal malabsorption, particularly in the adult, has continued in several centres in Holland. At Nijmegen, for example, dr. Cluysenaer, dr. van Tongeren and their associates have been involved in long-term studies of patients with intestinal disease for the past fifteen years. In this book they describe their experience of the investigation and treatment of fifty patients with the adult form of coeliac disease. Their monograph gives an account of the history, definition and incidence of the disorder, and then goes on to undertake a critical review of the pathogenesis of the coeliac lesion. Before embarking on the different patterns of malabsorption seen in adult coeliac disease, the authors describe the normal small intestine, its morphology and function. Coeliac disease is associated with a wide range of nutritional deficiencies and the authors have therefore concentrated not only on the more obvious intestinal lesion, but also on how vitamins and minerals are absorbed and on how deficiencies may arise in clinical practice. Their clinical experience enables them to define the widely different modes of presentation of the disease. They also describe the important association of coeliac disease with other disorders such as dermatitis herpetiformis. Treatment of malabsorption in the adult may be particularly difficult in those patients who do not respond to the withdrawal of gluten from their diet, a situation recognised by these authors who wisely separate this group of disorders from coeliac disease.

The understanding of human disease, from which successful treatment must stem, is based on observation and experiment. This monograph is an admirable example of careful clinical observation coupled with a detailed review of the experimental work upon which modern intestinal physiology and pathology are based. It is a further addition to the literature on intestinal malabsorption to which Dutch physicians have contributed so much.

C. C. Booth

ACKNOWLEDGMENTS

We gratefully acknowledge all persons who contributed to the realization of this monograph.

The assistance of the nursing staff of the gastrointestinal unit (head: miss A. M. Th. W. van der Belt; previously miss J. M. T. Dekkers), and of the out-patients' department (heads: miss Th. Th. M. Hoogenbosch, miss L. M. J. Schreppers and mr. G. C. Th. Delisse) is greatly appreciated. A great deal of work was done by the technicians of the laboratories for Clinical Chemistry, Haematology, Isotopic Investigations, Amino acids, Histochemistry and Bacteriology, for which the authors feel indebted. The dieticians miss H. A. van der Heijden and miss H. J. W. Lamers have provided much help.

We would like to express our thanks for the assistance of our colleagues from the departments of Pathology (Prof. dr. P. H. M. Schillings, drs. M. J. J. Koene-Bogtmans, dr. U. J. G. van Haelst, drs. K. J. M. Assmann), Radiology (dr. G. Rosenbusch) and Dermatology (dr. W. J. B. M. van de Staak, Prof. dr. J. W. H. Mali). Special thanks are due to ir. H. J. J. van Lier and drs. Ph. van Elteren for help with the statistical evaluation.

We are grateful to the authors and publishers who gave us permission to reproduce several figures. We personally admire the splendid illustrations by mr. H. M. Berris, and the photographs by mr. A. Th. A. Reynen and mr. Th. C. van Hout. Special thanks are due to mrs. B. J. R. Grootendorst-Lieve for her cheerful patience in typing the manuscript. The text was translated by mr. Th. van Winsen, for which the Jan Dekker and dr. Ludgardine Bouwman Foundations provided financial support. Dr. Adrian and mrs. June Roberts helped with grammatical corrections.

We greatly appreciated the help or advice of dr. J. T. M. Burghouts, miss W. C. A. M. Buys, drs. F. H. M. Corstens, dr. J. F. M. Fennis, dr. J. C. M. Hafkenscheid, dr. P. H. K. Jap, dr. R. A. P. Koene, dr. C. B. H. W. Lamers, dr. E. de Nobel, dr. J. M. F. Trijbels, dr. J. M. C. Wessels and dr. S. H. Yap.

This book is dedicated to all persons who have put accuracy, empathy and enthousiasm in their contribution.

CONTENTS

X

## CHAPTER 1

INTRODUCTION

1.1 HISTORY

The earliest descriptions of diseases of the intestine date back to ancient times. The clinical features of malabsorption were described in India as early as 15 centuries B.C. (41). The first European treatise was probably that of Aretaeus, during the second century of the Christian era (547), although his work may have been copied from an earlier author (33). It is a general description of patients with chronic diarrhoea, but some passages suggest that patients suffering from coeliac sprue were probably among them. In this respect it is notable that a female predominance was mentioned and that the condition was described as one of a chronic recurrent character, manifested by such symptoms as steatorrhoea, flatulence, borborygmi and chlorosis. It is also noteworthy that Aretaeus was the first to use the terms 'coeliac affection' and 'coeliacs' (547).

The next descriptions of the syndrome appeared during the 17th and 18th centuries. They were actually treatises on intestinal catarrh and malabsorption, and particularly on oral aphthae, and their causes. In 1669, for example, Vincent Ketelaer published a detailed description of stomatitis aphthosa (called 'spruw' in Dutch), and mentioned more or less casually that these aphthae could also be found in the intestine and give rise to severe diarrhoea which completely exhausts the patient (547). In the beginning of the 18th century about ten additional theses on aphthae appeared at the University of Leiden, which indicates an almost fashionable interest in this syndrome and its possible causes and implications. One of those who studied under Boerhaave in Leiden at that time was Hillary, who described stomatitis aphthosa in patients with malabsorption on Barbados in 1759. Reports on the association of aphthae and diarrhoea or malabsorption also came from other tropical regions (95, 114, 703).

The first accurate description of the clinical syndrome of coeliac sprue did not appear until 1888, when Gee published his treatise 'On the coeliac affection'. This description, the accuracy of which has so far scarcely been surpassed (305), has since been quoted in full or in part by several authors, to whose publications we refer (164, 234). It seems of importance to note that Gee believed he had encountered this syndrome in patients of all age groups, although the adults in whom he observed it had nearly always been in the tropics. It seems plausible, therefore, that most of these adults were actually suffering from tropical sprue. Another interesting point is that Gee already noted that in some cases the abdominal symptoms may be of minor importance, the clinical picture being dominated by marked cachexia and anaemia. Gee also pointed out the importance of restricting the amount of farinaceous ingredients in the diet of these patients, and he noted specifically that one of his young patients showed distinct improvement on a regimen which consisted of the best Dutch mussels.

The contribution which Herter (385) made by focusing attention on the growth retardation in coeliac sprue, found its reward in the fact that the disease was long known as Gee-Herter's disease. The name of the Dane Hess Thaysen (387) has also been linked with the syndrome as a result of the important monograph which he published on coeliac sprue. The currently most widely used designation – coeliac disease – dates back to the 1920's (597).

In the course of the past 25 years, two events have improved and facilitated both the diagnosis and the treatment of coeliac sprue. One was the identification of the pathological substrate of the condition; the other was the discovery of the importance of gluten. Post-mortem reports on patients with tropical sprue had already indicated (114) or described (58, 255, 554) morphological changes of the small intestine. For a long time, however, these changes were regarded as artefacts resulting from post-mortem autolysis (387). Paulley (663) is to be honoured as the first investigator to have demonstrated with certainty the mucosal abnormalities of coeliac sprue in tissue peroperatively obtained from the small intestine. Paulley's findings have been generally confirmed since the introduction of the peroral biopsy of the small intestine (185, 779). The knowledge since accumulated concerning the normal structure of the mucosa of the small intestine and its changes in coeliac sprue, has created an important objective method to establish the diagnosis and evaluate the course and prognosis of this condition.

Dicke's discovery that the cause of the abnormalities of the small intestine was to be sought in the presence of a toxic protein fraction from cereals in the diet, was published in 1950 (208). Dicke had suspected this for more than 10 years, but his revolutionary ideas had not been welcomed. The work of two other Dutch investigators – Van de Kamer (453) and Weijers (908) – which had actually been designed to prove the harmlessness of wheat once and for all, turned out quite definitely to corroborate Dicke's hypothesis

(455). Rational treatment of coeliac sprue has since become possible, and an end was put to the wide variety of often one-sided diets used for this purpose, e.g. the milk-protein diet (423, 749), the banana diet (346), fruit diet (261) and meat diet (124).

1.2 TERMINOLOGY

A large number of different terms are in current use to refer to the syndrome associated with idiopathic steatorrhoea and abnormalities of the intestinal mucosa (table 1.1). The use of so many different names would have been

Table 1.1. The various terms in use to denote patients with a sprue syndrome.

Coeliac disease	Gluten sensitivity
Adult coeliac disease	Gluten sensitive diarrhoea
Idiopathic coeliac disease	Gluten enteropathy
Coeliac affection	Gluten induced enteropathy
Coeliac condition	Gluten sensitive enteropathy
Coeliaca	Gliadin induced enteropathy
Coeliac syndrome	
Primary coeliac syndrome	Steatorrhoea syndrome
	Primary steatorrhoea
Coeliac sprue	Idiopathic steatorrhoea
Coeliac sprue disease	Adult idiopathic steatorrhoea
Sprue	
Sprue nostra	Malabsorption syndrome
Adult sprue	Primary malabsorption
Sprue syndrome	Primary malabsorptive disease
Idiopathic sprue	Intestinal insufficiency
Symptomatic sprue	Primary intestinal insufficiency
Temperate sprue	Chronic intestinal indigestion
Non-tropical sprue	
Idiopathic non-tropical sprue	Gee's disease
	Gee-Herter's disease
Atrophic jejunitis	Gee-Thaysen's disease
Idiopathic mucosal atrophy	Herter's infantilism

less confusing had the (usually ill-defined) criteria applied been less diverse (736). Fortunately, the tradition of introducing yet another name for this syndrome when publishing personal observations seems to have largely disappeared. Agreements on diagnostic criteria have greatly contributed to this (section 1.3). It has not been our intention to coin a new term for this disease in this monograph, but a choice had to be made between two names which have long been used by many authors: namely 'coeliac disease' and 'coeliac sprue'.

The adjective 'coeliac' comes from a Latin corruption of the Greek word 'koilia', which simply means abdomen. The significance of this adjective is clearly expressed in the anatomical nomenclature, e.g. coeliac artery, coeliac ganglion, etc. The designation 'coeliac disease' therefore does not mean much more than disease of the abdomen.

The noun 'sprue' is actually an anglicised version of the Dutch word 'sprouw' or 'spruw'. In 1880 Manson-Bahr adopted the word as a name for a malabsorption syndrome which he observed in patients in the tropics (481). In the former Dutch colonies in the Far East, this condition had long been known as native sprue or 'Indische sprouw' (95, 703). In fact the usage of the word 'spruw' is due to the frequent presence of one particular symptom in this malabsorption syndrome: aphthous stomatitis.

The word 'spruw' really means thrush. Etymologically it is thought to be related to sprinkling, and the original meaning is believed to have been sprinkling or spattering disease (930). The Dutch use the word not only for inflammation of the oral mucosa but also for inflammatory changes of other mucous membranes, e.g. those of the vagina. It therefore seems to be applicable also to inflammation of the mucosa of the small intestine.

In view of all these considerations we have a distinct preference for the designation 'coeliac sprue'. Additions such as idiopathic or primary seem to us superfluous, and adjectives such as adult or non-tropical incorrect. Further specification such as gluten-sensitive seems undesirable as long as the real identity of the harmful cereal protein and its exact role in the pathogenesis of the syndrome have not been established with certainty (section 2.2).

1.3 DEFINITION OF COELIAC SPRUE

It is difficult to define a syndrome when its true cause and pathogenetic mechanism are only partially known. In the case of coeliac sprue the difficulties are increased because of the many expressions of the condition, and the sometimes variable response to treatment. Manifestations of the disease can occur moreover in early childhood, but also at an advanced age. The symptoms may disappear rapidly and spontaneously, or persist and become worse. Yet it is evident that agreements will have to be reached concerning a definition in order to break the deadlock which has existed for some time. We need only think of the numerous names now being used with reference to various spruelike conditions (table 1.1).

This definition will have to account for a number of features or phenomena involved in this disease, e.g. malabsorption, villous abnormalities, and improvement during gluten withdrawal. One of the major difficulties, however, is that we do not know to what extent these features are conditiones sine qua non, while on the other hand the above mentioned phenomena may sometimes also occur in other diseases. This is evident so far as the malabsorption and the villous abnormalities are concerned, whereas some investigators have maintained that gluten abstinence can also be beneficial in affections of the small intestine other than coeliac sprue (54, 166, 724, 873).

In patients with a classical sprue syndrome, malabsorption is always evident and often extensive. Since it has become customary to do a jejunal biopsy on patients with dermatitis herpetiformis, it has been established that malabsorption needs certainly not be present in all patients with mucosal changes of the jejunum (section 10.2). Follow-up studies of individuals in whom coeliac sprue had been diagnosed in childhood, have confirmed this (573, 776), as well as investigations in relatives of coeliac patients (570, 709, 714). One may therefore distinguish a manifest (overt) and an occult type of coeliac sprue.

The presence or absence of villous abnormalities in coeliac sprue, and the question whether these are sufficiently marked to be called sprue lesions, are rather controversial subjects. In most cases one finds a flat, avillous mucosa; but less serious changes (e.g. a pattern consisting of convolutions) can also occur in coeliac patients. It has even been suggested that an increased lymphocyte count in the epithelial layer of the intestinal mucosa should be accepted as a criterion of abnormality (297). Experiments by Weinstein (901) have demonstrated that, in some patients with dermatitis herpetiformis, the apparently normal mucosa of the small intestine can become abnormal after administration of very large amounts of gluten. Such patients may be suffering from an atypical form of coeliac sprue for which Weinstein introduced the term 'latent sprue'. A few other investigators have also mentioned coeliac patients in whom mucosal abnormalities did not develop until after gluten provocation (129).

The response to a gluten-free diet can also vary widely: some patients show an excellent response to gluten abstinence, whereas others show only limited improvement. Several authors have suggested that this may be due to less than optimal adherance to the gluten-free diet, but no evidence has been presented to clinch this argument. Moreover, there are several well-documented case histories of patients who required glucocorticosteroids in addition to a gluten-free diet in order to produce a favourable turn in the course of their disease (section 9.3.4).

In spite of the above mentioned uncertainties, the general view is that, in principle, the following criteria should be fulfilled to establish a diagnosis of coeliac sprue:

a. the presence of morphological changes in the jejunal mucosa;
b. improvement of these changes upon gluten withdrawal;
c. exacerbation after reintroduction of gluten (90, 876).

Paediatricians have already reached agreement about such a definition (586), and for them the above mentioned definition seems to be workable. The situation in children differs from that in adults, however, in that improvement in response to a gluten-free diet is always complete. Moreover, provocation of jejunal mucosal changes by reintroduction of gluten after obtaining a remission is nearly always required in children to differentiate coeliac sprue from other diseases which can produce similar mucosal lesions. In children, this provocation rarely has serious consequences (876), but this does not apply to adults (141, 143). Routine gluten provocation in adult patients is therefore generally rejected, and resorted to only in exceptional cases (90, 164). Adults, unlike children, frequently show only an incomplete response to gluten withdrawal, particularly so far as the morphological changes of the jejunal mucosa are concerned (section 9.2).

In actual practice, therefore, the above mentioned diagnostic criteria are not always sufficiently met in adult patients. In clinical medicine it is not always possible or justifiable to collect all the parameters that are to be collected. Table 1.3 shows that, so far, no investigator has fully observed the above mentioned, so called basic definition. There is in actual fact a choice between two alternatives. One is to apply a very strict definition so that the number of 'true' coeliac patients remains very small and the 'unclassified' group is very large (736). In that case a discussion about variants of the villous morphology, symptoms, or response to treatment is superfluous with regard to coeliac sprue but relevant with regard to 'unclassified' sprue. This is in fact not much more than shifting the problem. The other alternative is to hold the view that coeliac sprue is a disease with a wide

Table 1.2. The different forms of presentation of coeliac disease, and their terminology.

CRITERION	PRESENT	ABSENT
Mucosal lesions	Coeliac sprue	Latent coeliac sprue
Malabsorption	Overt coeliac sprue	Occult coeliac sprue
Previous history	Coeliac sprue of childhood	Adult onset coeliac sprue
Improvement on diet	Responsive coeliac sprue	Refractory sprue
Relapsing on normal food	Permanent gluten-intolerance	Transient gluten-intolerance

variety of expressions (901), which do not always fulfil the above mentioned criteria (table 1.2).

The criteria so far applied by the various investigators to establish a diagnosis of coeliac sprue amount to five phenomena (table 1.3). As the table shows, all investigators have so far held that mucosal lesions should be present if the term coeliac sprue is to be applied. How severe or how char-

Table 1.3. The criteria for the diagnosis of coeliac sprue, as used by various authors.

CRITERION	BENSON et al. 1964	ROSS et al. 1966a	EK 1970	MEEUWISSE 1970	MANN et al. 1970	RUBIN et al. 1970	TRIER 1973	BARRY et al. 1974	BOOTH 1974	COOKE et al. 1974	CREAMER 1974	DISSANAYAKE et al. 1974	SHINER 1974	STEWART 1974	WEINSTEIN 1974	CERF et al. 1975	MODIGLIANI et al. 1975
MUCOSAL LESIONS	*	*	*	*	*	*	*	*	*	*	*	*	*	*	*	*	*
MALABSORPTION																	
unspecified								*			*			*			
clinical		*	*														*
biochemical		*	*			*							*				*
radiological		*	*														
PREVIOUS HISTORY		*										*					
IMPROVEMENT ON DIET																	
unspecified		*	*									*					
clinical				*	*	*	*	*						*	*		
biochemical	*				*	*										*	
morphological	*			*	*			*	*	*			*	*	*	*	
RELAPSE ON NORMAL FOOD																	
unspecified																	
clinical																	
biochemical																	
morphological				*						*			*				

acteristic these mucosal lesions should be, however, is still a controversial question. Many investigators restrict the term coeliac sprue to patients whose jejunal biopsy specimen is completely flat (128, 164, 182, 553, 601, 668, 736). In our opinion, this attitude does not adequately account for patients with a convoluted mucosa. In any case it is advisable that patients with a flat mucosa but without signs of crypt hyperplasia should not be included in the group of coeliac patients unless several other criteria warrant the diagnosis (section 11.4). The symptoms of malabsorption can be clinical as well as biochemical. Radiological changes, which some investigators use as diagnostic criterion (247, 724) are in our opinion too unspecific to be of much use. A history of a malabsorption syndrome in early childhood has to be very typical (section 9.1) to be used as an argument in establishing the diagnosis. The effect of introducing or discontinuing a gluten-free diet can be evaluated on the basis of clinical, biochemical or morphological parameters, or on a combination of them. In our opinion there are no arguments to regard patients as non-coeliacs who require other dietary restrictions or glucocorticosteroids in addition to a gluten-free diet.

A diagnosis of coeliac sprue is usually accepted if a patient fulfils at least two of the criteria mentioned in table 1.3 in addition to the presence of an abnormal jejunal mucosa. This seems sufficient to us to justify presentation as such for the time being. As long as our knowledge of the exact nature of the aetiology and pathogenesis of the disease is as limited as it is, it seems ill-advised to apply excessively strict definitions. It is advisable however, to specify in each publication exactly which criteria were applied, and to apply strictly the standards chosen.

1.4 INCIDENCE

Symptoms of coeliac sprue can occur at any point in a lifetime. The majority of patients develop symptoms at an early age, usually a few months to a year after introduction of cereal products (i.e. of gluten) in the daily diet (581). In some 50% of the cases the disease is diagnosed prior to the second year of life (358, 581). The symptoms disappear quickly after gluten withdrawal and often do not return when the gluten-free diet is discontinued after a few years (776, 875). Even without gluten withdrawal the symptoms often disappear spontaneously after a few years (section 9.1). Follow-up studies have shown, however, that unmistakable mucosal changes persist in all children and adults in whom the diagnosis has been made on sound evidence (573, 614, 776, 936). It can be maintained, therefore, that the maxim 'once a coeliac, always a coeliac' (233) is certainly valid, even though some investigators do not want to exclude the possibility of transient gluten intolerance (584, 883). Many patients do get a recurrence of symptoms even after a lengthy remission (53, 776).

Careful questioning of patients in whom coeliac sprue is diagnosed in adult life, reveals that some 25% indicate having had symptoms suggestive of coeliac sprue in childhood (53, 60, 159). We personally found anamnestic indications of childhood coeliac sprue in two-thirds of our patients. For the time being it remains a moot question whether the remainder of the adult patients have really acquired the disease later in life or have suffered from an asymptomatic or latent form of the disease in childhood and ever since.

In view of the above considerations, the incidence of coeliac sprue does not diminish after the first few years of life but remains constant or may even show a slight increase. The incidence of clinical symptoms does show two peaks, however (fig. 1.1): one during the first few years of life, and the

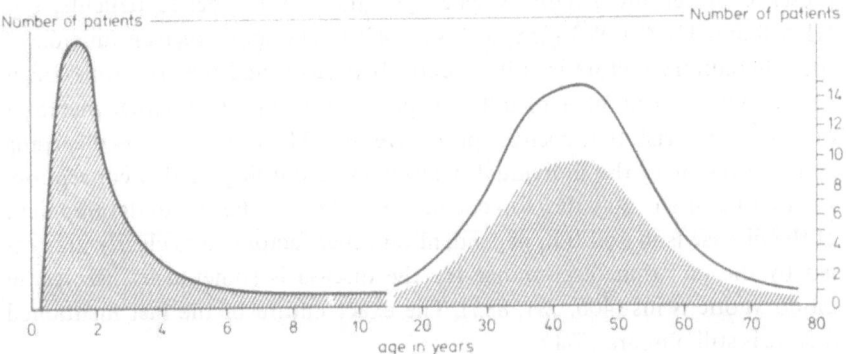

Fig. 1.1. The incidence of clinically manifest coeliac sprue. On the left the age distribution at the time of diagnosis in children is given (Hamilton et al., 1969; Young et al., 1971), while the age distribution of our 47 adult patients at the time of diagnosis is drawn on the right. The unshaded area in the right figure represents the percentage of patients without a history of childhood symptoms.

other during the fourth and fifth decades. Which of these two peaks is higher seems to vary regionally (14, 24, 569), and probably depends on the type of medical care available or on the knowledge of and interest in this syndrome.

It has been known for some time that coeliac sprue can occur in several members of a family. Extensive studies, focused on the familial occurrence

9

of coeliac sprue, have confirmed the suspected higher incidence (126, 625, 844). Most investigators found that some 10% of the first-degree relatives of coeliac patients examined showed unmistakable mucosal changes consistent with coeliac sprue (537, 570, 709, 821). Some found a frequency of almost 20% (31). However, in none of the above mentioned studies were biopsies done in all family members, and the percentages given may therefore be slightly exaggerated. Individuals with health complaints are probably more willing to undergo a jejunal biopsy than those who feel well. This suspicion seems to be confirmed by the fact that Rolles et al. (714) found a frequency of 5.5% in a study in which *all* family members were examined.

Familial occurrence of a disease can be based on environmental as well as on genetic factors. It seems unlikely, however, that the increased familial frequency of coeliac sprue is determined largely by environmental factors, because an increased probability in marital partners, school children or military recruits has never been established. The role of genetic factors in this context seems more important. This is also suggested by the frequent presence of certain hereditary leucocyte antigens in coeliac patients, e.g. HLA 8 and HLA-DW3 (258, 363, 475, 820). The mode of transmission of these hereditary factors is still obscure. It is suspected that transmission is determined by a number of different genes, each of which either increases or reduces the risk that coeliac sprue develops. The number of predisposing factors present in the individual determines, according to this conception, whether he or she may develop coeliac sprue (709). The actual development of the disease is in addition dependent on other factors, as is clearly illustrated by the fact that discordance for the disease is sometimes observed in monozygotic twins (406, 581, 885). The exact nature of the last mentioned factors is still obscure (571).

It looks as if coeliac sprue occurs in particular in Europe, North America and Australia, but the number of cases reported from other continents has increased in recent years (398, 599, 881), although it represents only a fraction of the incidence as for example in Europe. The incidence in Sweden is estimated to be 1:3000 births (247); British estimates range from 1:1850 (571) to 1:1100 (582). The calculated frequency in Switzerland is as high as 1:900 (785) and that in Ireland 1:300 (625). Data on the incidence in The Netherlands have not yet been published. On the basis of the annual number of hospitalised infants under the age of 1 with coeliac sprue reported to the Dutch Foundation for Medical Registration, an incidence of 1:6250 is obtained when dividing these registered coeliacs by the total number of infants (healthy or ill) in that age category (672). In view of the fact that only

15-35% of infants with coeliac sprue are identified as such during the first year of life (358, 581, 936), the true incidence of coeliac sprue is probably 3-6 times as high, i.e. roughly 1:1500. Another possible way of estimating the incidence in The Netherlands is by dividing the national consumption of gluten-free flour, being approximately 14.000 kgs a year (670) by the average consumption per patient estimated at 65 kgs a year for an adult. This calculation yields a total number of merely 215 patients on a gluten-free diet, i.e. a incidence of 1:60.000. The total membership of the Dutch Coeliac Society is even slightly greater (126 children, 251 adults; 671). It should be emphasized, however, that calculations on the incidence of coeliac sprue cannot be anything but very inaccurate.

The rate of detection of the disease is dependent on the familiarity of the attending physician with the many manifestations of coeliac sprue. We have the strong impression that the knowledge of the symptomatology of coeliac sprue is still very imperfect. In the Netherlands, some physicians are heard to state that they have never seen a case of coeliac sprue in the course of their career, whereas others detect a number of new patients every year. The fact that in our adult patients the mean interval between onset of symptoms and diagnosis was some 13 years (!) indicates that the diagnosis is only too often being overlooked. The true incidence of clinically manifest coeliac sprue, therefore, is probably much higher than the above mentioned calculations suggest; to say nothing about the hardly detectable cases of occult coeliac sprue. It is consequently difficult to escape the impression that the differences in the reported incidence of coeliac sprue are in part based on differences in medical care and diagnostic acumen. In Asian children living in England, for example, the disease is found as frequently as in English children (631), although coeliac sprue is reportedly rare in India (881).

There are several other possible explanations for the discrepancies in the reported incidence of coeliac sprue. For example, the frequency of HLA 8 – the leucocyte antigen present in 60-90% of coeliac patients (13, 258, 416, 820) – proves to differ widely in different parts of the world. HLA 8 is most frequently present in Caucasians who seem to have also the highest probability of coeliac sprue. Histocompatibility testing has shown that the frequency of HLA 8 is low in the peoples of Asia or Central and South America (395), where coeliac sprue seems scarcely to occur, if at all. Another possible determinant of the differences in incidence is the mean amount of cereals (gluten) contained in the diet of certain population groups. Black (74) found a higher incidence of coeliac sprue in that socio-economic group of the population of Scotland which had a greater per-capita consumption of bread. However, the incidence of coeliac sprue in the various countries correlates only moderately with the mean per-capita consumption of wheat (582). This may be due to differences in methods of baking bread (679) or the use of other wheat strains. Many publications indicate differences in baby-feeding habits as a cause of the variable incidence of coeliac sprue (581). There are, however, no objective data on the possible influence of the time of gluten introduction in the diet on the development of coeliac sprue in children. As with other possible determinants, this argument remains speculative.

## CHAPTER 2

PATHOGENESIS OF COELIAC SPRUE

2.1 INTRODUCTION

Although the coeliac sprue syndrome was accurately described almost 100 years ago (305), little is known with certainty about its aetiology and pathogenesis at the present time. On the other hand it cannot be denied that – particularly in the past 25 years – unmistakable advances have been made in this respect. An important event in this context was the discovery that the presence in the diet of a protein fraction from certain cereals caused the symptoms of coeliac sprue (208, 209). On the other hand, the detection of villous abnormalities and inflammatory changes in the mucosa of the small intestine (663) and the introduction of a simple and elegant method of obtaining biopsy specimens from the intestinal mucosa (185, 779) facilitated as well as stimulated research into the nature of this disease and its pathogenesis. Another important advance was made with the recent introduction of facilities for culturing mucosal biopsies, on the basis of which research into the pathogenesis of the disease is possible in vitro (109, 446, 859).

The causative factor and a few theories on the pathogenesis of coeliac sprue will be discussed in the following sections.

2.2 CAUSATIVE FACTOR

Research into the causative factor in coeliac sprue did not really begin in earnest until after the discovery of the noxious influence of gluten by Dicke (208, 209). On the basis of clinical experiments this investigator was able to demonstrate that the factor noxious to coeliacs was contained in the protein fraction of wheat and rye flour. In addition he noted that this factor continued to be present after treatment of this protein with a diluted salt solution and that, according to the definition of Osborne (652), it had therefore to be gluten.

On the basis of its solubility in ethanol, gluten can be separated into a soluble gliadin fraction and an insoluble glutenin fraction. At further chemical analysis, both fractions prove to consist of different subfractions (459). For many years, several investigators have concerned themselves with attempts at further fractionation and determination of these subfractions. It was found that the method of electrophoretic separation could be regularly improved, as a result of which subfractions initially regarded as pure were later found to consist of several components (254). Moreover, differences were found according to the origin and purity of the wheat strains involved. As a result of these circumstances investigators have long been disagreeing about the number of fractions, their nature and their nomenclature (254).

On the basis of several observations it seems likely, for the time being, that α-gliadin – one of about 40 different gliadin components (459) – is the fragment which determines the noxious influence of gluten (260, 374, 459). This α-gliadin probably has a coiled, fibril-like structure and a molecular weight of some 30,000. Its amino acid composition is now partly known. In particular it contains many consecutive molecules of glutamine and glutamic acid beside a relatively large number of proline molecules (459). Further breakdown of α-gliadin with the aid of trypsin yields a fraction with a molecular weight of 18,000, which is believed to carry the toxic properties of α-gliadin (375).

According to Phelan et al. (679), the noxious effect of gliadin is not localized in a particular peptide fragment but determined by the presence of carbohydrates bound to this gliadin. According to their observations, the toxic properties of gliadin disappear after decomposition of these compounds with the aid of carbohydrases.

It is to be noted, meanwhile, that flour made of cereals other than wheat and rye can sometimes also be harmful for coeliac patients (section 9.2.1). The protein fractions from these other cereals differ from gliadin not only in name but also in structure (39). This may stimulate further research into the causative factor, as does the fact that there are also nutrients with glutamine-bearing peptides (e.g. meat, eggs, rice and corn), which cause no changes or complaints (454).

It is evident that, despite extensive research by many investigators, there is as yet no certainty about the precise nature of the factor in the gluten fraction of wheat and rye flour or in the protein fraction of other cereals, which causes the lesions of the small intestine and the clinical symptoms in patients with coeliac sprue.

2.3 PATHOGENESIS

2.3.1 Peptidase deficiency theory

The first investigator to suggest that coeliac sprue might be caused by an enzyme deficiency was Frazer (288, 290). His hypothesis was based on the observation that gliadin, after incubation with fresh intestinal mucosa of hogs, lost its toxicity. This theory has been tested by several other investigators (89, 231, 854).

It postulates that a coeliac patient is suffering from a primary deficiency of one or several intestinal peptidases which normally ensure complete decomposition of gliadin. This deficiency is believed to result in accumulation of a given toxic peptide in or near enterocytes, which peptide damages the cell by disrupting the lysosomes (705).

Several observations have seemed to confirm this theory, for deficiency of dipeptidases in the mucosa of untreated coeliacs has been demonstrated by several authors (150, 224, 231, 516). In addition it was found that, when incubated with a half-digested gluten solution, jejunal mucosa specimens from untreated patients released fewer amino acids such as proline and glutamine than did normal jejunal biopsy specimens (168, 230).

According to this theory the favourable effect of gluten withdrawal is quite understandable, and the influence of corticosteroids can be explained by their stabilizing effect on the lysosomal membrane (89).

During treatment with a gluten-free diet, however, the jejunal mucosa resumes normal peptidase activity (231, 285), and this phenomenon is one of the principal arguments advanced by opponents to reject this theory: the diminished peptidase activity is apparently not a primary but a secondary phenomenon. A similar phenomenon is the decrease in lactase activity in the jejunal mucosa of untreated coeliacs. This lack of activity also disappears during treatment with a gluten-free diet (191, 231, 285). The only possibility to uphold this theory is to assume the existence of a primary deficiency of an enzyme not so far identified. However, suggestions in this direction (150, 454, 489) have not yet been confirmed or proven to be unlikely (926).

2.3.2 Immunological theory

At this time, the theory which aims to explain the abnormalities in coeliac sprue in immunological terms, has more advocates than the peptidase deficiency theory. The principal arguments advanced in support of an immunological pathogenesis are: the altered proportions of immunologically competent cells in the lamina propria of the intestinal mucosa (alterations which differ according to various investigators; 172, 232, 738, 810); changes in the serum immunoglobulin levels, e.g. increased IgA and decreased IgM (28, 76, 396, 810); and the presence of antibodies against gliadin (12, 267, 465, 472) and against reticulin (17, 107, 252, 501, 544, 766) in the serum of coeliac patients. Other arguments are the regular finding of an atrophied reticulo-histiocytic system (561, 568), and the fact that administration of glucocorticosteroids has proved to be an effective aid in combating the disease symptoms. Moreover, identical mucosal lesions have been found in some patients with acquired immunodeficiency (108, 166, 246) and in test animals which were rendered immunodeficient (269).

The immunological theory postulates that coeliac sprue patients have an intolerance to gliadin which may be based on inability to develop normal tolerance to gliadin antigen, normally acquired by production of local antibodies (268). As a result, the presence of gliadin in the jejunal lumen gives rise to a local hypersensitivity reaction. For the time being, however, both the nature of this local reaction and its mechanism of action remain obscure (29, 222, 397, 781).

There are several conceivable ways in which this immunological reaction might be produced. It may be that gliadin binds itself to enterocytes and then attracts anti-gliadin antibodies. The enterocytes would consequently be destroyed, either directly (antibody mediated cytotoxicity) or via a cellular immune response (cell mediated toxicity). On the other hand, gliadin could prompt the production of certain local antibodies in the jejunal mucosa, followed by local formation of an antigen/antibody complex which causes damage to the enterocytes. Finally, it is not inconceivable that, in coeliac patients, abnormal lymphocytes circulate which bind the gliadin penetrating the intestinal epithelium and so give rise to tissue damage (29, 270, 826).

Apart from the above mentioned arguments, observations made by Shiner and Shmerling (781, 782) also corroborate the immunological theory. These investigators found that, after gluten provocation in treated coeliacs, first the endothelial cells of the capillaries in the lamina propria begin to swell, and that subsequently the basement membrane becomes thicker and the number of plasma cells in the lamina propria increases. This increase in plasma cells is accompanied by increased local synthesis of immunoglobulins against gliadin peptides (259, 260, 520). The serum complement level also falls (223, 725); this is caused by precipitation of complement in the basement membrane of the mucosa (223, 781). Finally, it is a striking phenomenon that the intestinal epithelial layer in coeliac sprue patients shows a marked increase in interepithelial lymphocytes (266, 297, 412, 782).

16

2.3.3 Other theories

On the basis of purely theoretical considerations (77) and of experience gained with experimental animal models (616, 708), other theories on the pathogenesis of coeliac sprue have been evolved. In this context it does not seem useful to discuss these theories and hypotheses in detail. An exception may be made for the lectin theory recently advanced by Weiser et al. (904). These investigators postulated that enterocytes in coeliac sprue patients function abnormally and are prematurely destroyed because of the fact that gliadin, or a fraction of it, attaches itself to the cell membrane of the enterocytes, thereby acting as a lectin, which reaction initiates cell toxicity. This attachment is believed to be effected as a result of the presence of abnormal glycoproteins in the cell membrane, or as a result of deficient hydrolysis of gliadin (904).

CHAPTER 3

MORPHOLOGY OF THE SMALL INTESTINE UNDER NORMAL CONDITIONS AND IN COELIAC SPRUE

3.1 GENERAL INTRODUCTION

In the small intestine as in nearly every other organ, form and function are related. And in this case, too, interaction is bidirectional. On the one hand, the function of the small intestine is determined by its structure, and on the other hand the structure of the small intestine seems to be subservient to the function which this organ is expected to fulfil. This interdependence prevails in normal circumstances as well as in diseases. For a better understanding of the function of the small intestine, we believe it is useful first to present a few remarks on the architecture and structure of the small intestine, and on the changes to which they are subject in patients with coeliac sprue. It is not our intention to give a detailed description of the morphology of the small intestine. More detailed data can be found in textbooks on anatomy or in other publications (775, 783, 857).

3.2 THE NORMAL SMALL INTESTINE

3.2.1 Macroscopic anatomy

Reports on the length of the small intestine range from 3.5 m to 7 m (860). One of the factors which influence its length is the muscle tonus, by which the length during operation and post-mortem examination exceeds that found at radiological examination for example. At post-mortem examination, the length of the small intestine varies, from hardly 2.5 m to some 8 m (843), while during intubation a length of 2.16-3.37 m has been found (75). This fairly long bowel lies coiled up in the abdominal cavity, which is made possible by a rather summary fixation to the posterior abdominal wall. Only the duodenum, of which the proximal part is localized retroperitoneally, and the terminal loop of ileum are more or less fixed. The jejunum and ileum ly in a double-layered, loosely draped mesenterial membrane, and can move freely. In between the layers of the mesentery are localized the arterial

18

and venous vessels, the lymphatic vessels and the autonomic nerve fibres.

The small intestine is divided into duodenum, jejunum and ileum. The duodenum is 12 inches long and its junction with the jejunum is characterized by a bend (the duodenojejunal flexure) at the level of the ligament of Treitz. On the distal side the end of the jejunum is not sharply defined, and no real demarcation indicates its transition to the ileum. The boundary between jejunum and ileum is arbitrarily taken to be localized at two-thirds of the total length of the small intestine (860). The jejunum differs from the ileum in that it has a larger diameter and a thicker wall.

The wall of the small intestine consists of the following layers, from the outside to the inside: serosa, lamina muscularis propria (of which the outer part contains muscle fibres with a longitudinal, and the inner part with a circular course), submucosa and mucosa. The mucosa is characterized by marked plication, especially in the proximal jejunum; more distally the number of plicae slightly diminishes. These folds, the so-called plicae circulares (valvulae conniventes or Kerckring folds) are reduplications of the mucosa which are kept together by the submucosa. Their course is usually not quite circular but they extend to halfway or two-thirds of the circumference. They remain present also as the bowel distends (775). In addition there are irregular folds, created by the peristaltic contractions.

The mucosa of the small intestine is covered with finger or tongue shaped projections, which are called villi. These are present throughout the small intestine, and only just visible with the naked eye. They give the mucosa a velvet-like appearance. For better evaluation of the length and shape of the villi, a magnifying-glass or dissecting microscope has to be used.

3.2.2 Stereomicroscopic aspect of the mucosa

Our current knowledge of the structure of the villi of the small intestine dates back to the time when it became possible to take biopsy specimens from the small intestine perorally (185, 779). The mucosa of the small intestine has since been examined in many situations, and one of the findings was that the shape of intestinal villi can vary rather widely (fig. 3.3). The normal villi are cylindrical, finger-like structures with a length of 0.5-1 mm. They are usually described as finger-shaped. However, their shape varies as widely as their length, and differs locally within the intestine, per individual, and probably also per geographic region (42). Especially in the duodenum, the villi are often of a different shape, i.e. they are less slender, more broadened, and thus more reminiscent of leaves or tongues than of fingers. Distal to the duodenojejunal flexure, these leaf-shaped villi are observed only sporadically. The villi in the ileum are usually somewhat shorter and also more widely interspaced. Nevertheless, the villi are as a rule lying so closely together that the crypt openings are not readily recognizable.

3.2.3 Microscopic morphology of the mucosa

The histological section of a peroral biopsy specimen from the small intestine as a rule shows not much more than the mucosa. In some cases, also part of the submucosa can be observed beneath the lamina muscularis mucosae. The mucosa consists of an epithelial layer of cylindrical cells called enterocytes, which covers the lamina propria on the side of the intestinal lumen (fig. 3.1). The lamina propria constitutes the interior mass of

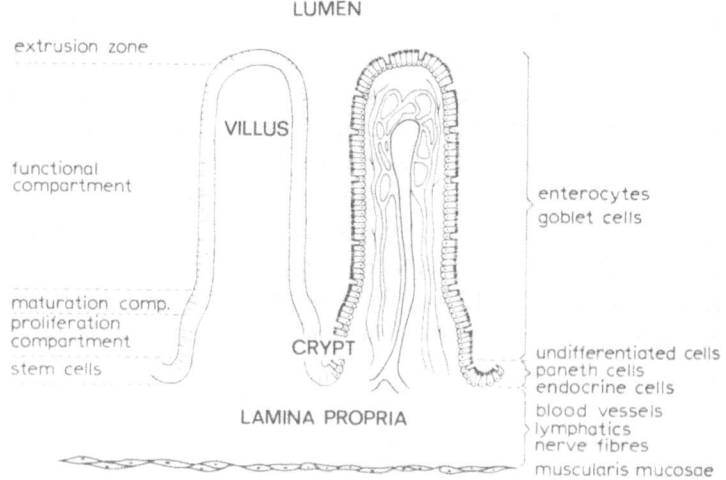

Fig. 3.1. Diagram of the anatomical organization of the small intestinal mucosa. The kinetic cell compartments are given on the left, while the main histological elements are summarized on the right.

the villi of the small intestine. It is within this lamina propria that the small blood vessels, lymphatics and nerves extend. In addition the lamina propria contains smooth muscle fibres, reticulin fibres, elastin filaments and various cells, chiefly lymphocytes, plasma cells, macrophages and eosinophilic cells. The presence of these cells is indicative of the important role which the lamina propria plays in the defence of the intestinal wall against microorganisms and toxic substances from the lumen.

Villi and crypts are readily recognizable in a well-cut histological section.

The villi vaguely resemble coniferae, owing to the corrugated course of the epithelial layer which probably results from fixation of the tissue or from contraction of the smooth muscle tissue. The cylindrical enterocytes show no signs of degeneration at the tip of the villus, where they are ultimately extruded, at the so-called extrusion zones. Interspersed with the enterocytes one observes occasional goblet cells, and in addition lymphocytes or even granulocytes are sometimes found in the epithelial layer (297, 757). The villi are lined with functionally mature enterocytes. Maturation and production of these cells take place in the Lieberkühn crypts. These crypts, which extend within the lamina propria as far as the muscularis mucosae, are actually short tubules which supply the enterocytes for the lining of the intestinal villi (fig. 3.1). In the histological sections the crypt epithelium is often observed to continue in the epithelial layer of the intestinal villi, but some crypts show no continuity (fig. 3.3.b). In the past, these features have been ascribed to tangential cutting of the jejunal biopsy specimen, but analytical studies by Cocco et al. (146) have shown that these apparently separate tubules may communicate with each other as well as with the villi. Particularly in the jejunum, the crypts may consist of several tubules, whereas in the ileum one usually finds only one crypt tubule per villus (146).

The crypts contain at the bottom the so-called undifferentiated cells which, through mitosis and differentiation, supply both the enterocytes and the goblet cells. In addition one finds endocrine cells and Paneth cells. The function of the latter has so far remained obscure. Apart from their role in cell production, the crypts of the small intestine are possibly also important in some secretory processes of the mucosa of the small intestine, e.g. the secretion of mucus, intestinal hormones and probably also of fluids and electrolytes (378).

The crypts can be divided into a proliferative compartment, where cell production takes place, and a maturation compartment which consists of cells that gradually differentiate to fully developed, mature enterocytes (fig. 3.1). These enterocytes are pushed up and line the intestinal villi. The enterocytes of the intestinal villi as a whole are called functional compartment (894) (fig. 3.1).

3.2.4 Ultrastructure of the enterocyte

The cylindrical, functionally mature enterocytes carry their nucleus in the basal part, while the other cell organelles are contained in the apical half (fig. 3.2). These organelles include the mitochondria, the Golgi apparatus, the smooth and the rough endoplasmic reticulum, the ribosomes and the

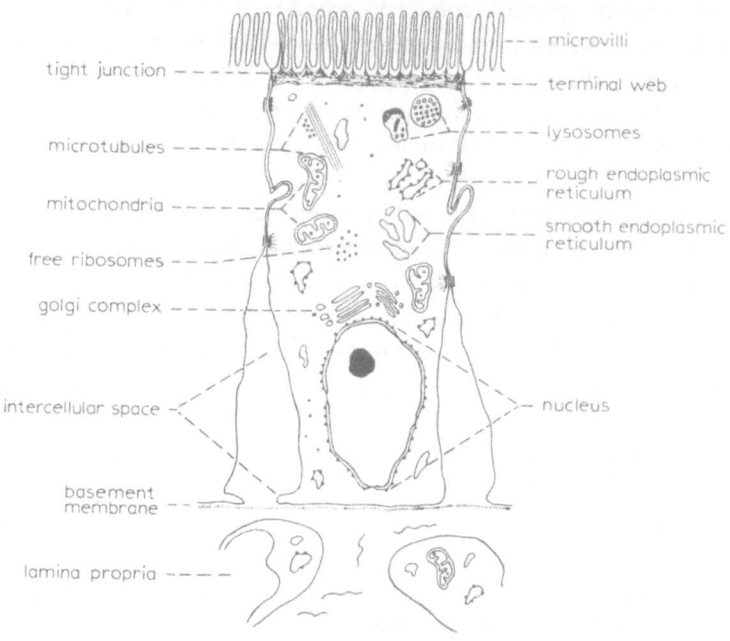

Fig. 3.2. Diagram of a normal enterocyte, showing the arrangement of the various intra-cellular structures (Redrawn from Trier et al., Gastroenterology 49: 575, 1965; with permission of the author and publishers).

lysosomes (860). On the side of the lumen the cell membrane forms the so-called brush border – a collection of finger-shaped cell extensions called microvilli. These microvilli contain some central supporting fibres which arise from a firm network beneath the brush border: the terminal web. It is probably from these fibrous structures that the enterocytes derive the firm-ness of their apical wall. The terminal webs of adjacent cells connect through the so-called tight junctions. On the side of the intestinal lumen these junctions seal the intercellular spaces almost hermetically while still permitting them to distend fairly freely. The microvilli enlarge the surface area of the interface between enterocytes and intestinal lumen by about factor 30 (860). On top of the brush border lies the so-called fuzzy coat, a layer which, because of the amount of glycoproteins contained in it, is sometimes called glycocalyx. The glycocalyx is formed by the enterocytes themselves and, by virtue of the enzymes which it contains, is believed to play an important role in membrane digestion (860, 866).

22

3.3.1 Macroscopic anatomy

In coeliac sprue, lesions of the mucosa of the small intestine develop in response to the presence of gluten in the diet. The pathological changes are usually confined to the mucosa, while the remainder of the intestinal wall is normal. At laparotomy a distension of the loops of the small intestine and a dough-like consistency of the intestinal wall are occasionally found. The not uncommon presence of enlarged mesenteric lymph nodes will be discussed elsewhere (section 6.5.4).

3.3.2 Stereomicroscopic aspect of the mucosa

When examining the mucosa of the small intestine from untreated coeliac patients with the aid of a magnifying-glass or dissecting microscope, no normal villi are observed. The shape of the villi depends on the severity of the mucosal damage. In the most severe form, a flat mucosa is seen in which no villi or villous remnants are visible. In such a mucosa only the crypt openings can be distinguished (fig. 3.3.g). One is regularly struck by the presence of polygonal local elevations in this otherwise flat surface, which have been compared with cobble-stones or mosaic pieces (86). Less severe mucosal damage produces a pattern of convolutions: gyrate structures in which individual villous remnants have merged (fig. 3.3.e). Finally, there are also unilaterally broadened, tongue-shaped villi, which are sometimes so broad as to resemble a ridge rather than a tongue (fig. 3.3.c).

The mucosal features in coeliac sprue patients generally vary with the site from which the biopsy specimen is taken. The changes in the proximal segment are usually more marked than those at more distal levels; this is probably related to the gluten concentration in the intestinal lumen (734).

Examination of biopsy specimens with the aid of a magnifying-glass or dissecting microscope has the advantage that an impression of the severity and extent of the mucosal lesion can be instantly gained (86, 733). Observed local abnormalities can be taken into account moreover when cutting the histological sections.

The terminology and classification of the various villous appearances in the literature vary. Personally we have always, after painstaking examination of biopsy specimens and registration of the villous types observed, classified specimens according to the predominant type in four categories: normal villi, slightly abnormal villi (tongues and ridges), a convoluted type, or a flat mucosa (fig. 3.3).

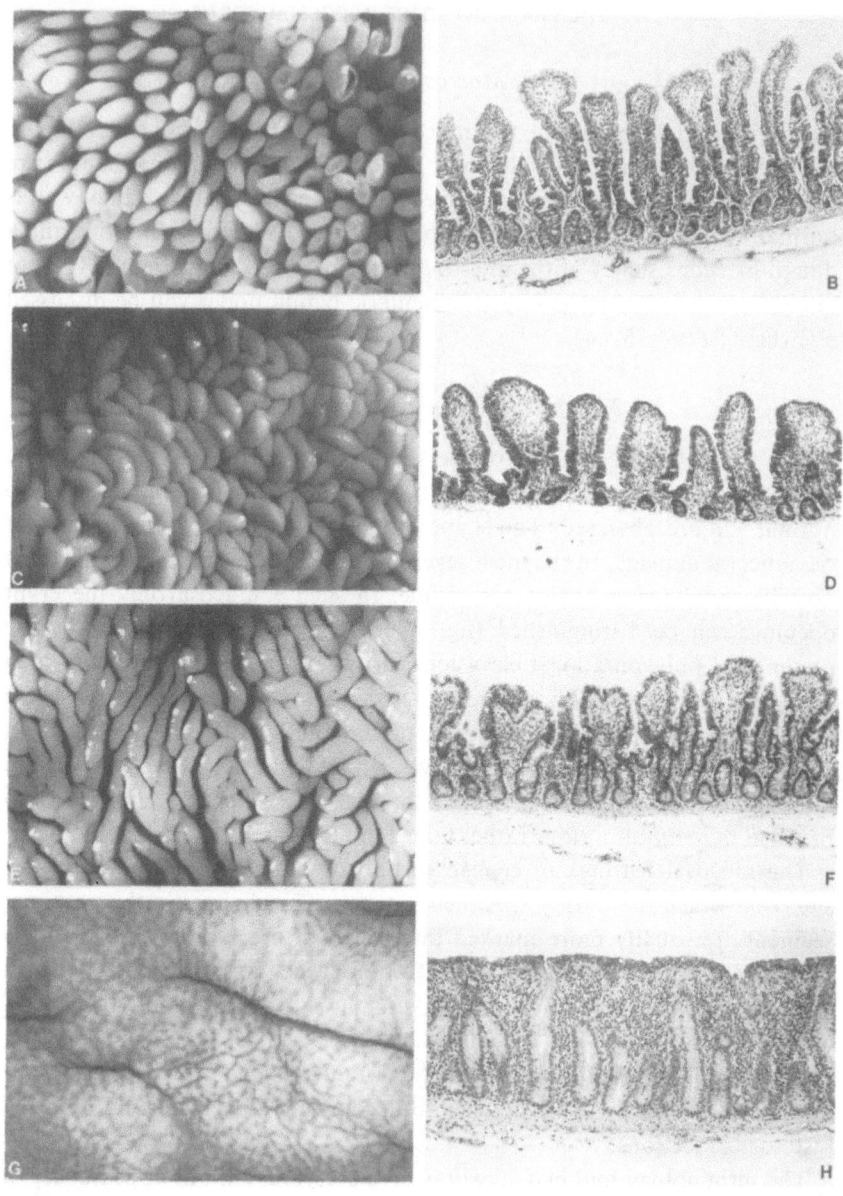

Fig. 3.3. The various appearances of the jejunal mucosa, as seen under the dissecting microscope (on the left) or at histological examination (on the right). The illustrations show normal finger-shaped villi (*a, b*), leaf-shaped villi (*c, d*), convolutions (*e, f*), and a flat mucosa (*g, d*).

For a sophisticated form of stereomicroscopic examination it is now possible to make use of the scanning electron microscope (562). More details of the mucosal surface can be observed in this way. Apart from reproductions of excellent quality, however, this sophisticated technique of examination has so far failed to add important supplementary data.

3.3.3 Microscopic morphology of the mucosa

Doniach and Shiner (228) were the first to publish a classification of the various mucosal changes observed at microscopic examination of biopsy specimens from the small intestine in coeliac sprue patients. They described the shortening or disappearance of intestinal villi respectively as partial and subtotal villous atrophy. Efforts have since been made to stop the use of the term atrophy, which most investigators consider to be inappropriate.

In the histological section the mucosa, which shows no villi on stereomicroscopy, is bounded by a horizontal to slightly sloping surface epithelium which consists of cubical to flat enterocytes (fig. 3.3.h). Their nuclei are pyknotic and vary in shape, size and localization (859). In such biopsy specimens the crypts have markedly increased in length, and sometimes also in width. They often show several ramifications which may have been cut tangentially. The cells in the crypt basis show numerous mitoses. The basement membrane is often more readily visible than is normally the case, and may contain some collagen interspersed with the connective tissue fibres in and beneath this membrane (755). A pronounced increase in cellular infiltration is always observed in the lamina propria. In particular the number of plasma cells producing immunoglobulin IgA and IgM is increased (232). Lymphocytes and eosinophilic granulocytes are also increased in number, if less markedly so. Moreover many lymphocytes are found in the surface epithelium, in between the enterocytes (266). In the smooth muscle cells of the muscularis mucosae and muscularis propria, finally, a brown pigment is sometimes visible around the nucleus, which consists of accumulated ceroid (847).

3.3.4 Ultrastructure of the enterocyte

Electron microscopic examination of the mucosa of the small intestine in coeliac sprue patients invariably reveals marked abnormalities of the microvilli: not only are there fewer microvilli, but those present are shorter and of irregular shape, as well as chaotically rather than neatly arranged. Changes of the brush border are usually the first to appear in the case of enterocyte damage (783). The brush border can ultimately disappear almost completely.

Histochemical examination shows that the brush border also contains fewer enzymes. This is demonstrable by enzyme staining of histological sections (655) as well as by quantitative determination in cell homogenates (191).

Most intracellular structures present a swollen appearance, e.g. Golgi apparatus, mitochondria and lysosomes. The amount of endoplasmic reticulum seems to be diminished. In addition large fat globules and vacuoles are often observed in the enterocytes (655, 783, 859).

The above described changes are observed only in the enterocytes on the villous remnants or on the mucosal surface. The enterocytes in the crypts nearly always remain normal (655, 859).

3.4 MORPHOGENESIS OF THE COELIAC MUCOSA

The epithelium of the intestinal mucosa consists of rapidly dividing cells which have a short life-span. The life-span is varyingly estimated, ranging from 2-4 days (178) to 4-6 days (536). The worn-out enterocytes (which are not identifiable as such either morphologically or histochemically) are extruded at the villous tips, at the so-called extrusion zones. The production of enterocytes takes place in the crypts. The enterocytes therefore migrate from

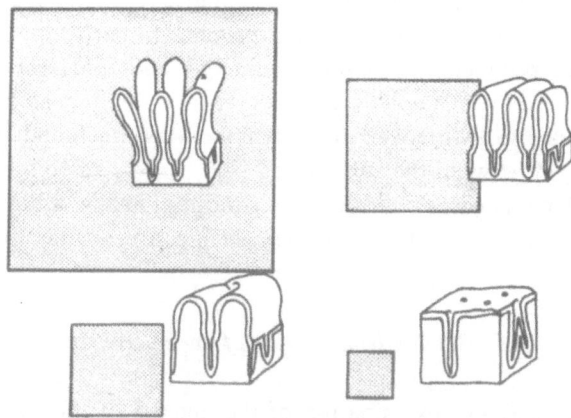

Fig. 3.4. Diagram of the comparative surface areas (stippled squares) of functional enterocytes covering various villous shapes. (Reproduced from Creamer, in Postgraduate Gastroenterology: 18, Baillière, Tindall and Cassell, 1966; with permission of the author and publishers).

the crypt basis to the villous tip and this distance comprises their life-span (859). The exfoliation of enterocytes is believed to be a primary process, for it continues even when mitosis is experimentally inhibited (775).

The existing dynamic balance between cell production and exfoliation determines the number of enterocytes available for lining the mucosal surface. The size of this surface seems to determine the degree of evagination of the mucosa or, in other words, the number and shape of the villi (fig. 3.4). One of the determinants of this dynamic balance is the rate of production. A decreased production of enterocytes in the intestinal crypts is observed after irradiation of the small intestine or administration of cytotoxic drugs, as well as in the presence of malignant processes (52, 706, 710). In refractory sprue, too, the mitotic activity in the crypts is certainly decreased (section 11.3).

In coeliac sprue, the life-span of the enterocytes is greatly reduced. Experiments involving perfusion of intestinal loops have demonstrated markedly increased cell exfoliation, up to 4-6 times the normal (178, 184). In response to this, the intestinal crypts attempt to compensate the enterocyte loss by increased mitotic activity, via a feed-back system not yet understood (300, 301). In fact the number of mitoses in the crypts is found to be greatly increased (655, 894). In addition one observes hyperplasia of the crypts, which become longer as well as wider, and show increased ramification (587, 894). The rate of migration of enterocytes from crypt to surface also increases (859). As a result, the enterocytes may lack sufficient time to mature to differentiated absorptive cells, and consequently the mucosal surface in coeliac patients may be lined with functionally immature cells

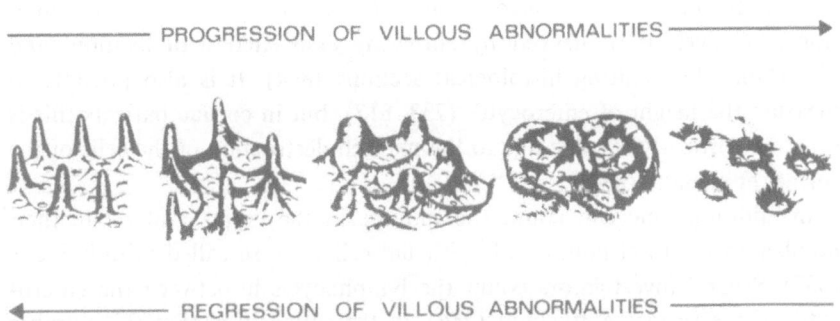

Fig. 3.5. Diagrammatic representation of the sequential changes in the villous appearances from normal villi to a flat mucosa, or vice versa. (Reproduced from Loehry et al., Gut 10: 11, 1969; with permission of the authors and publishers).

(655, 707). Due to the decreased number of surface cells in coeliac sprue, it is hardly possible to provide sufficient covering for normal villus formation (fig. 3.4). In addition, the inflammatory reaction with oedema and cellular infiltration in the lamina propria probably also plays a role in the morphogenesis (757). Experiments with gluten instillation have shown that a subepithelial inflammatory reaction actually comes first and that as a result the aspect of the villi changes characteristically within a few hours (734, 782). The morphology of the intestinal mucosa depends on the severity of this inflammatory reaction and the degree of cell exfoliation. This is why stereomicroscopic examination of biopsy specimens from the small intestine can reveal a variety of features. In the case of minor mucosal damage rather short, leaf-shaped villi or ridges will be visible. A convoluted mucosa indicates rather serious damage. The most severe lesions are associated with an entirely flat mucosa (fig. 3.5).

3.5 MORPHOMETRY OF THE MUCOSA

There is an increasingly urgent need for quantification of the morphological characteristics of the intestinal mucosa. This is based on the need for methods to differentiate between normal and abnormal on objective grounds, which at the same time make it possible to detect minor changes. Without quantitative data, one must rely too heavily on subjective impressions, and be too dependent on the shortcomings of such impressions so far as minimal changes are concerned.

Several phenomena can be quantified. The height as well as the width of the villi can be measured, and the same applies to the depth of the crypts and the thickness of the mucosa (543). The accuracy of these determinations, however, is influenced by shrinking associated with fixation, and distortion while cutting histological sections (894). It is also possible to measure the height of enterocytes (733, 817), but in coeliac patients this is often not properly feasible due to the marked destruction of the cells of the surface epithelium (894).

In addition, one can count the mitoses in the crypts and relate their number to the total number of epithelial cells: the so-called mitotic index (655). Several investigators count the lymphocytes in-between the enterocytes of the surface epithelium (266), in the supposition that this number correlates well with the severity of the mucosal damage caused by gluten (297). It is also possible to determine the number of inflammatory cells in the lamina propria (412).

Finally, many methods have been devised to measure the surface area of the intestinal mucosa (123, 134, 239, 543, 733). Despite various, very ingenious techniques it has not been possible to include the third dimension in these determinations, which are all carried out in two-dimensional, histological sections.

Although all the above mentioned techniques have their drawbacks, they also have the advantage of objectivity and of the possibility to demonstrate minimal changes. Apart from the research done to demonstrate the validity of these various methods, however, they have so far scarcely been applied.

## CHAPTER 4

PHYSIOLOGY OF THE SMALL INTESTINE

4.1 GENERAL INTRODUCTION

Food, once ingested, becomes fragmented by chewing and mixed with saliva to facilitate swallowing. Saliva contains the enzyme α-amylase, which degrades the starch in the food. After passing through the oesophagus the food bolus enters the stomach, where it is further kneaded by vigorous contractions of the gastric wall and mixed with gastric juice, which contains pepsinogens and hydrochloric acid. The secretion of gastric juice is regulated by nervous and hormonal factors, especially by gastrin. The stomach serves as a temporary store for the food ingested. By periodic relaxation of the pyloric muscle, small amounts of the chyme are passed into the duodenum. The mode of evacuation of the stomach is dependent on the volume of stomach contents, the osmotic pressure and fat content of the meal, and the acid concentration (192). In addition to nervous reflexes, intestinal hormones probably also play an important role in the evacuation of the stomach.

In the duodenum, the chyme comes into contact with pancreatic juice and bile. The pancreatic juice contains many proteolytic enzymes and lipases in addition to amylases. The optimal pH for intestinal digestion is much higher than the pH which prevails in the stomach; hence the importance of secretion of bicarbonate by the pancreas. The pancreatic secretion is regulated mainly by the intestinal hormones secretin and cholecystokinin (pancreozymin). The former induces in particular the water and bicarbonate secretion, while the latter effects the release of digestive enzymes. In addition, nervous factors play a part in the regulation of pancreatic secretion. One of the functions of bile is to emulsify the fatty substances in the chyme in order to facilitate hydrolysis by lipases, and to form micelles. Release of bile by the gall-bladder is effected by nervous and humoral stimuli, particularly by cholecystokinin. During the passage of the chyme through duodenum and jejunum, further degradation of carbohydrates, protein and fats takes place. The digestive juices degrade not only food constituents but also physiological substances released in the small intestine. These so-called endogenous substances include protein-rich fluid leaking from the intestinal wall, mucus, exfoliated enterocytes and the digestive juices themselves. The intestinal wall is protected from the influence of these proteolytic enzymes by the layer of mucus secreted by the goblet cells. Digestion is usually sufficiently advanced in the proximal jejunum to facilitate absorption.

The complex process of absorption of digested food constituents takes place during the slow transport of the chyme through the small intestine. The motility of the small intestine, which serves not only the propulsion of the chyme but also the mixing with digestive juices and the homogenization of the mass, is a process controlled by the autonomic nervous system. Absorption of most food constituents is completed in the proximal jejunum. Bile acids and vitamin B_{12} are absorbed in the ileum only. The absorbed substances are transported further via the blood stream, while lipids mainly pass via intestinal lymphatics.

The undigested, unabsorbed chyme residue ends up in the colon, where bacterial degradation of fibrous food constituents takes place, along with some absorption of water and electrolytes. The ultimate residue is eliminated from the body by defaecation.

4.2 MOTILITY

The small intestine is in constant motion. This process, which in actual fact involves several phenomena, is called motility. Its function is to mix the chyme properly with digestive juices, homogenize it, bring it into contact with the absorptive surface, and finally to evacuate the ultimate residue.

The movements of the small intestine are executed by the smooth muscle fibres contained in the intestinal wall. The muscular coat of the small intestine consists of an outer layer of longitudinal smooth muscle fibres, and an inner layer of circular fibres. At some sites bundles of fibres probably pass from the one layer to the other. The mucosa is separated from the submucosa by a thin layer of smooth muscle fibres, the so-called lamina muscularis mucosae, which likewise consists of a longitudinal and a circular layer. From this muscularis mucosae bundles of muscle cells extend into the valvulae conniventes (Kerckring's folds) and the individual villi as well (138).

So far, little has been established with certainty concerning the motility of the small intestine. One of the reasons is that investigation is hardly practicable without drastically changing normal physiological conditions.

Motility actually consists of a collection of muscular contractions of separate intestinal segments, which seem to be induced by electrical im-

31

pulses from a more proximal level; these impulses are also known as basic electrical rhythm, pacesetter potential, electrical control activity, or slow waves (748). It is suspected that the pacemaker of these electrical impulses is localized in the duodenum, immediately below the outlet of the common bile duct. It is also possible, however, that this electrical impulse is an illusory phenomenon consisting of the depolarization waves of muscle cell groups in consecutive intestinal segments. These depolarizations probably occur in the outer longitudinal muscular layer, according to an intrinsic rhythm. Due to the influence on the time of depolarization in the adjacent intestinal segment the depolarization seems to propagate itself. Only this second hypothesis can explain why, after transection of the small intestine, depolarization waves continue to occur in the distal fragment (138). The intrinsic rhythm of the depolarizations in the various parts of the small intestine varies slightly: the frequency is 10-12 per minute in the proximal part, and 8 per minute in the distal small bowel (840).

Intestinal peristalsis in the proper sense of the word consists of segmental muscular contractions which occur very locally over a distance of 1-2 cm, at intervals of 4-8 cm. These contractions are also known as fast activity, spike bursts, or electrical response activity (748). They do not move but disappear after a few seconds, to be replaced by contractions at other sites, usually exactly between the preceding localizations (fig. 4.1). The segmental mus-

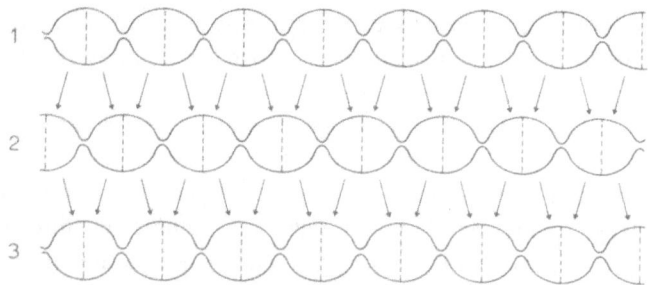

Fig. 4.1. Diagram of the segmental contractions of the small intestine. The sequence of rhythmic segmentations is indicated by lines 1-3. The arrows show from where the chyme of the new segments originates, the dotted lines the regions of division. (Redrawn from Hightower, in Handbook of Physiology section 6 IV: 2001, American Physiological Society, 1968; with permission of the author and publishers).

cular contractions can occur only during the depolarization phase of the basic electrical rhythm. This rhythm, therefore, does not itself produce segmental contractions but only dictates the moments at which these are possible.

32

The segmental contractions push the chyme away in several directions, cranially as well as caudally (fig. 4.1). The fact that the chyme ultimately does move caudally therefore remains a mystery. Perhaps the explanation is that the frequency of the segmental contractions is higher at proximal than at distal levels (840).

Apart from the above mentioned segmental contractions, some other types of movement of the small intestine have been registered, such as circular contractions which propagate themselves over a small distance. The origin and purpose of these contractions have so far remained obscure. In addition, some motor activity can appear or disappear due to irritation of the mucosa or to stimulation of the afferent nerves, as in the reflexes of Bayliss and Starling and the intestino-intestinal inhibitory reflex (138).

The activity of intestinal motility is influenced by many factors, and in particular by neurogenic impulses. Stimulation of the parasympathetic receptors gives rise to contractions. Activation of the sympathetic nerve causes the contractions to diminish. In addition, some intestinal hormones perhaps also exert an influence on motility. The basic electrical rhythm of duodenum and jejunum is believed to be stimulated by cholecystokinin/pancreozymin and inhibited by secretin (345). Peristalsis is believed to be promoted by 5-hydroxytryptamine, which is produced by the APUD cells in the mucosa of the small intestine (240). The type of nutrition and the bacterial flora may also influence motility.

On a smaller scale, too, movements occur in the small intestine. The intestinal mucosa shows ever-changing plications due to contractions of the lamina muscularis. The intestinal villi are also in constant motion: they make pendular and pumping movements. These movements are stimulated by mechanical stimuli; the candidate hormone villikinin may also play a role in this respect. It is suspected that these micro-movements of the villi of the small intestine are of importance in reducing the unstirred layer (section 5.1.5) and in propelling the absorbed substances from the villous core to the submucosa (771).

4.3 INNERVATION

The innervation of the small intestine can roughly be described as an intrinsic local nervous system, localized in the wall of the intestinal tract and operating relatively independently, with in addition a number of extrinsic nerves which transmit the impulses from the central, the sympathetic and the parasympathetic nervous system.

The intrinsic part of the innervation consists of an enormous number of neurons and nerve fibres, localized in the intestinal wall in certain layers which are called plexuses. The most prominent of these are the myenteric plexus (Auerbach's plexus) and the submucosal plexus (Meissner's plexus); the former is localized between the longitudinal and the circular muscular layer of the intestinal wall, and the latter between the circular muscular layer and the lamina muscularis mucosae (532). Further examination probably reveals several other distinguishable plexuses (138). Both above mentioned plexuses consist of a dense network of neurons and unmyelinated nerve fibres, which can be efferent, afferent or associative (fig. 4.2). The efferent part comprises the neurons which innervate above all the musculature of the intestinal wall, and in addition also the muscle cells of the blood vessels in the intestinal wall. The efferent sympathetic and parasympathetic fibres which partly synapse with these neurons, are likewise regarded as belonging to this efferent part. The afferent part consists of neurons which receive sensory impulses from the (sub)mucosa. Their fibres synapse, either locally with efferent neurons or centrally in the sympathetic or parasympathetic ganglia near the spinal cord. The associative neurons govern the extensive connections between the neurons in the same plexus or between those of both plexuses (138, 532). It is not impossible that several other types of nerve elements are localized in the plexus (138).

The efferent and afferent fibres of the sympathetic and parasympathetic nervous system extend between the intestinal wall and the spinal cord. They synapse in the two plexuses with the motor and sensory neurons of the intestinal wall proper.

The nerves of the gastrointestinal tract play an important role in the diges-

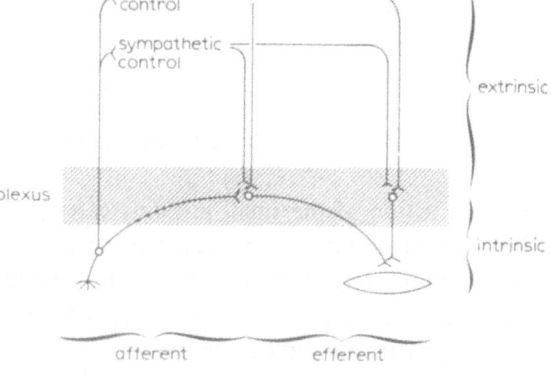

Fig. 4.2. Diagram of the autonomic nervous control of the small intestine. In addition to the local intrinsic reflex arc, the pathways of the extrinsic nerves are indicated (Design adapted from Lundgren, 1972).

tion and absorption of food in that they influence motility, blood supply and secretory processes. In actual fact this regulation is achieved in interaction with intestinal hormones. These interactions are so closely interlocked that it is impossible to assess the role of every separate nervous or hormonal factor (548).

The neural regulation of motility, blood supply and secretion probably takes place largely on a local level. Afferent stimuli from the intestinal lumen or the intestinal wall can produce effects via a direct reflex arc. The extrinsic (i.e. sympathetic or parasympathetic) efferent nerve fibres can produce effect, if necessary, by facilitation or inhibition of the reflex or by direct stimulation of the effector cell (fig. 4.2). Similar effects can be produced by the release of intestinal and other hormones.

The motility of the small intestine is extrinsically influenced by both the parasympathetic and the sympathetic nerves. The parasympathetic fibres can directly stimulate the smooth muscle cells of the intestinal wall (fig. 4.3.a) but

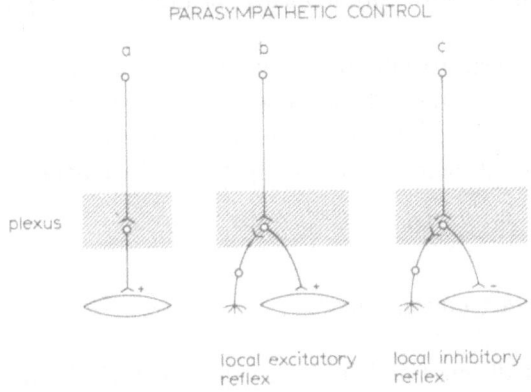

PARASYMPATHETIC CONTROL

a   b   c

plexus

local excitatory reflex   local inhibitory reflex

Fig. 4.3 Diagram of the extrinsic parasympathetic control on the intestinal wall musculature and the local intrinsic reflex arc (Reproduced from Lundgren, in Pathophysiology: 617, Lippincott, 1972; with permission of the author and publishers).

they can also exert an indirect excitatory influence on local excitatory and inhibitory reflexes (fig. 4.3.b and c). The sympathetic fibres, on the other hand, inhibit spontaneous intrinsic motility and abolish the effect of the parasympathetic (fig. 4.4.a and c). Motility, on the other hand, can also diminish due to an increase in the catecholamine concentration (fig. 4.4.b) (532).

The stimulation of motility concerns in particular the segmental contractions, which become both more frequent and more vigorous. Perhaps the pacesetter potential is also influenced by nervous factors (548).

The blood supply to the wall of the small intestine (the muscular layer as well as the submucosa) is subject to the extrinsic influence via the sympathetic nerves. The efferent sympathetic fibres cause vasoconstriction by stimulation of the smooth muscle fibres in the arterial wall. There are no indications

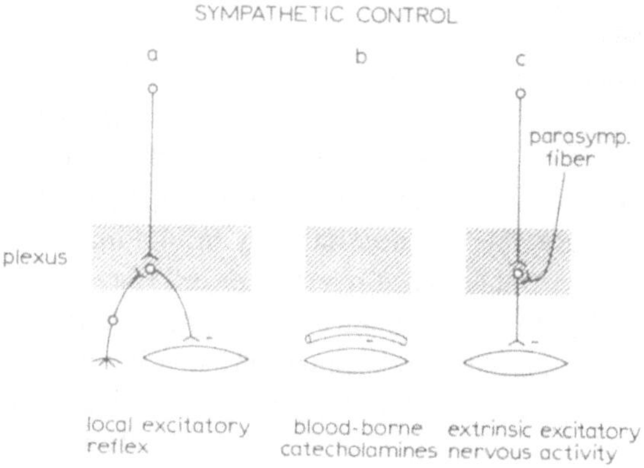

SYMPATHETIC CONTROL

Fig. 4.4. Diagram of the extrinsic sympathetic control on the intestinal wall musculature and the local intrinsic reflex arc (Reproduced from Lundgren, in Pathophysiology: 618, Lippincott, 1972; with permission of the author and publishers).

so far that the parasympathetic exerts any influence on the blood supply (532).

Secretion in the stomach is extrinsically stimulated by the parasympathetic, partly by direct stimulation of the cells of the gastric wall, but also via its influence on the gastrin production. There are vague indications that secretion in the pancreas is likewise stimulated by the parasympathetic system (548).

4.4 CIRCULATION

The blood supply to the small intestine is covered almost entirely by the superior mesenteric artery. This artery communicates, however, with the coeliac artery via the pancreaticoduodenal arteries. The superior mesenteric artery produces a total of 10-16 branches, which in turn divide or combine to form a sort of network between the membranes of the mesentery. At the interface between mesentery and small intestine, the vasa recta arise which extend on either side around the intestine. These semicircular blood vessels produce smaller branches which penetrate all layers of the intestinal wall. They also anastomose abundantly and form plexuses at various levels in the intestinal wall. The arterioles which supply blood to the intestinal villi arise from such a vascular network in the submucosa (fig. 4.5). The stroma of each intestinal villus contains a small central arteriole which rises perpendicularly to the apex, where it divides into a number of capillaries that extend down on the outside of the villous stroma and, on their way, ramify in such a manner that an extensive capillary network is formed immediately

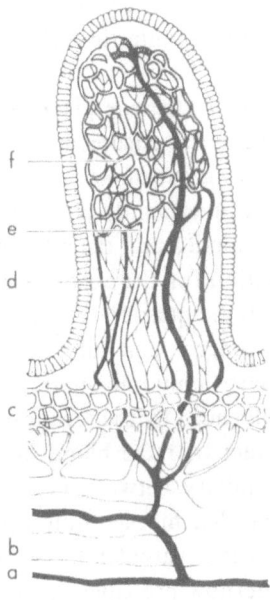

Fig. 4.5. Diagram of the vascularisation of the intestinal villus. Depicted are the submucosal artery (*a*) and vein (*b*), the submucosal venous plexus (*c*), main villous arteriole (*d*) and venule (*e*), and capillary network (*f*). (Reproduced from Sessions et al., in Progress in Gastroenterology I: 252, Grune and Stratton, 1968; with permission of the authors and publishers).

beneath the epithelial layer of the villus. These capillaries connect with small venules which open up into veins that largely follow the pattern of the arterial vascularization. At the base of the villi there are probably direct anastomoses between arterioles and venules so that, when intestinal activity is low, the circulation in the villi can be short-circuited (533, 771, 775).

The arterial blood supply to the small intestine serves the function of providing it with the nutrients and the oxygen which it needs to fulfil its functions, such as absorption, secretion and motility. The venous system takes care of the removal of the substances absorbed.

During the process of digestion and absorption, the blood flow through the small intestine is increased by 100-200%. This is made possible by vasodilatation which occurs as a reflex action in response to mechanical stimulation of the mucosa of the small intestine by food (66). Moreover, the blood flow can be stimulated by the intestinal hormones secretin and cholecystokinin, which are released in response to chemical stimulation of the mucosa (262). Finally, metabolites of the intestinal motility process may also play a role in vasodilatation (649). The extrinsic autonomic nerves play no significant role in dilatation of the intestinal blood vessels. It seems likely that

37

only sympathetic nerve fibres innervate the intestinal vasculature, giving rise to only brief and transient vasoconstriction (532). However, within some minutes a so-called autoregulatory escape mechanism is activated by the release of local vasodilatators or by reduced sensitivity of the sympathetic receptors (772). This mechanism ensures that the intestinal villi are supplied with a sufficient amount of blood at all times.

The circulation in the mucosa of the small intestine plays an important role in intestinal absorption. Not only because it ensures rapid removal of the absorbed nutrients, but also in supplying substances required for the metabolism of the absorbing enterocytes. Consequently there seems to be a correlation between the amount of blood supplied and the intestinal absorption (527). The importance of the circulation for the absorptive process is also emphasized by the fact that about three-quarters of the total blood supply to the small intestine goes to the mucosa and submucosa, whereas the musculature of the intestinal wall receives only one-quarter (532).

It seems plausible that absorption is influenced by the arrangement of the blood vessels in the villi (fig. 4.5). The fact that the blood in the central arteriole and that in the subepithelial capillary network flow in opposite directions makes it hypothetically possible that marked differences in concentration of solutes are built up along these vascular loops. This is explained on the basis of the so-called counterflow principle, analogous to the situation in the kidney in the loop of Henle (120). Exchange of water between arteriole and venule at the base of the villus could give rise to marked hyperosmolarity in the villous tip, both in the arteriole and in the surroun-

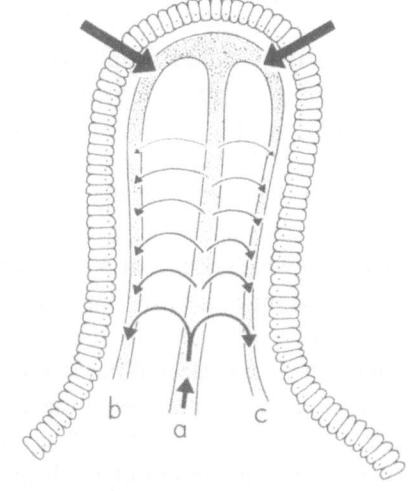

Fig. 4.6. Diagram of the functional implications of the postulated countercurrent exchange in the intestinal villus. The curved arrows represent the flux of water from the main villous arteriole (*a*) to the capillaries (*b* and *c*), producing a gradual buildup of the ion concentration towards the villous tip. The straight broad arrows indicate the flux of water and solutes from the intestinal lumen, resulting from local osmolar differences.

ding tissue (fig. 4.6). Water from the intestinal lumen may be attracted, and with it solutes via the so-called solvent drag (section 5.1.6). With the result that substances can be absorbed against a concentration gradient. Another result of the possible cross diffusion of water at the villous base is haemoconcentration in the upper half of the villus. Due to a decreased flow rate, the time for exchange between epithelial layer and the villous capillaries may be prolonged. Experimental observations seem to support this counterflow hypothesis (120, 533).

The lymphatic system of the small intestine consists of an extensive network of lymphatics with delicate extensions in each villus. These extensions – variously known as central, terminal or initial lacteals – are in fact the 'blind' starting-points of the lymphatic system. Apart from extracellular tissue fluid they also transport chylomicrons, so that the term 'lacteals' is more appropriate than 'lymphatics'. The wall of the lacteals consists of a thin layer of endothelial cells. At several sites this wall shows valve-like cell junctions which are usually firmly closed but can open to accommodate the passage of lymph. This endothelial layer is probably covered by a fragmentary basement membrane and besides surrounded by a network of reticulin fibres (450).

The initial lacteals connect with the larger lymphatics in the submucosa, which at some sites communicate with lymph follicles or aggregates of lymphoid tissue in the intestinal wall like the so-called Peyer plaques in the ileum. The lymphatics form an extensive system of ramifying and anastomosing vessels, merging into larger collecting vessels, which extend circularly as well as longitudinally in the muscular layers of the intestine. As the diameter of the lymphatics increases, their wall becomes firmer due to the presence of fibres and muscle cells. Except in the most minute lymphatics, valves are found at regular intervals in the lumen. In the mesentery, the lymphatic vessels roughly follow the pattern of the mesenteric blood vessels. At several sites along this route one finds lymph nodes, which are arranged in groups at the origin of the superior mesenteric artery. The large lymphatic vessels which arise here combine to form the gastrointestinal trunk, ending in the cisterna chyli. From this cisterna arises the thoracic duct, which empties into the left subclavian vein (450).

Via the lymphatic system, fluid and substances are transported which originate partly from the tissues and partly from the intestinal lumen. Extracellular tissue fluid results from the flux of water and other plasma constituents on the arterial side of the capillaries. Most of this tissue fluid is usually taken up again by the veins. However, macromolecular substances such as immunoglobulins, proteins, chylomicrons produced by the enterocytes, as well as the immunocytes from the lymph follicles cannot be readily taken up through the venous wall. The lymphatic system transports these macromolecular substances and the immunocytes. In addition, the lymphatics can assist in transporting smaller molecules, should the blood circulation insufficiently cope with these (286).

It is assumed that chylomicrons and macromolecular substances are taken up via the valve-like inlets in the wall of the initial lacteals. Passage through these valves is made possible by an increase of pressure in the villous stroma around the lacteal as a result of accumulation of fluid and plasma constituents effused from the blood stream, and of substances absorbed from the intestinal lumen (fig. 4.7.a). After taking up fluid, (macro)-

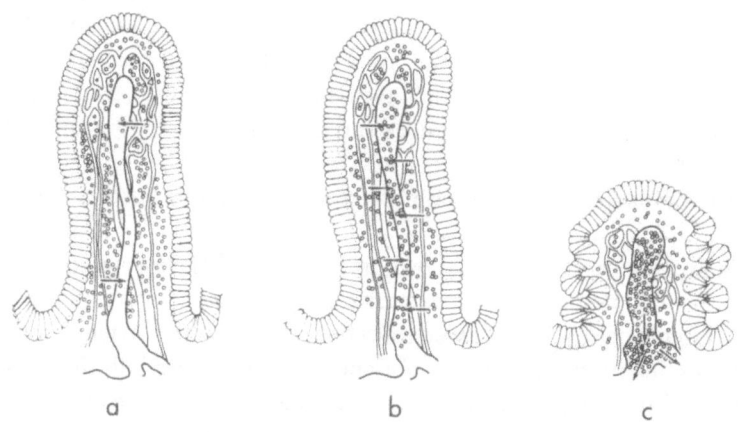

a   b   c

Fig. 4.7. Diagram of the uptake and transport of chylus by the initial lacteal. Arrows show the postulated movement of chylous particles from the interstitial tissue into the lacteal (*a* and *b*) and their subsequent ejection when the villus contracts (*c*). (Reproduced from Sessions et al., in Progress in Gastroenterology I: 254, Grune and Stratton, 1968; with permission of the authors and publishers).

molecules and particles, the lacteal will become dilated. In consequence the pressure within the lymphatic vessels exceeds that outside the vessel, with the result that the valves close. As a result of the tension generated in the circular fibres around the basement membrane, the dilated lacteal will attempt to expel the amount of chylus and lymph taken up (286).

An important contribution to the transport of lymph from the lacteal to the submucosa is probably made by the muscle fibres in the villous stroma, which can cause both transverse and longitudinal contraction of the villus, thus milking the lacteal empty, so to speak (fig. 4.7.c). Perhaps this milking is done in coordination with contractions of the muscularis mucosae and the musculature of the intestinal wall (771). The somewhat larger lymphatics have themselves a small number of muscle fibres in their walls, giving them the possibility to contract independently. It cannot be excluded, however, that the drainage of lymph is further assisted by arterial pulsations, changes of pressure in the abdominal cavity or movements of the mesentery. The direction in which the lymph flows is otherwise determined by the presence of valves in the medium-sized and large lymphatic vessels (286).

4.6 DIGESTIVE SECRETIONS

4.6.1 Introduction

The degradation of food in the intestine is ensured by enzymatic and chemical processes. The enzymes and other substances required for this purpose are supplied by the digestive juices secreted in the gastrointestinal tract. These include saliva, gastric juice and pancreatic juice. For the emulsification of lipids and micelle formation, bile is secreted. The digestive juices play an important role in the absorption of food constituents in that they change these constituents to a form which permits rapid and efficient absorption.

4.6.2 Gastric secretion

Gastric juice consists of several constituents, each originating from certain cell types in different parts of the stomach (192). The most important area of gastric juice production is the corpus ventriculi which, like the fundus, contains glands which produce hydrochloric acid (HCl), pepsinogens and intrinsic factor. The production takes place in the parietal (or oxyntic) cells, which secrete intrinsic factor as well as hydrochloric acid (400), while the chief (or zymogenic) cells produce pepsinogens. At the junction between the glandular ductules and mucosal surface are localized the so-called mucous neck cells, probably precursors of the chief cells, which secrete mucus and

41

perhaps also pepsinogens (746). Mucous cells are otherwise found everywhere between the parietal cells and the chief cells in the glands.

The tubular glands in the antrum produce mucus, with some pepsinogens, but no HCl. In addition the antral glands also contain gastrin-producing cells (577). The glands of the cardia produce only mucus. The whole surface of the gastric mucosa is lined with epithelial cells which produce mucus.

Stimulation of gastric acid production can take place in three ways (phases) (888). In the cephalic phase this comes about extrinsically via the vagus nerve, which is stimulated when food is seen, smelled or tasted. During the gastric phase the local receptors in the wall of the stomach are stimulated, while in the intestinal phase acid production is caused by stimuli which originate from the duodenum or jejunum. Throughout all these phases, gastric acid secretion is provoked by acetylcholine or gastrin, often in combination with each other (888).

Gastric acid production is probably inhibited in as many different ways, such as by acidification of antrum or duodenum, and by inhibiting the release of gastrin. In response to the entrance of fats, acids or hypertonic solutions in the duodenum, cholecystokinin and secretin are released. These hormones are suspected of inhibiting the gastric acid production, but this is by no means certain (888). The pepsinogens, of which seven types are known so far (746), are secreted as inactive zymogens. Pepsinogen is turned into active pepsin by detachment of some peptide groups, caused by gastric acid and already activated pepsin. These pepsins are important proteolytic enzymes, maximally effective between pH 1 and pH 3. The secretion of pepsinogens is stimulated in the same way as that of gastric acid, apart from the fact that secretin, believed to stimulate pepsin production, probably inhibits acid production (888).

4.6.3 Pancreatic secretion

The pancreas produces several digestive enzymes such as α-amylase, lipases, cholesterol esterase and phospholipase, pro-carboxypeptidase A and B, pro-elastase, chymotrypsinogen and trypsinogen, along with some less well-known enzymes. The proteolytic enzymes are secreted as inactive zymogens. Trypsinogen is activated in the duodenum by enterokinase, which requires the presence of calcium ions. Activated trypsin activates other enzymes such as chymotrypsinogen, pro-elastase and phospholipase, while all activated enzymes autocatalytically activate their precursors. The enzyme α-amylase is secreted in an active form, just like the lipases. In addition, the pancreas secretes a fluid which contains large amounts of bicarbonate, sodium and potassium ions in concentrations more or less equal to those in plasma, and small quantities of chloride, calcium and magnesium (238).

Pancreatic secretion is stimulated by the presence of food in the stomach or duodenum. The secretion is regulated by hormonal as well as nervous factors. Of the intestinal hormones, secretin in particular stimulates the pancreas to secrete water and bicarbonate. The release of digestive enzymes is incited particularly by cholecystokinin and, in lesser degree, by secretin. Enzyme secretion is believed to be stimulated also by the parasympathetic nerves (101).

Like gastric juice, pancreatic juice is released in several ways or phases. In addition to the cephalic phase there is a gastric phase, in which the pancreas is stimulated in response to mechanical irritation of the stomach through local reflex arcs. There exists also an intestinal phase in which local intestinal hormones are released and perhaps the parasympathetic system is stimulated as well (101).

The synthesis of enzymes by the pancreas can be influenced by the composition of the diet. There seems to be some sort of adaptation, in that enzyme synthesis is adjusted to the requirements (206).

4.6.4 Bile secretion

Bile is produced by hepatocytes and in part also by epithelial cells in the bile ducts. The hepatocytes mostly secrete bilirubin and bile acids, along with cholesterol and phospholipids; the bile duct cells secrete in particular sodium and bicarbonate. Water and solutes go passively along with the active secretion of the above mentioned organic and inorganic ions. Secretion by the bile duct cells is believed to be controlled by some intestinal hormones such as secretin and cholecystokinin (9).

The bile is collected and concentrated in the gall-bladder which, if necessary, can release a large amount of bile all at once. Concentration is effected by absorption of water, together with sodium, chloride and bicarbonate.

Efflux of bile to the duodenum is normally prevented by the sphincter of Oddi. This sphincter relaxes in response to cholecystokinin which also causes the gall-bladder to contract vigorously. This hormone is released when lipid substances enter the duodenum.

The bile acids are synthesized in the hepatocytes from cholesterol. By alterations in the steroid skeleton, cholic acid and chenodesoxycholic acid are produced. They are conjugated to glycine or taurine and so secreted in the bile. This conjugation is absolutely necessary for their function, which is to form micelles (210). Having served as vehicles for lipid substances in the lumen of the small intestine, the bile acids are reabsorbed in the terminal ileum. This is effected by an active transport process which accounts for the reabsorption of almost 95% (235), while the remainder is degraded by bacteria in the colon to deoxycholic acid and lithocholic acid, which are in part eliminated with the faeces. Relatively much of the deoxycholic acid, but only a small fraction of the lithocholic acid is reabsorbed. The reabsorbed bile acids are returned, degraded or not by bacteria, to the liver via the portal circulation and recovered by the hepatocytes. The bile acids are again secreted in bile, after renewed conjugation to glycine or taurine, if necessary. In actual fact, synthesis of bile acids has only to compensate for their loss via the faeces. This loss is estimated to be 0.2-0.5 g per day, but can be many times as large in the case of disease or resection of the terminal ileum (9).

4.7 INTESTINAL HORMONES

Hormones of different types are produced in the digestive tract. Several organs of this tract contain endocrine cells in such amounts that, all in all, the gastrointestinal tract is one of the largest endocrine organs (666). In the past, these endocrine cells were known as clear cells ('helle Zellen') (273), but also as enterochromaffin, argentaffin or argyrophilic cells because they are able to precipitate silver salts and are thus to be identified in histological specimens. The name currently preferred is APUD cells, which denotes the various properties of these cells, e.g. the presence of *A*mines and their capability of amine *P*recursor *U*ptake and *D*ecarboxylation. They are localized mainly in the crypts of the small intestine. These cells contain hormone granules in their basal part. Using electron microscopic and especially immunofluorescence techniques, several types of endocrine cell have been identified. According to the hormone produced by them, these cells are called A-cell (glucagon), G-cell (gastrin) and S-cell (secretin). In addition, several other cells have been identified of which the significance has so far remained obscure. In the small intestine, only a few of these endocrine cell types are present (666). All APUD cells secrete in addition to a particular hormone or hormone-like polypeptide one or several amines, like 5-hydroxytryptamine or serotonin. The function of this 5-hydroxytryptamine is still unexplained. Perhaps it promotes motility or even circulation in the small intestine (240).

The intestinal hormones influence the function of stomach, bowels, pancreas and gall-bladder, and perhaps in addition also processes outside the digestive tract. Purified or even synthetic preparations of these hormones have become available only a few years ago, making it possible to study their influence on processes in the gastrointestinal tract. The possibility of demonstrating physiological (i.e. usually minute) quantities of hormone in body fluids by means of radio-immunoassay has also been of great importance for further research into the presence and activities of intestinal hormones. Effects of these hormones on absorption and secretion in the small intestine, on fluid and enzyme secretion in stomach and pancreas, and on motility and tissue growth of the digestive tract, have been described by several investigators (341). Not infrequently, however, these effects could be produced only with extremely large, so-called pharmacological doses of hormones which, moreover, often were not pure or obtained from a different animal species. Another disadvantage in studying the effect of a given hormone is that other hormones are sometimes secondarily released or that its effects are masked by simultaneous action of other hormones (341).

It has been established with certainty that at least three hormones are formed and operating in the small intestine: secretin, cholecystokinin (CCK-PZ) and gastrin. In addition, several 'candidate hormones' have been described, i.e. polypeptides of which it is not yet certain that they exert any influence on the gastrointestinal tract, or that their effect is not produced secondarily via other hormones. This group encompasses such substances as enteroglucagon, gastric inhibitory polypeptide (GIP), vasoactive intestinal polypeptide (VIP), motilin, pancreatic polypeptide and somatostatin (342, 699).

Gastrin is known to be present in several components (889). It is formed in the G-cells, which are mainly localized in the antrum of the stomach and in the duodenum (637). Gastrin is released via stimulation of the vagus nerves or in response to the presence of food in the stomach (485). This stimulation is inhibited by the presence of acid in the stomach (889). In physiological concentrations, gastrin can probably only stimulate gastric acid secretion, activating the pepsinogens as a secondary effect (440).

Secretin, too, occurs in a number of variants, which usually have a higher molecule weight than secretin proper (80). Secretin is produced by the S-cells which are found in great numbers in the duodenum (591). The hormone is released after reduction of the pH in the duodenum due to the entrance of gastric juice and, in lesser degree, of food (699). Stimulation of the vagus nerve causes no release of secretin (828). The principal and under physiological conditions probably only effect of secretin is stimulation of water and bicarbonate secretion by the pancreas (426). Perhaps other hormones such as CCK-PZ or VIP contribute to this effect (342). The increased secretion of pancreatic enzymes observed after administration of secretin, is probably

45

based on a so-called wash-out effect (814). The blood flow to the small intestine through the superior mesenteric artery probably increases (262). The motility of the small intestine and the intestinal absorption of water and sodium, however, are believed to be inhibited by secretin (441).

The hormone cholecystokinin, also known as pancreozymin in view of its influence on the pancreas, is produced by certain not yet identified cells in the mucosa of the small intestine. The concentration of CCK-PZ attains its maximum in the jejunum, but substantial concentrations are present also in the duodenum and ileum (79). CCK-PZ is released in response to the presence of food (more specifically amino acids and fatty acids) and in lesser degree to the presence of hydrochloric acid in the duodenum and jejunum (251, 314). Cholecystokinin stimulates the gall-bladder to contract and probably also promotes bile production (445). In addition, this hormone is believed to stimulate the pancreas to secrete enzymes (815), bicarbonate (623) and insulin (868). The intestinal motility is probably also promoted by CCK-PZ (370), as well as the blood flow via the superior mesenteric artery (97, 262). Finally, absorption of sodium chloride and potassium in the jejunum is believed to be inhibited by CCK-PZ (441).

As pointed out, it is not certain whether the 'candidate hormones' exert any influence on the digestive tract, or produce an effect only via the stimulation of other hormones. Some of these 'candidate hormones' are polypeptides which are isolated from the mucosa of the small intestine, while the presence of other 'candidate hormones' is assumed merely in order to explain certain physiological phenomena (343). In view of the uncertainty about their existence and activities, these 'candidate hormones' will not be further discussed in this context.

The effect of hormones on their target cells (e.g. the parietal cell of the stomach or the pancreatic acinar cell) occurs through stimulation of receptors in the cellular wall. The nature or affinity of the receptor determines whether a hormone can produce any effect and, if so, which effect occurs (341). The target cells probably have several types of receptor, both for the various hormones and for the neurotransmitters.

The effect of a hormone on a target cell is produced – at least in some cases – via a mediator: cyclic AMP. If so, the hormone is the first messenger, which informs the target cell of the desirability of a certain effect, and cyclic AMP is the second messenger (829). Alteration of the amount of cyclic AMP in the cell, caused by a given hormone, is believed to produce the desired effect in the target cell. This change in the AMP concentration results on the one hand from enzymatic conversion of ATP in the cytoplasm by the enzyme adenylcyclase, bound to the cell membrane and localized close to the

46

hormonal receptor site (829). On the other hand, the intracellular concentration of cyclic AMP is also determined by the rate at which AMP is degraded by enzymes, which are also localized near the cell membrane and influenced by hormones (513).

4.8 INTESTINAL MUCUS

Like most of the epithelium lining the digestive tract, the mucosa of the small intestine contains mucus producing cells: the so-called goblet cells. These differ from the other cells of the intestinal epithelium in that they are specialized in the production and secretion of mucus. Goblet cells evolve from undifferentiated cells in the crypts of the intestinal mucosa. The mucus is produced in or near the Golgi apparatus. Continuous synthesis and polymerization of mucus takes place throughout the life-span of these goblet cells, which is estimated to be 4-6 days. It takes an average to two hours for mucus to be synthesized from its basic elements and to become visible in the apical part of the goblet cell. Subsequently, secretion into the intestinal lumen takes place within a few hours via apertures in the apical cell membrane (518). The secretion of mucus is promoted by stimulation of the sympathetic nerve fibres, resulting from the contact between the food and the mucosa of the small intestine (192). The intestinal hormones probably play no role in the secretion of intestinal mucus.

Mucus has a number of special physical properties. Since it can form a gel, its viscosity is high. It also has a marked adhesive power, and the ability to form film-like layers. The basic elements which make up mucus consist of glycoproteins (mucoproteins), i.e. proteins with carbohydrates on the side chains. The composition differs slightly from one individual to another. So little as these basic elements are influenced by chemical or physical changes, so unstable is the three-dimensional structure of intestinal mucus (762). As a gel, mucus is made up of a large number of basic elements which, through the electrical forces of the charged side chains and terminal groups, can form large spatial structures (16). When these electrical forces are lost, due to a decrease in pH or the attachment of certain ions, the structure of the mucus changes. The gel becomes fragmented and begins to liquefy before dissolving in the intestinal lumen (762). Usually there is continuous degradation of mucus by gastric juice, enzymes and bacteria. Under normal conditions production of mucus can keep pace with its destruction so that a dynamic equilibrium exists.

The function of intestinal mucus is partly determined by its physical properties (762). The mucus secreted by the goblet cells forms a continuous layer covering the epithelial cells of the gastrointestinal tract, which probably protects the intestinal wall from the influence of proteolytic enzymes, bacteria, etc. Perhaps bacteria are even killed in this layer of mucus (664). It is not inconceivable that this covering of the enterocytes can also influence absorption from the intestinal lumen, either because the mucous gel acts as a kind of filter, or as a result of the fact that certain ions become bound to the mucus during the absorptive process (762).

This protective coating of mucus secreted by the goblet cells should not be confused with the so-called glycocalyx on the brush border of the enterocytes, which likewise partly consists of glycoproteins. This layer is probably secreted by the underlying enterocytes, and forms an integral part of their outer wall. The glycocalyx contains many enzymes and may therefore play a role in the digestion of food (511).

4.9 EXFOLIATION OF ENTEROCYTES

The mucosa of the small intestine is covered by an epithelial sheet consisting of cells which have only a limited life-span. There is constant production of epithelial cells in the crypts of the intestinal mucosa. The cells produced are moved up and meanwhile continue to differentiate. Later, as functional, mature enterocytes, they make up the lining of the intestinal villi. Once moved up to the apex of the villus, the enterocytes are extruded at the so-called extrusion zones (fig. 3.1). Exfoliation is believed to be necessary because the enterocytes are exhausted or worn out (section 3.2.3). This means that the epithelial lining of the intestinal villi is in a process of constant regeneration. Each epithelial cell is extruded a few days after its production. The life-span of the enterocyte is varyingly estimated, ranging from 2-4 days (178) to 4-6 days (537). It follows that one-sixth to one-half of the total number of enterocytes is shed each day. The exfoliated cells are estimated to amount to 250 g per day (186, 507). Under normal conditions the exfoliated cells are rapidly degraded in the intestinal lumen. The cell constituents are probably for the greater part reabsorbed. Under normal conditions, therefore, little material is lost to the body (179).

4.10 ENTERIC PLASMA PROTEIN LOSS

The occurrence of protein leakage from the tissues into the lumen of the digestive tract was first observed in 1957. The discovery was made in a patient suffering from hypoproteinaemia, caused by protein loss via the gastric wall as a result of hypertrophic gastritis (140). In subsequent years, more or less serious protein loss in the gastrointestinal tract was demonstrated in a wide variety of conditions (431, 850, 879). The possibility of measuring the protein leakage in so many situations was created by marked simplification of the measuring procedure. The method currently regarded as the simplest and most accurate is that of labelling plasma proteins with ^{51}Cr (848). The widely used designation plasma protein leakage resulted from the observation that this process entails a loss of all plasma proteins, which from the blood stream enter the intestinal lumen via the intercellular fluid. This protein loss often gives rise to a decreased plasma protein concentration. It was established with the aid of the above mentioned method that some protein loss in the gastrointestinal tract also occurs in healthy subjects, although in a much lesser degree than the loss found in patients with gastrointestinal disorders (437). The phenomenon per se is not abnormal, therefore, but only its degree. It seems useful to point out that, through leakage of tissue fluid, several constituents of this fluid other than proteins also enter the intestinal lumen. This has been demonstrated by, among other things, analysis of fluid recovered after intestinal perfusion (179).

Little has so far been established concerning the underlying mechanism of this enteric protein leakage in normal subjects. The epithelial layer which lines the wall of the gastrointestinal tract is usually a tight, continuous layer. Leakage of tissue fluid might take place at the apex of the villus, at the so-called extrusion zone, where the worn-out enterocytes are shed so that a temporary breach occurs in the continuous row of epithelial cells. It is conceivable that, during this exfoliation of enterocytes, a minute quantity of tissue fluid from the villous stroma enters the intestinal lumen. Some investigators suggest that the protein loss occurs via the intercellular spaces in the epithelium (437, 879). Using autoradiography after administration of labelled albumin, Brooks et al. (105) were in fact able to demonstrate that albumin accumulated in these intercellular spaces particularly in those parts of the epithelial layer localized at the villous tip or resting over capillaries. The albumin did not seem to enter the intestinal lumen from these spaces, however, perhaps as a result of the tight junctions which firmly connect the enterocytes at their apical side. Perhaps the albumin also partly enters the enterocytes proper (e.g. by pinocytosis) and finds itself in the intestinal lumen only after their exfoliation (105).

Protein which leaks into the intestinal lumen is bound to be largely degraded and reabsorbed. One of the factors which determine the degree of degradation and reabsorption is the site where the leakage occurs. Protein leaked into the distal part of the small intestine is probably subject to a less marked degree of degradation and reabsorption than protein which enters the proximal jejunum. The enteric leakage of protein, therefore, does not always have to be associated with an equally large loss of protein or protein degradation products in faeces or urine.

4.11 INTESTINAL FLORA

Even under normal conditions, the human intestine harbours a world of micro-organisms. These in principle exogenous micro-organisms enter the body with the food, and it is from this constant supply that the human intestinal flora is selected (73). Only very specific bacteria are able to maintain themselves in the gastrointestinal tract; the majority of micro-organisms are destroyed or excreted. Determinants of the ability of bacteria to maintain themselves in the human intestine are the requirements of these micro-organisms as well as the characteristics of the environment which accommodates them. This natural selection determines the particular nature of the bacterial flora in the intestinal tract, which is usually fairly stable and self-regulating. Only in the upper part of the digestive tract can a variable bacterial flora be present as a result of the ever-repeated ingestion of common as well as less common micro-organisms (237). The faeces, too, contains a variable population of micro-organisms, including the bacteria which failed to 'take'. In the small and large intestine, however, a fairly stable bacterial flora prevails which usually resists any change. The micro-organisms conventionally found in the intestine have become accustomed to the particular conditions in the intestine. New micro-organisms still have to develop these properties but often are not given the chance or the time to adjust. An important factor for maintenance in the intestine is that the micro-organisms develop the ability to propagate by slow instead of by rapid division (311).

The nature of the bacterial flora prevalent in the intestine is largely determined by the interactions between the various types of micro-organisms. These include competition with regard to available nutrients or enzyme proteins, the influence on pH or oxygen pressure, the production of growth-inhibiting or growth-promoting substances, and the possible transfer of resistance to antibiotics (226). In addition, the composition of the bacterial flora in the small intestine is determined also by some factors unrelated to these interactions. Important factors in this respect are the peristalsis, which ensures constant removal of micro-organisms, and the presence of gastric juice and bile acids (237). Many investigators suspect that as yet unidentified inhibitors of bacterial growth are also present in gastric juice, pancreatic secretion, bile or intestinal fluid (226). The intestinal wall itself functions as an effective barrier against invasion of micro-organisms from the intestinal lumen. The mucosa is probably enabled so to function by its coating of mucus and by local synthesis of antibodies (copro-antibodies). All the above mentioned factors keep the growth of intestinal bacteria under control in normal circumstances. It has been calculated that, in the absence of any inhibition of growth, the micro-organisms in the digestive tract would be so numerous within 24 hours, that the total amount of necessary nutrients would exceed the body mass of an average human individual (311).

The small intestine normally contains few bacteria in its proximal part: as a rule less than 10^4/ml. Some of these are micro-organisms from the food or the oral cavity, which are en route. The autochthonous flora of the proximal small intestine largely consists of Gram-positive aerobic or facultative anaerobic micro-organisms such as streptococci and lactobacilli. Small numbers of enterobacteria or strictly anaerobic bacteroides can also be present (322). In the distal part of the small intestine the population of micro-organisms is much larger, usually some 10^5-10^7/ml. The bacterial flora at this level is also more varied and stable, and in addition to streptococci and lactobacilli comprises about equally large numbers of enterobacteria and bacteroides (237, 322). A faecal flora usually prevails in the lower ileum. It comprises bacteroides, bifidobacteria and non-spore-forming anaerobes, along with many other micro-organisms. As many as 37 species of micro-organism have been isolated from faeces, which probably contains still many more bacterial species (605).

The bacterial flora in the small intestine largely determines the internal environment via its influence on many processes in the intestinal lumen such as digestion, absorption and degradation of food constituents, vitamins, enzymes, medicinal agents, etc. Some micro-organisms are even able to synthesize certain vitamins. It has been stated that, in terms of metabolic activity, the bacterial flora of the digestive tract in its totality is equivalent to the liver (918). However, since under normal conditions the bacterial flora in the small intestine comprises only a limited assortment and small numbers of micro-organisms, it probably plays only a minor role in the absorption and degradation of food constituents (226, 237). A different situation prevails in the colon, where the cellulose-rich vegetable food constituents are partly degraded by bacteria (419). The question, however, is to which extent these degradation products are still absorbed. The same applies to the vitamins synthesized in the colon (923). Some pharmacological agents, e.g. salazosul-phapyridine, depend on bacterial conversion for release of their active metabolites (918). The presence of an intestinal flora is also of great importance in preventing truly pathogenic micro-organisms from settling down. This is achieved via the creation of a particular environment in which no suitable conditions prevail for these pathogenic micro-organisms (237). Due to the presence of micro-organisms in the intestine the human organism is constantly immunized against the bacteria commonly found in food.

## CHAPTER 5

INTESTINAL DIGESTION AND ABSORPTION

5.1 GENERAL INTRODUCTION

5.1.1 Surface

The interaction between the contents of the lumen and the mucosa of the small intestine takes place at and via the membrane which separates one from the other. Their interface is greatly enlarged by the presence of mucosal folds (valvulae conniventes of Kerckring), intestinal villi, and microvilli. This surface enlargement is quite pronounced, particularly in the proximal segment of the small intestine (921). The total area of the interface between the enterocytes and the intestinal lumen has been estimated to equal that of a lawn-tennis court (180, 808). It is not quite clear why this surface area should be so large. An obvious suggestion would seem to be that it is required for optimal absorption. However, experience gained with patients after resection of a large portion of the small intestine contradicts this. The available surface area is evidently substantially larger than would be strictly necessary; there is, it seems, a considerable functional reserve. This is also apparent from the large amounts of food which the human organism is able to absorb. This has been demonstrated for several food constituents such as fat, the absorption of which is still normal at a daily intake of some 600 g (460), and for protein, of which amounts up to 600 g/day can likewise be absorbed (701). Perhaps the large surface area of the small intestine should be viewed as a vestige of man's remote past, when meals were less regular and food was taken when the hunt was successful, often after a fast of several days.

5.1.2 Mucosal contact time

The absorption of each substance increases as the increase in duration of exposure to the absorbing surface. The propulsion of the food bolus in the small intestine, therefore, should not be too rapid if adequate absorption is

53

to be ensured. The average speed of intestinal contents is estimated to be 1.5-2 cm/minute while fasting, and is believed scarcely to increase after ingestion of a modest meal. After food consumption, the intestine distends if necessary in order to pass more food without accelerating its transit. This adaptation of the diameter of the intestinal lumen to the amount of ingested food, together with the above mentioned functional reserve of absorbing surface, is an important aid in coping with a sudden supply of large amounts of food (808).

5.1.3 Digestion

The ingested food is largely digested before it is absorbed in the small intestine. Degradation is required to obtain fragments sufficiently small to be absorbed. Dietary proteins are thereby sufficiently altered to lose their antigenic properties. Experience shows, however, that very large molecules such as haem and polyglutamate, can be adequately absorbed without degradation (44, 157). It has also been found that some protein molecules are able to pass the intestinal wall without any preceding degradation, thus retaining their antigenic properties (891). Another explanation of the use of intraluminal digestion is perhaps that fragments can be more quickly absorbed because they pass through the cell membrane more easily (121). Absorption, however, does not always prove to be faster as the fragments become smaller. Oligopeptides, for example, are absorbed at least as quickly as amino acids (173, 791).

It has long been assumed that food constituents are completely degraded in the intestinal lumen before they are absorbed. It has gradually come to be established, however, that digestion of proteins, fats and carbohydrates in the intestinal lumen is usually incomplete (567). It is probable that digestion also takes place to an important extent in the brush border of the enterocytes (866), and even intracellularly (673). The brush border therefore has a function beyond merely that of enlarging the absorbing surface. It contains many enzymes for food digestion and also carriers for the transport of degradation products, as well as ATPase to obtain the energy from ATP required for active transport (807). The notion has developed that the side-by-side presence of digestive enzymes, carriers and energy suppliers in the brush border ensures rapid and efficient absorption of food constituents (414).

5.1.4 Translocation

It is difficult to imagine how the digested nutrients pass through the intestinal wall during the translocation process, because the cell membrane of the enterocyte consists largely of lipids. Only the passage of fat-like substances poses no problems because they can – more or less – diffuse through this membrane. For all other ions and for water, translocation would theoretically seem to be almost impossible. In actual practice, however, these substances prove to pass through the cell membrane without difficulty. There are only two conceivable ways in which this can take place.

One possible way is via water-filled pores in the enterocyte membrane, otherwise known as aqueous channels. Perfusion studies with solutions of molecules of different size would seem to warrant the conclusion that, in the jejunum, most of these pores have a diameter of 0.8 nm, versus about 0.3 nm in the ileum. In addition, a small number of wider pores are believed to be present through which larger molecules can pass (282). It is conceivable that these pores are not only found in the enterocyte membrane but also at the tight junctions between the enterocytes (284).

Another possibility is that non-lipid substances pass through the cell membrane by means of so-called transport carriers which are believed capable of carrying these substances through the cell membrane. These carriers have been conceived of as a kind of rotating ticket-window or turnstile, taking up substances on the luminal side of the cell membrane, and releasing them intracellularly (175). The exact nature of these carriers is unknown, for they have never been isolated or visualized. Yet their existence is plausible, for phenomena such as active transport, facilitated diffusion and congenital disorders in intestinal amino acid transport could hardly be explained without this carrier concept.

5.1.5 Unstirred layer

The absorption of substances from the intestinal lumen is expected to be influenced by the phenomenon of the so-called unstirred layer (213). This term refers to the fact that there exists no direct contact between the lipid enterocyte membrane and the aqueous solution in the intestinal lumen. There is a kind of liquid intermediate layer present, called unstirred layer, which differs in composition from the remainder of the intestinal contents. Its thickness should range from 10 to 1000 μm, dependent on the nature of the lipid membrane and the flow of intestinal contents. At the villous tips this layer is much thinner than near the crypts. The unstirred layer impedes the absorption of various substances, particularly of hydrophobic molecules. It prevents a direct contact between luminal contents and intestinal wall. Changes in the intestinal contents are not demonstrable in the unstirred layer until after some time, and often in a lesser degree. The rate at which nutrients are absorbed, therefore, can be largely determined by the quality of the unstirred layer (213).

5.1.6 Absorption

The fundamental process which underlies absorption in its totality is based on the characteristic property of all epithelial cells, including enterocytes, to maintain a certain intracellular sodium concentration (659). The cells of the intestinal wall maintain a sodium concentration, which is comparatively low. The sodium is pumped out of the enterocytes, into the intercellular space via the lateral cell membrane. This transport usually takes place against an electrochemical gradient, and therefore requires energy. For this purpose the lateral cell membrane contains Na^+-K^+-activated ATPase (797), which can convert the ATP synthesized by the enterocytes to energy (fig. 5.1.a;

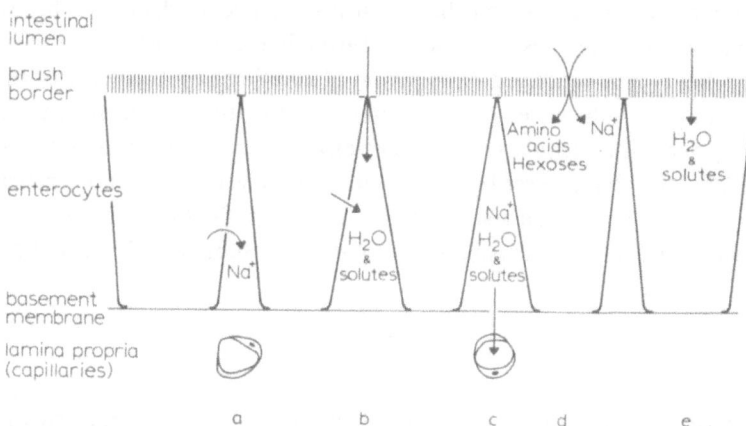

Fig. 5.1. Diagram of the various components of the intestinal absorption process of fluid and electrolytes.
a. the sodiumpump at the lateral cell membrane
b. the solvent drag into the intercellular space
c. the emptying of the intercellular space
d. the transepithelial carrier transport mechanism (coupled translocation of sodium and amino acids or hexoses)
e. the solvent drag into the enterocyte

659). In this way, hyperosmolarity is created in the intercellular space, and water is attracted. It has not been established whether this water is attracted from the enterocytes via their lateral cell membrane and/or from the intestinal lumen via the tight junctions. This water flux takes along solutes by means of convection, a process known as solvent drag (fig. 5.1.b). In this way, certain ions can even be transported against a concentration gradient.

There is an additional absorptive mechanism operating in the brush border membrane. The translocation of various substances by means of carriers is believed to take place here. These carriers, which in some respect are specific for the substance to be absorbed (567), seem to be able to function only if sodium can be translocated along with the molecule or ion in question. In fact the sodium translocation is probably the primary process. Since the intracellular sodium concentration is low, as sodium is continuously being pumped to the intercellular space (fig. 5.1.a), the sodium from the intestinal lumen can enter the enterocyte with the concentration gradient, in a transport process which requires no energy. On the 'pillion-seat' of the carrier, the sodium takes along other substances such as glucose or amino acids into the cell (fig. 5.1.d; 175, 763). Just as sodium stimulates the absorption of glucose and amino acids, the latter two substances stimulate the absorption of sodium (284). It follows from the above that translocation of sodium is of fundamental importance for all absorption processes in the small intestine.

The translocation of sodium and other substances over the brush border membrane also attracts water, which creates a solvent drag (fig. 5.1.e).

In addition to active transport, passive transport can take place through the cell membrane. This passive transport, otherwise known as diffusion, is possible only with the concentration gradient or electrochemical gradient. If diffusion takes place with the aid of carriers, it is called facilitated diffusion.

All absorbed substances enter the intercellular spaces, be it as a result of diffusion, solvent drag, or active transport. The accumulation of absorption products causes dilatation of the initially narrow intercellular spaces (284). As a result of the high hydrostatic pressure thus produced, water and solutes are pressed through the basement membrane into the lamina propria, where they are taken up by the capillaries (fig. 5.1.c).

5.1.7 Secretion

Apart from absorption, secretion of water and ions also takes place in the small intestine. In fact there are two opposite fluxes over the intestinal wall: one from the intestinal lumen to the blood stream, and the other from the blood stream to the intestinal lumen. The phenomenon of secretion was detected when, in perfusion studies of the small intestine, a larger amount of water or solutes was occasionally recovered from the perfusate than had been initially instilled. Moreover, intravenously administered isotopes also proved to be demonstrable in the perfusate after a while.

In some types of diarrhoea, particularly in cholera, this secretion is quite substantial (802). The extent of the intestinal secretion under normal conditions, however, has not yet been established with certainty. Some authors maintain that the amounts secreted cannot be considerable (284), whereas others (659, 680) suspect them to be very large.

The mechanism of secretion in the small intestine is likewise still largely unknown. In principle, secretion could take place via the same routes as absorption, albeit in opposite directions. A passive secretion of water and electrolytes would be readily possible in the jejunum if it had sufficiently large epithelial pores. Active secretion is possible moreover, as suggested by the presence of ATPase in the brush border (284). Some investigators suspect that secretion is effected by the enterocytes in the crypts of the intestinal mucosa, whereas the enterocytes of the villi serve only the absorption (378). The intestinal hormones seem to exert no influence on the nature and extent of the secretion (284).

Finally, it is not clear either why secretion takes place in the small intestine at all. It could be the result from osmotic attracting forces from the intestinal lumen (284). This attraction of fluid and electrolytes, which probably takes place especially in the proximal part of the small intestine, might be required to render the hypotonic or hypertonic intestinal contents isotonic, thus facilitating their absorption (284, 659). Another possibility is that sodium is deliberately and constantly secreted into the intestinal lumen to ensure a sufficient intraluminal sodium concentration. For the presence of sodium in the intestinal lumen is required for the translocation of several important nutrients, and probably for that of all nutrients (fig. 5.1.d; 175, 763).

Due to secretion, the small intestine actually absorbs more than it would seem to do at first sight. This is why a distinction is sometimes made between net absorption and total absorption. Net absorption is defined as the resultant of absorption and secretion, or the difference between oral intake and faecal loss. Total absorption encompasses this net absorption as well as the indiscernible absorption of water and electrolytes, which were released by secretion (659, 802).

5.2 WATER AND ELECTROLYTES

The human organism largely consists of water and electrolytes. Their amounts have to be kept within certain limits to ensure proper body function. Continuous loss of fluid and electrolytes takes place via the skin, lungs, urine and faeces. The amount lost depends on physical activity, environmental temperature and humidity, and on metabolic factors. The excretion of water and electrolytes via the skin, lungs and intestine is less dependent on the oral intake than the excretion by the kidneys. The kidneys can largely regulate the amount excreted. They have to excrete a minimum amount of fluid under all circumstances, however, in order to eliminate such substances as urea, etc. There are therefore certain water and electrolyte requirements which have to be met by oral intake. These requirements show interindividual differences as well as intraindividual variations. The human organism obtains its sodium and chloride partly from meat, fish and dairy products. By far the largest amount is added to the food as taste corrigent. The daily food intake contains a total of 6-18 g sodium chloride (700), and this is usually more than sufficient. The potassium requirement is estimated to be about 2.5 g/day (700). Potassium is contained in virtually all foods, e.g. potatoes, milk, vegetables, meat and bread.

The amounts of water and electrolytes presented for absorption in the small intestine are many times larger as the oral intake. This is caused by the large amounts of endogenous water and electrolytes released, for example, with the digestive juices and the secretion via the intestinal wall (section 5.1.7). The extent of this intestinal secretion cannot be readily established (284). It is suspected that the total amount of water and electrolytes presented for absorption per 24 hours (i.e. the sum of oral intake, digestive juices and secretion via the intestinal wall) amounts to about 10 litres of water, containing 1000 mmole sodium chloride (799). The maximum capacity of the small intestine is probably at least twice as large (526).

The role which the stomach plays in the absorption of water and electrolytes is merely to serve as storage space for food. The stomach is virtually impermeable to water and sodium (147), and consequently the gastric contents can long remain non-isotonic in relation to the blood (281). In the duodenum, whose wall is freely permeable to water and sodium, the food bolus is quickly rendered isotonic. This is effected by attraction of water via an osmotic gradient, while sodium chloride moves into the lumen via a concentration gradient (281) (fig. 5.2). As a result of the events in the duodenum, the food bolus is isotonic – so far as the aqueous phase is concerned – at the moment it reaches the jejunum (281). In the duodenum itself, probably no significant absorption of water and electrolytes occurs; but immediately after, absorption becomes maximal. Water and sodium absorption largely take place in the proximal jejunum (91). Perfusion studies have shown that efficient absorption of water and sodium requires the presence of other substances such as glucose (798), galactose (283), maltose (579) and some amino acids (4). It is assumed that these substances are effective in that they stimulate the translocation of sodium over the cell membrane (section 5.1.6).

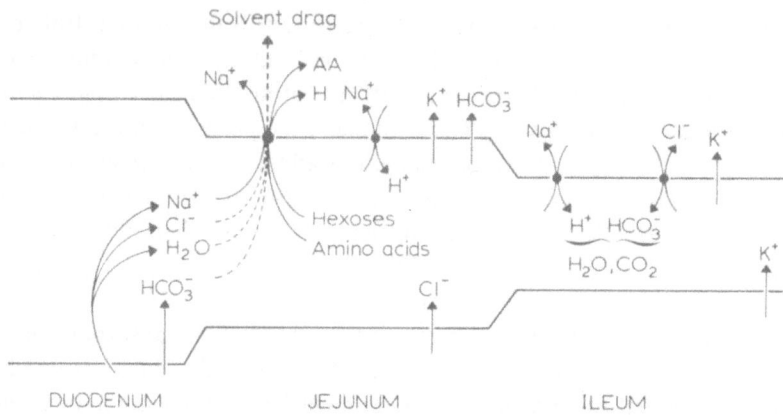

Fig. 5.2. Diagram of the localization and mechanisms of electrolyte absorption in the small intestine.

The chloride ion probably always accompanies the sodium ion, for as much chloride as sodium is absorbed. In addition, some chloride is perhaps secreted in the jejunum (680).

In the jejunum, bicarbonate is probably absorbed against a concentration gradient. An alternative possibility is that the bicarbonate, together with the hydrogen ions secreted into the lumen, forms water and carbon dioxide; for secretion of hydrogen ions is believed to occur in exchange for absorption of sodium ions. By trapping the hydrogen ions, the bicarbonate stimulates the secretion of hydrogen and, secondarily, the absorption of sodium (283). Perhaps the bicarbonate secreted by the pancreas promotes by this mechanism the absorption of water and sodium (802).

Potassium passively disappears from the jejunum, either by diffusion to the plasma (680) or by solvent drag (864).

The absorption of water and electrolytes in the ileum is quite different from that in the jejunum. This is probably due to the fact that most of the substances which stimulate absorption of water and sodium, such as sugars, amino acids and bicarbonate, have already been absorbed in the proximal jejunum (91). Absorption in the ileum largely consists of an exchange between different ions. For example, sodium is absorbed in exchange for hydrogen secretion, and chloride is absorbed in exchange for the secretion of bicarbonate (863). The hydrogen and bicarbonate ions secreted in the lumen of the ileum are osmotically inactive, probably because they form water and carbon dioxide. In the ileum, more chloride than sodium seems to be absorbed (207). It is not yet quite clear how potassium is absorbed in the ileum, but this is probably passive, by diffusion (864). Perhaps some secretion of potassium also occurs in the ileum (243).

In the colon, too, an important amount of water and electrolytes is still absorbed, as shown by the marked quantitative and qualitative changes to which the contents of the terminal ileum are subject before leaving the body as faeces (681). The processes of absorption and secretion in the colon are roughly the same as those in the ileum (207), but there are also some important differences. For example, bacterial degradation of food roughage produces large amounts of organic anions, so that some chloride can still be absorbed (731). Another difference is that passage through the colon takes about ten times as long as the transit time through the ileum, so that there is more time for the various processes of absorption and exchange. An important feature of the colon in this respect is its relatively low permeability, which enables marked concentration gradients to be built up (68).

The absorption of water and electrolytes is influenced by several hormones. Absorption in the proximal jejunum, for example, is inhibited by secretin and CCK-PZ, perhaps in order to keep intestinal contents liquid for a longer time in order to facilitate digestive processes (609). Calcitonin causes increased secretion of water and electrolytes (336). Aldosterone, finally, increases the absorption of water and sodium in the colon, and also the secretion of potassium in the colon (514).

5.3 CARBOHYDRATE

Carbohydrates are important for the human organism as a source of energy. About 50% of the caloric requirements are covered by carbohydrates, of which about 300-400 g are ingested per day. The carbohydrates ingested largely consist of starch (60%, of which one-fifth is amylose and four-fifths is amylopectin), and sucrose (30%). Only 10% is in the form of lactose, while trehalose and various monosaccharides are consumed in only very small quantities (335).

The digestion of starch is catalysed by the enzyme α-amylase, from saliva and especially pancreatic juice. Due to the fact that almost 10 times as much α-amylase as is thought necessary is probably available (335, 633), conversion to maltose, maltotriose and α-dextrin is fairly well completed in the duodenum (189) (fig. 5.3).

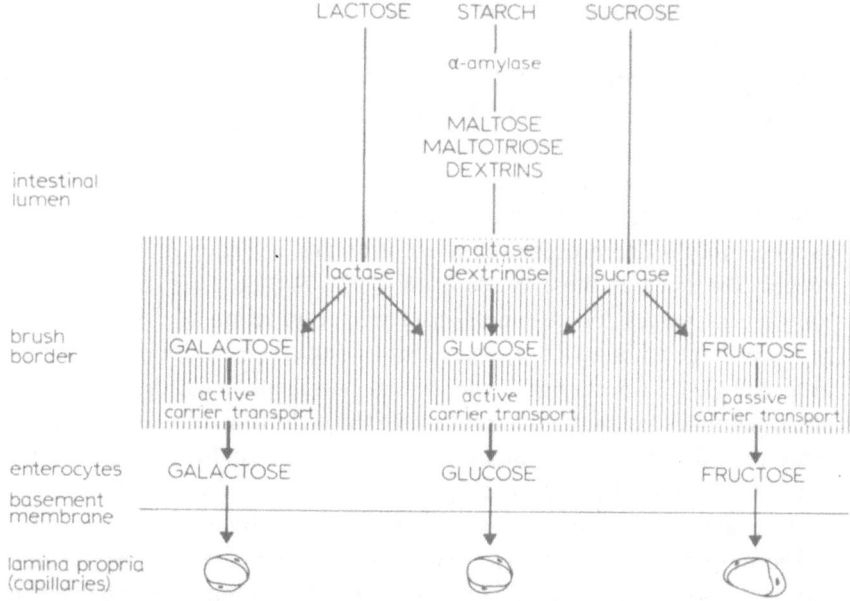

Fig. 5.3. Diagram of the digestion and absorption of dietary carbohydrate.

The second phase of carbohydrate digestion, the degradation of disaccharides, takes place at the brush border of the enterocytes. The brush border membrane contains several disaccharidases such as five types of maltase, but also enzymes which split lactose (two lactases), sucrose (sucrase) and trehalose (trehalase) (596). It may be that these disaccharidases are not localized in the brush border but just on the outside, in the glycocalyx (439). The amounts of the different disaccharidases present in or near the brush border vary substantially. Normally, the ratio between the amounts of maltase, isomaltase, sucrase and lactase is 8:2:2:1. This ratio is constant throughout the whole length of the small intestine. The absolute amounts of the various disaccharidases, however, vary. Enzyme activity, while low in the duodenum, is maximal the proximal jejunum and decreases in the distal jejunum and the proximal ileum (632). The maltases convert maltose and maltotriose into glucose, to which also the dextrins are degraded. The lactases split lactose into galactose and glucose, and sucrase converts sucrose into glucose and fructose (fig. 5.3).

62

Whereas abundant data are available on carbohydrate digestion little is known with certainty about absorption of carbohydrates. They are probably absorbed only in the monosaccharide form. Since the monosaccharides are absorbed more quickly than a simple diffusion process could explain, transport carriers are likely to be involved in their absorption. Transport of monosaccharides over the cell membrane is linked to the translocation of sodium (section 5.1.6). It has not yet been established whether there are separate types of carrier for glucose and galactose, or whether these two make use of the same carriers. Fructose is probably absorbed, not by active transport but passively, by means of carriers (the so-called facilitated diffusion) (327). The carriers and disaccharidases are probably localized close together so that, after the splitting of the disaccharides, the fragments can be passed on to the carriers (414). This explains why the absorption of disaccharides is about as rapid as that of monosaccharides (205, 333).

The degradation and absorption of carbohydrates is effected quickly and efficiently. The absorption is usually already completed in the jejunum (91). The rate at which carbohydrates are absorbed by the enterocytes is dependent on the speed of the carrier transport. The rate of lactose absorption, however, is determined by the rate of degradation, i.e. by the amount of lactase available.

5.4 FAT

5.4.1 Introduction

The fat in the human diet, usually 60-100 g/day, covers about one-third of the energy requirement. In addition, fat serves as a vehicle for the fat-soluble vitamins. Some 95% of the nutritional fat consists of triglycerides. In addition to triglycerides, the human diet contains 0.5-1 g cholesterol and an even smaller amount of phospholipids (754).

The triglycerides consist of a glycerol skeleton to which three fatty acids are coupled. These fatty acids have a carbon chain which can differ in length. According to the length of their chain, a distinction is made between long-chain triglycerides (LCT, with chains of 12-20 carbon atoms), medium-chain triglycerides (MCT, with chains of 6-10 carbon atoms), and short-chain triglycerides (SCT, with chains of 2 or 4 carbon atoms). The triglycerides in the diet comprise about 90% LCT and 10% MCT (335). Fatty acids are not essential for the human organism, with the exception of linoleic acid. Deficiency of this essential linoleic acid causes severe skin lesions (151, 361, 851).

63

The cardinal point in the absorption of fats lies in the solubilization, so that they are finely dispersed in the aqueous intestinal contents. Only in that way is efficient absorption by the enterocytes possible. Three processes actually play a role in this respect: emulsification, lipolysis and solubilization (micelle formation) (335, 754).

5.4.2 Triglycerides

The emulsification of triglycerides is in fact started by the mastication of food in the mouth and by the kneading in the stomach. Apart from these mechanical processes, emulsification is mostly effected chemically, by various emulsifiers such as lecithin from bile, and monoglycerides. Most of these emulsifiers are only available in or beyond the duodenum. In its emulsified form, fat consists of particles with a diameter of 0.3-1 μm (754).

Lipolysis, or hydrolysis of triglycerides is effectuated by various lipases. Gastric juice, for example, contains a lipase which hydrolyses especially the MCT-triglycerides (149). In the duodenum, several lipases (glycerol ester hydrolases) are released which have been produced in large amounts by the pancreas. These lipases detach the two outer (1-, 3-) fatty acids from the triglyceride molecules so that free fatty acids and (2-) monoglycerides remain (fig. 5.4). Most of the monoglycerides is not further hydrolysed but absorbed as such (467).

To be adequately absorbed, the triglyceride degradation products have to be dispersed in a particular way. This is effected with the aid of bile acids which form globular aggregates called micelles. An important factor for the formation of these aggregates is the molecular structure of the bile acids, with on the one side a highly polar end (which is hydrophilic), and on the other side a non-polar hydrocarbon group (which is hydrophobic). Only above a certain concentration (the so-called critical micellar concentration) do these bile acids form micelles. The orientation of these globular bile acid aggregates is such that the hydrophilic poles are on the outside, while the lipophilic poles are at the centre.

In the interior of this micelle, highly hydrophobic products such as cholesterol and fat-soluble vitamins can be carried. More on the outside of the aggregate, between the polar ends of the bile acids, more hydrophilic products such as monoglycerides, fatty acids and phospholipids are carried (fig. 5.4). The micelles ensure that the fat degradation products, cholesterol and fat-soluble vitamins are solubilized and finely dispersed so that ample contact with the brush border of the enterocytes is possible. At the transition from emulsion to micellar form, the diameter of the fat particles is reduced

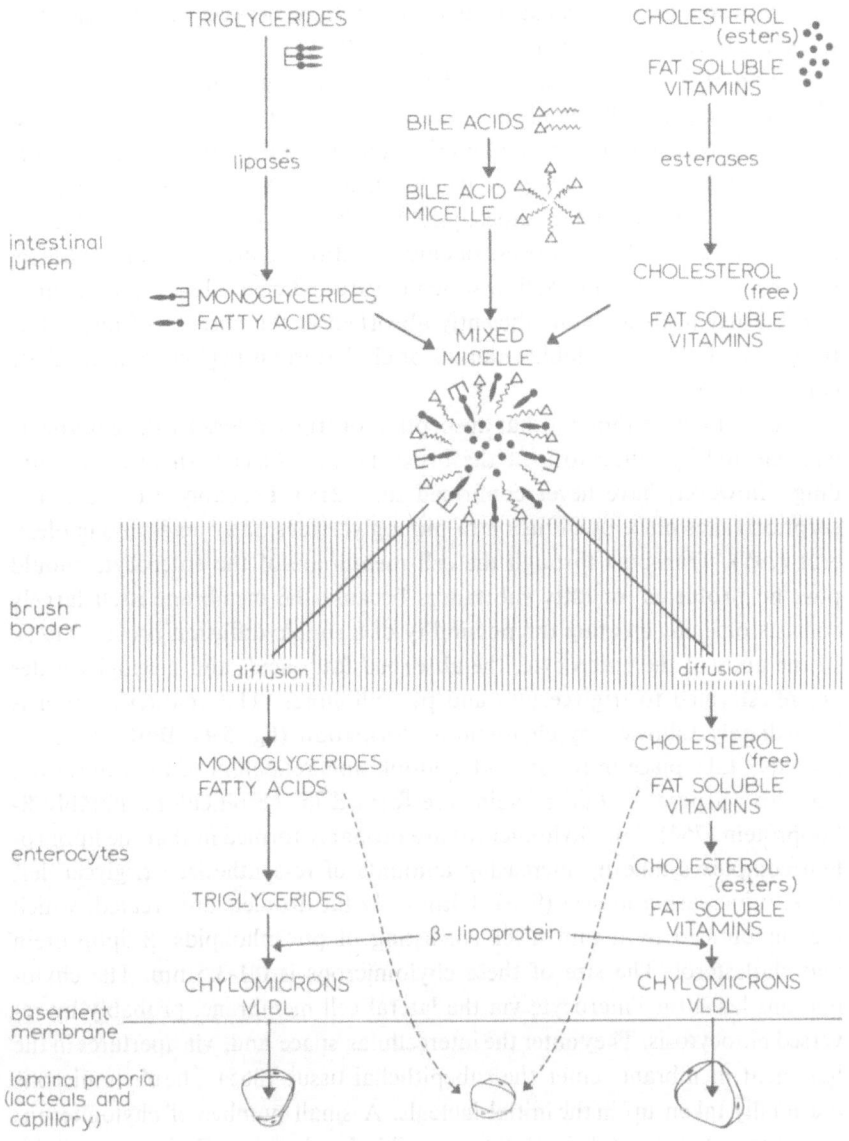

Fig. 5.4. Diagram of the digestion and absorption of dietary lipid.

by factor 100-200, and consequently the interface between fat particles and intestinal fluid increases by factor 10,000-40,000 (525).

During their passage through the small intestine, the lipid food constituents are gradually emulsified and degraded. The degradation products are in turn good emulsifiers, and on the other hand degradation occurs more readily if the lipids are already well emulsified. The degradation products are taken up by the available unoccupied micelles, or wait until they become available. The combined process of emulsification, hydrolysis and solubilization is an integrated interaction which ensures efficient absorption of lipids (408). Fatty acids are still efficiently absorbed in the absence of bile, while the absorption of fat-soluble vitamins or cholesterol is negligible under these conditions (690).

It has long been thought that absorption of triglycerides by the enterocyte was effected by pinocytosis at the brush border. Electron-microscopic findings, however, have never confirmed this (219). Probably, therefore, absorption takes place by diffusion of monoglycerides, fatty acids and cholesterol (735). Transport through the cell membrane of the enterocyte should pose no problems for fatty substances because the membrane itself largely consists of lipids creating the possibility of a simple diffusion process (192). In the apex of the enterocyte, the absorbed fatty acids and monoglycerides are re-esterified to triglycerides and phospholipids. This re-esterification is immediately followed by chylomicron formation (fig. 5.4). Both processes probably take place in the smooth endoplasmic reticulum of the enterocyte. For this purpose, certain proteins are formed in the reticulum, notably β-lipoprotein (754). The chylomicrons are probably formed in that the lipoprotein complexes take up increasing amounts of re-synthesized triglycerides, thereby increasing in size (865). Ultimately fat droplets are created, which are surrounded by a thin layer consisting of phospholipids, β-lipoprotein and cholesterol. The size of these chylomicrons is 0.1-3.5 nm. The chylomicrons leave the enterocyte via the lateral cell membrane, probably by reversed pinocytosis. They enter the intercellular space and, via apertures in the basement membrane, enter the subepithelial tissue (865). The chylomicrons are finally taken up in the initial lacteals. A small number of chylomicrons directly reach the portal circulation, possibly by shunting. Endogenous lipid, however, is transported in the very low density (pre-β) lipoproteins (754).

The medium-chain triglycerides (MCT) are more rapidly degraded in the intestinal lumen by lipase than LCT. Moreover, their absorption requires no preceding hydrolysis, because degradation can also take place in the enterocytes. Most medium-chain fatty acids are transported via the portal circulation without preceding re-esterification.

5.4.3 Cholesterol

The human diet as a rule contains but little cholesterol: about 0.5-1 g/day, mostly consumed as eggs, meat and dairy products (754). However, the human organism itself synthesizes large amounts of cholesterol from acetates, particularly in the liver and in the epithelial cells of the digestive tract (212). Cholesterol found in the intestinal lumen therefore originates from several sources, such as food, exfoliated cells (estimated to amount to 0.25-0.40 g/day) and bile (1-2 g/day) (192). Cholesterol is required for the synthesis of steroid hormones, vitamin D and bile acids. In addition it probably has other, not yet identified functions as indicated by its high concentration in several organs such as the brain.

So far as it is present in esterified form, cholesterol is hydrolysed by cholesterol esterase, an enzyme secreted by the pancreas but found also in the brush border of the enterocytes (855). The pancreatic cholesterol esterase is activated by bile acids. Due to its poor solubility in water, cholesterol can virtually only be dissolved by incorporation in micelles. In the absence of bile, therefore, virtually no cholesterol is absorbed (690). Cholesterol absorption probably takes place by diffusion (793), followed by re-esterification in the enterocyte (192). Cholesterol enters the lymph pathways with the chylomicrons, and so reaches the blood stream. Under normal conditions, only 20-40% of the ingested cholesterol is absorbed (93), mainly in the proximal jejunum (92). It is believed that 1-3 g cholesterol, from food, bile and exfoliated intestinal epithelial cells on the one hand, and from the cholesterol pool in the intestinal epithelial cells on the other, is transported daily via the lymph pathways (192).

Since the cholesterol level is usually more or less constant, it is evident that the synthesis, degradation and elimination of cholesterol are adjusted to each other by a control mechanism. When cholesterol absorption diminishes, its synthesis in the liver increases. Cholesterol synthesis in the epithelial cells of the digestive tract is partly determined by absorption of bile acids. Absence of bile acids from the intestinal lumen causes a substantial increase in cholesterol synthesis (212). The height of the serum cholesterol level is otherwise influenced by various hormonal, genetic and age-linked factors (196).

5.4.4 Phospholipids

In addition to triglycerides and cholesterol, food also contains a small amount of phospholipids, which are found in meat and eggs. Otherwise the phospholipid requirement is largely fulfilled by their de-novo synthesis in the liver, small intestine, muscles and brain. The human organism needs these phospholipids for a normal functioning of cell membranes, mitochondria and neurons. Phospholipids in food facilitate the emulsification of triglycerides and the incorporation of cholesterol and fat-soluble vitamins in the micelles.

Hydrolysis of phospholipids is effectuated by phospholipase A, an enzyme secreted by the pancreas and activated by bile acids. The hydrolysis products become soluble by incorporation in micelles. After absorption by the mucosa, the phospholipids, too, are re-synthesized and incorporated in the chylomicrons (754).

5.4.5 Fat-soluble vitamins

5.4.5.1 Introduction

Absorption of the fat-soluble vitamins A, D, E and K takes place in roughly the same way as cholesterol absorption. Like cholesterol, these vitamins consist of relatively large molecules which, like all non-polar lipids, have a very poor solubility in water. For their absorption, therefore, micelle formation is essential. The vitamin-ester complex is abolished by hydrolysis, exactly as in the case of cholesterol. The enzymes required for this purpose originate from the pancreas and possibly also from the brush border of the enterocytes (302). Absorption takes place in the proximal part of the small intestine (88). After absorption, vitamins A and D are mostly re-esterified within the enterocyte. After incorporation in chylomicrons fat-soluble vitamins are transported with the lymph. A small amount directly enters the portal circulation (842).

5.4.5.2 Vitamin A

Vitamin A (retinol) is contained in many foods such as milk, eggs, meat and fish. Its precursors, the carotene pigments, are found especially in green vegetables, carrots and yellow-red fruits such as apricots and peaches. Vitamin A is synthesized from this carotene in the human and animal intestinal wall. Since the liver has very large vitamin A reserves, deficiency does not become manifest until after months or years. The symptoms of vitamin A deficiency are: night-blindness, xerophthalmia, keratomalacia and keratosis follicularis. A low vitamin A level is found not only in the case of a deficient diet or malabsorption but also in some patients with infectious diseases, anaemia, hepatitis or cirrhosis of the liver. Its occurrence in these cases has so far not been elucidated (448).

5.4.5.3 Vitamin D

The human organism can partly fulfil its vitamin D requirement by synthesizing a pro-vitamin which is converted to vitamin D_3 (cholecalciferol) by solar light on the skin. This vitamin D_3 can also be acquired via food. In less sunny climates, and as result of the wearing of clothes, this supply with the food is very important. Fish liver in particular contains large amounts of vitamin D_3. In much smaller amounts, it is also present in liver, eggs and dairy products (700). After absorption in the intestine, vitamin D_3 is first hydroxylated to 25-OH-D_3 in the liver, and then to 1,25-OH-D_3 and 24,25-OH-D_3 in the kidneys. The question remains whether the various vitamin D metabolites have their own particular functions. By far the most effective metabolite seems to be 1,25-OH-D_3, which induces the synthesis of a protein for calcium transport in the enterocytes (250). In addition to a stimulating effect on calcium absorption in the small intestine, vitamin D also enhances the degradation of bone tissue. Moreover, it inhibits renal excretion of calcium and phosphate, possibly by means of parathormone (691).

Vitamin D deficiency causes disorders of mineralization in bone tissue (rickets or osteomalacia). It is not only associated with a deficient diet and malabsorption but can also occur as a result of renal diseases or vitamin D resistance.

5.4.5.4 Vitamin E

Vitamin E (tocopherol) actually consists of a group of vitamins of which α-tocopherol is the most active. Vitamin E is found in virtually all foods, particularly in cereals, vegetable oils, green vegetables, eggs, butter and meat (especially liver). Nevertheless, vitamin E deficiency due to a wrong choice of food seems to be possible (805). Vitamin E deficiency can also develop as a result of malabsorption (69). The consequences of vitamin E deficiency are unknown. Vitamin E is believed to inhibit oxidation of lipids in the cell membrane, and it is consequently regarded as important for the proper functioning of cell membranes. In infants haemolysis has been described, and changes in the muscles and in the reproductive function have been observed in test animals (196). The presence of ceroid pigment in the muscle tissues of various organs has been ascribed to vitamin E deficiency (69, 847).

5.4.5.5 Vitamin K

Vitamin K is a term applied to several vitamins, of which only vitamin K_1 (phytomenadione) is of clinical significance. This vitamin is found in particular in green vegetables. In addition, it is endogenously synthesized by bacteria in the colon, mainly by Escherichia coli (328). Vitamin K deficiency due to a deficient diet has been observed only in association with simultaneous use of antibiotics (292). The body's vitamin K reserves seem to be small, and are exhausted after 3-4 weeks. The function of vitamin K concerns blood coagulation, as indicated by its designation ('K' stands for 'Koagulation').

Vitamin K stimulates the production of the clotting factors II, VII, IX and X in the liver. The presence of this vitamin can be determined only indirectly, by measuring the concentration of the above mentioned coagulation factors. This is usually done with the aid of the prothrombin time (PTT), thrombotest or normotest. Since these coagulation factors are synthesized in the liver, disorders of liver function can exert a negative influence on these determinations too.

5.5 PROTEIN

The human organism is continuously degrading its protein store. The mechanism and the site of this degradation are only partly understood (730). If a positive nitrogen balance is nevertheless to be maintained, then this loss has to be replenished via the food. The amount of protein normally required for this repletion is estimated to be about 45 g/day (700). The usual daily diet contains about twice this amount, mainly in meat, fish, eggs and dairy products. Cereals and legumes also contain substantial amounts of protein. The human organism can digest and absorb large amounts of protein. In experimental situations, daily amounts up to 600 g were found to be adequately absorbed (701).

The digestion of dietary protein begins in the stomach, which secretes several types of pepsinogen, i.e. enzyme precursors which the gastric juice converts into active pepsins (911). The principal role of the stomach, apart from its function as storage space, is so to denature dietary protein with the aid of gastric juice and pepsins as to facilitate, and therefore accelerate, its degradation in the small intestine. This role is not such a very important one, as demonstrated by the fact that malabsorption of protein usually does not occur in treated pernicious anaemia.

The lion's share in protein digestion is taken by the proteolytic enzymes secreted by the pancreas. Pancreatic secretion of these enzymes is stimulated by the intestinal hormone CCK-PZ, which is synthesized by cells in the mucosa of the duodenum and the proximal jejunum, and released after stimulation of these cells by e.g. food rich in fat or proteins (section 4.7). There are several types of proteolytic pancreatic enzyme, each with a specific effect which is determined by their access to the link between certain amino acids. A distinction is thus made between the endopeptidases trypsinogen, chymo trypsinôgen and pro-elastase, and the exopeptidases such as carboxypeptidase A and B (334). The former break certain peptide links within the protein molecule, while the latter break only the terminal peptide link at the carboxyl side of the molecule (fig. 5.5).

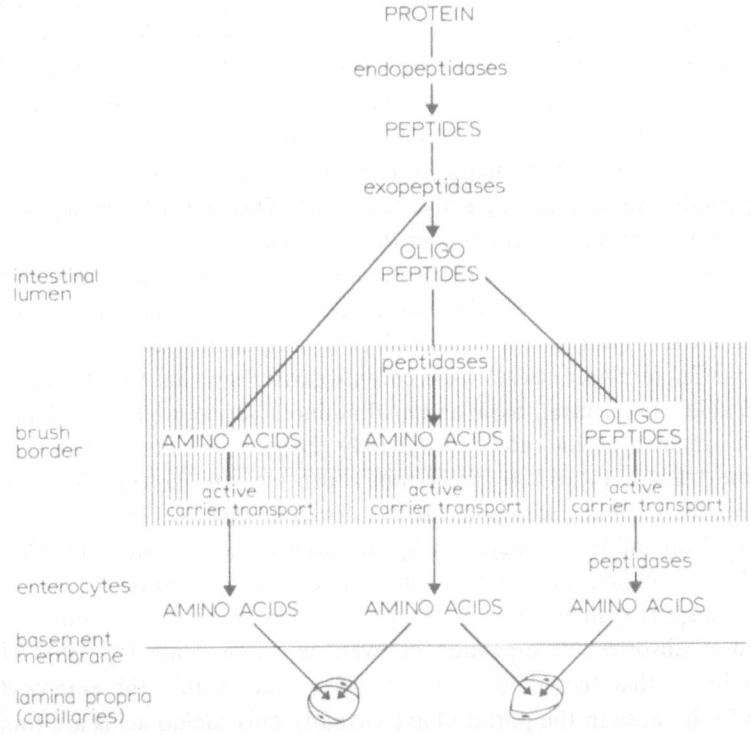

Fig. 5.5. Diagram of the digestion and absorption of dietary protein.

Most pancreatic proteolytic enzymes are secreted as inactive precursors. An important factor for activation of these precursors is enterokinase, an enzyme likewise synthesized by the duodenal mucosa (642). This enterokinase converts trypsinogen into trypsin, while trypsin in turn activates the precursors of the other enzymes. In addition, each activated enzyme catalyses its own inactive precursor. Under normal conditions the amount of enzymes secreted by the pancreas is quite excessive in relation to the amount of protein contained in the food (334).

It is generally assumed that protein is not completely degraded to amino acids in the intestinal lumen, as it was believed to be in the past (567). An important part of the protein digestion takes place at the brush border of the enterocytes or in the enterocytes themselves (fig. 5.5). The brush border contains a large amount and wide variety of peptidases, each of which is relatively specific (377). In addition the brush border is believed to carry a considerable amount of pancreatic enzymes which, as it were, become glued to the mucosa (316). The brush border of the enterocytes consequently has a great protein-splitting capacity. The degradation at this site is sometimes referred to as 'membrane digestion'. Ugolev (866), who introduced this term, holds the rather extreme view that virtually the entire degradation of protein takes place at the brush border of the enterocytes.

The absorption by the enterocyte of all these amino acids, dipeptides or oligopeptides, takes place by active transport. This transport is dependent on the translocation of sodium over the cell membrane (section 5.1.6). The reverse also seems to be true: absorption of sodium and water is stimulated when amino acids or dipeptides can be absorbed simultaneously (4, 376). This active transport probably takes place by means of transport proteins or carriers. There would seem to be several carrier systems for the various amino acids, the neutral, basic and acid amino acids, as well as carriers for proline, hydroxyproline and glycine (334, 567). There are probably also separate transport carriers for certain dipeptides (6, 7) (fig. 5.5). The existence of so many different carriers for individual or grouped amino acids and dipeptides, is suggested by the occurrence of various hereditary disorders of amino acid transport which are evidently based on the lack of a given transport system (598). It seems likely that a substantial amount of protein is absorbed as dipeptide or even as oligopeptide (5, 638). This would imply that further degradation takes place within the enterocytes (fig. 5.5), because in the portal blood virtually only amino acids are found (634, 673). According to Peters (673), peptidase activity is for the most part localized within the enterocyte rather than outside. When absorbed as oligopeptide, more amino acids enter the circulation per unit of time than would be the case if the same amino acids were offered in a completely hydrolysed form (173, 790). This finding suggests that the rate of absorption is determined largely by the total number of transport carriers available.

Absorption of minute quantities of undigested protein also takes place. These proteins are found unchanged in lymph and portal blood (882, 891).

This phenomenon, still unexplained, plays no essential role in protein absorption in its totality.

Absorption of dietary protein is believed usually to be completed in the proximal part of the small intestine (91, 638). However, this is not corroborated by observations reported by other investigators who, in perfusion studies, were able to recover substantial quantities of protein and protein degradation products from the perfused intestinal loops, sometimes many hours after instillation (5). Protein from food is usually efficiently and almost completely absorbed by the small intestine, however. The faeces as a rule contains no more than 2 g nitrogen (192, 291, 701), half of which originates from endogenous and metabolic losses (700). This demonstrates that the total faecal loss of unabsorbed protein is less than 10% of the amount of dietary protein available for absorption.

In addition to protein from food, a substantial amount of endogenous protein released in the small intestine has to be absorbed. The exact amount of endogenous protein involved cannot be estimated with any certainty, and estimates have so far been very disparate (181, 621). The endogenous protein fraction consists of digestive ferments and mucus, with probably about 8 g protein per meal (638), exfoliated cells of the intestinal wall up to about 10 g/day (188), and plasma protein leakage through the intestinal wall, which accounts for about 1 g/day. It has been maintained that, as a result of this supply of endogenous protein, the amino acid concentrations in portal blood only partly reflect the intermittent supply of dietary protein (312, 627), so that, through the day, the supply of amino acids to the liver would be relatively constant – a fact of importance for an efficient and optimal synthesis of protein. Hardly any data in support of this hypothesis have so far been presented, however (377).

5.6 CALCIUM

The human organism contains a substantial amount of calcium, estimated to be 20-25 g/kg fatless tissue. About 99% of all calcium is found in the skeleton. The remaining 1% plays an important role in cell membrane function, the muscle cells and nerve synapses, in blood coagulation and in a variety of enzyme reactions. For the purpose of all these functions the calcium concentration in the various body compartments must be kept within certain, rather narrow limits (691). There is always some loss of calcium in urine and faeces. Under special circumstances calcium is lost also in other ways, e.g. during pregnancy and lactation. To replenish this loss, some calcium has to be absorbed from the food. The amount of calcium in the daily diet of Europeans and Americans is estimated to be about 1000 mg, which is usually ample to cover requirements. Some 50% of this calcium is ingested as milk or dairy products (except butter) (641), and the diet of persons who take no dairy products is therefore sometimes relatively poor in calcium. Other dietary calcium sources are green vegetables, potatoes, meat and bread (196, 422).

The presence of free hydrochloric acid is required to solubilize several calcium salts from food (427). In addition, certain food constituents precipitate free calcium ions or form less soluble complexes with them, such as the phytates (920), oxalates, carbonates and phosphates (468) or saturated LCT fatty acids (11). Other substances form readily soluble complexes with calcium ions and thus enhance calcium solubility; these substances include sugars, amino acids (411) and bile acids (898). In brief: several intraluminal factors influence the amount of calcium available for absorption.

The absolute amount of calcium absorbed from food varies less than the amount of soluble calcium contained in it. Relatively more calcium is absorbed at a low intake, up to twice the amount absorbed at a high calcium intake (812). Hence it can be maintained that the composition of the diet and the form in which calcium is supplied generally do not influence the amount of calcium absorbed (607). The same applies to the influence of gastric acid production or the release of bile and pancreatic juice.

Apart from the ingested calcium, an amount of so-called endogenous calcium (i.e. calcium released in the intestine) is available for absorption. This calcium enters the intestinal lumen via the bile and pancreatic juice, or as a result of secretion from the enterocytes and of exfoliated cells. The amount of this endogenous calcium has not so far been accurately calculated, but is estimated to be 200 mg (641) or 400-1000 mg per day (691).

Absorption of calcium by the intestinal wall takes place by active transport; besides some passive transport by diffusion probably occurs (691). Active transport probably takes place by means of a transport carrier (887). Important factors for active transport are the presence of a calcium-binding protein (892) as well as of ATP and ATPase to supply the energy required (202).

The capacity of the small intestine to absorb calcium is maximal in the duodenum (71, 906). This does not necessarily imply, however, that most of the calcium is actually absorbed there. The time available for absorption is probably equally important, for calcium absorption takes a relatively slow course (411). Hence the distal part of the small intestine normally absorbs a probably important amount of calcium (174, 556).

Calcium absorption is influenced by numerous factors, of which vitamin D is by far the most important. The presence of this vitamin is essential for a normal calcium absorption, as clearly demonstrated by the negative calcium balance due to extremely large faecal losses in rickets (364). Vitamin D repletion improves calcium absorption in these cases, but only after several hours or days. This interval can be explained by the time required to convert the vitamin D administered to a metabolically active form (section 5.4.5.3), and on the other hand by the time which elapses before the effect of the $1,25$-OH-D_3 on the enterocyte becomes manifest. This effect is believed to consist of stimulation of the synthesis of calcium-binding protein (892) and/or the formation of ATPase for active transport (202). Other factors also influence calcium absorption, such as parathormone (606). Parathormone is effective only in the presence of vitamin D, perhaps because it stimulates synthesis of active vitamin D metabolites (303). Growth hormone, too, is believed to stimulate calcium absorption (789). The effect of corticosteroids is not quite clear, but they probably reduce calcium absorption (640). The same applies to thyroid hormone (158). Although the above mentioned hormones can virtually influence calcium absorption it remains questionable – apart from vitamin D – to which extent this normally occurs.

The amount of calcium absorbed in the small intestine is adapted to individual requirements (71). The regulating mechanisms have so far not been identified. Perhaps they involve an influence on the conversion of vitamin D into 1,25 dihydrocholecalciferol in the kidney (203) or on the capacity of the active transport system (411). Under normal conditions active transport takes place only in the proximal part of the small intestine (751), but if the calcium intake is low it also occurs more distally (71). Regulation of calcium absorption is required in view of the fact that intestinal absorption plays an important role in calcium homeostasis. Other regulators of this homeostasis are bone turnover and renal excretion; together they ensure that the amount of calcium in the human organism is kept within certain limits.

5.7 MAGNESIUM

So far, relatively little is known about magnesium absorption. This is probably due to the fact that the significance of magnesium for the human organism has long been uncertain. It has been established quite recently that magnesium deficiency can give rise to behaviour disorders, convulsions, ataxia, vertigo, tremors, muscular weakness (359) and tetany (869). It is obvious, therefore, that magnesium plays an important role in the normal functioning of the neuromuscular system. It seems essential moreover for the activation of certain enzymes (505, 877). The function of magnesium resembles that of calcium in many ways. The same applies, to some degree, to the absorption of the two minerals.

There is usually some loss of magnesium with urine and faeces. To compensate this loss, some magnesium has to be absorbed from food. It is believed that, to maintain a positive magnesium balance, the daily intake should be about 4 mg/kg body weight (443). The normal diet usually contains sufficient magnesium. Rich sources are bread, potatoes and green vegetables (196). The absolute amount of magnesium absorbed from food varies – like that of calcium – less than the amount of magnesium in the diet, for relatively less is absorbed from a high-magnesium diet than from a low-magnesium diet (330). This is one of the control mechanisms by which the amount of magnesium in the organism is kept constant. Another, likewise important role is played by the kidneys, which normally excrete about one-third of the oral intake but release only minimal quantities into the urine in the case of a magnesium-deficient diet (47). Marked variations in the magnesium concentrations in serum and body cells are otherwise prevented by the large magnesium stores in the skeletal system, in which about half the total amount of 21-28 g magnesium is contained (877). As a result of these reserves and the marked re-absorption in the kidneys, manifest magnesium deficiency due exclusively to a low-magnesium diet has never been observed (877).

The amount of magnesium absorbed is partly dependent on the degree of solubilization of the magnesium ions, which determines their availability for absorption. In this respect, the form in which magnesium is present in food, and the composition of the diet in general, are important (877). The same probably applies to the presence of gastric juice.

Apart from the dietary magnesium, endogenous magnesium is also released in the intestine, in amounts estimated to be 25 mg/day. This magnesium originates from digestive juices and exfoliated enterocytes (192).

The absorption process of magnesium takes a very slow course, as demonstrated in experiments with labelled magnesium. Radioactivity is demonstrable in the circulation only after an interval of one hour, while maximum radioactivity is measured after 2-8 hours. This suggests that absorption probably takes place throughout the length of the small intestine (330). The mechanism of absorption is largely unknown, but it is probably active, with the aid of a transport carrier. This would explain why absorption relatively diminishes as the amount of magnesium in the food increases (330). Some investigators postulate that the magnesium carrier is the same as the one involved in calcium transport, because administration of large amounts of calcium has a negative effect on magnesium absorption (15). Unlike the situation with calcium, magnesium is not more avidly absorbed when a deficiency prevails in the organism (192). Magnesium absorption is probably influenced by several hormones. So far, data are available only on the influence of parathormone and aldosterone, both of which are reported to inhibit magnesium absorption. Vitamin D probably enhances the absorption (877).

5.8 HAEMATOPOIETIC FACTORS

5.8.1 Iron

The human organism contains about 4-5 g iron, of which 2-3 g is contained in haemoglobin, while 1 g is stored in the iron stores (liver, spleen and bone marrow). The remainder is contained in the myoglobin of the muscle cells (400-900 mg), and the enzyme systems of all body cells (100 mg). Only 4 mg iron is bound to transferrin and is present in the circulation as serum iron (604). Particularly with a view to the role which iron plays in cellular metabolism (oxygen transfer), it is of importance that the amount of iron is kept within certain, fairly narrow limits. This implies that the small loss of iron with the faeces, urine, via the skin or during menstruation, has to be compensated by absorption from food, which on the other hand should not exceed the iron loss. The normal diet contains about 10-15 mg iron per day (110), mostly in meat, cereals, potatoes, vegetables or fruit (196, 422). These food constituents contain iron both in inorganic and in organic form.

When discussing iron absorption it is best to distinguish between the 'intraluminal' phase, meant to change dietary iron to a form suitable for absorption, and the 'mucosal' phase, which refers to absorption in the strict sense. The intraluminal phase comprises all processes which, after ingestion of iron, take place in the stomach, duodenum and other parts of the small intestine. These are in fact a series of chemical reactions which differ in accordance with the type of food and the form in which the iron is contained in it. A number of reactions play a fundamental role in this intraluminal phase. First, there exists always an equilibrium between the divalent ferrous and the trivalent ferric ions; their concentrations depend on the nature of the iron salts as well as on the presence of reducing or oxidizing substances and on the pH of the luminal contents. A second point is that iron is also capable of forming co-ordination bonds, which virtually cannot be broken if organic substances are involved and if the pH is basic (110).

In addition to these fundamental reactions, various other factors play a role in the solubility (i.e. availability for absorption) of iron. Of importance in this respect is the presence of substances, such as ascorbic acid, which reduce iron, and of substances which form stable, readily soluble compounds with iron, such as citrate, gluconate, lactate, succinic acid, mannitol, sorbitol, fructose and some amino acids. All these substances stimulate iron absorption. On the other hand, there can be factors with a negative influence on absorption because they form insoluble compounds with iron. Examples are the phytates, oxalates, carbonates, phosphates and certain pharmaceutical compounds such as EDTA, magnesium trisilicate and cholestyramine (110).

It looks as if the influence of the stomach and pancreas on iron absorption is essentially determined by their ability to alter the pH and, therefore, to alter the solubility of iron (110). The question is whether the stomach also exerts other influences on iron absorption, e.g. by forming a stimulating factor known as intrinsic factor (482) or an inhibitory factor known as gastroferrin (197). On this point, the findings reported by different authors are controversial (110). At any rate it has been established in patients with achylia that absorption of inorganic iron (if dissolved in an acid milieu) and of haemoglobin iron is always normal in the absence of gastric juice (264, 373). Nor are there sufficient clues to warrant the hypothesis that pancreatic juice or bile should contain factors which influence iron absorption (110).

The above mentioned factors seem to be of no importance for the solubility of organic iron (429). Both haemoglobin and myoglobin are stripped of their protein fraction by proteolytic enzymes in the small intestine. Subsequently the haem is absorbed intact, without further conversion or degradation (157).

An average of only 5-10% of dietary iron is absorbed, significantly less than the percentage of an oral dose of iron which fasting test subjects absorb (428). Absorption varies widely with the type of food that contains the iron. Moreover, the other constituents of the meal can also influence iron absorption. Eggs, for example, prevent the absorption of iron from food other than meat (122), and iron from vegetables is more readily absorbed if ingested together with veal (564). Due to the enormous diversity of possible interactions, iron absorption from a meal cannot be accurately predicted (110).

Normally, iron absorption takes place largely in the duodenum and proximal jejunum (645). The remainder of the small intestine is as such also able to absorb iron, but less efficiently than the proximal part. In the case of iron deficiency, the absorption in the distal part of the small intestine is quantitatively considerable (909). The absorption process actually comprises three phases: absorption of iron on the luminal side of the enterocyte, transport and storage in the enterocyte, and exchange of iron on the serosal side. The uptake on the luminal side is based on an active process (550), probably involving transport carriers (313). The chemical form in which iron is taken up is unknown. Perhaps it is bound to a suitable chelating agent such as an amino acid or sugar (428). Intracellular transport in the enterocyte probably also takes place after combination with a carbohydrate (136), amino acid (551), protein (927) or carrier (428), since it is unlikely that the active iron ion is present as such in the enterocyte (428). Part of the iron absorbed is bound within the enterocyte to the protein apoferritin, thus producing ferritin. From this ferritin, only a minute quantity of iron is later released into the circulation. The bulk remains in the enterocyte as ferritin. After exfoliation, it enters the intestinal lumen with the enterocyte and is excreted with the faeces or re-absorbed after cell degradation (155, 276, 428).

Haem is as such absorbed by the enterocyte (157), and degraded intracellularly (903). The iron ion released then follows the same metabolic pathways as the other ionized iron (428).

The transfer of iron from the enterocyte to the blood stream is probably also effected by active transport (550), involving a specific transport carrier (684).

Iron absorption actually takes a biphasic course. Isotope studies have shown that there is a rapid phase, during which 40-60% of the total absorbable iron fraction appears in the circulation within two hours. In addition there is a slow phase which lasts about 24 hours, during which a small proportion of the iron primarily stored in the enterocytes, is released into the blood stream (263). Normally, about half the iron absorbed (35-70%) remains sequestered in the enterocytes as ferritin (81). After exfoliation of these enterocytes, some of this ferritin iron can again be absorbed after digestion of the cell and degradation of the compound. This also explains why the faecal elimination of labelled iron given by mouth, continues for a few weeks after its administration (155, 276).

Apart from the factors which influence iron solubility in the intestinal lumen, the requirement of the organism is an important determinant of the absorption of iron from food. The degree of iron absorption is inversely proportional to the size of the iron reserves in the organism (369). Iron absorption exceeds the normal in the case of iron depletion or increased erythropoiesis for example (902). On the other hand, iron absorption is evidently less when the iron reserves are repleted. This regulation, however, is not entirely adequate, for after protracted oral administration of large doses of iron, the organism can retain too much iron ultimately (111). Both the nature of the control mechanism and the manner in which it is informed about the individual's iron status, have so far remained obscure (110).

5.8.2 Vitamin B_{12}

Vitamin B_{12} has an essential function in various elementary metabolic processes, such as the nucleic acid synthesis and folic acid metabolism. The name vitamin B_{12} actually covers a group of biologically active cobalamins, all of which probably serve a similar function as coenzyme constituent. The qualitatively and quantitatively most important vitamin B_{12} analogue is deoxyadenosyl cobalamin (= coenzyme vitamin B_{12}). Virtually all cobalamin, both in the human organism and in the food, is synthesized by bacteria. In man vitamin B_{12} synthesis largely takes place in the colon. Hardly any of this endogenous vitamin B_{12} is absorbed. One must therefore rely on the vitamin B_{12} contained in the normal diet, which supplies an average of 16 μg (range 1.2-75.6 μg) per day (139). This is usually more than the recommended dietary allowance, which is estimated to be 3-4 μg (196). Rich vitamin B_{12} sources are food of animal origin such as meat, fish, eggs, milk and cheese (422). The human organism has relatively substantial vitamin B_{12} reserves (about 2 mg) in the liver; this is sufficient to meet daily requirements for a few years (490).

In the food, vitamin B_{12} is usually bound to proteins, from which it is detached by cooking or through the action of pepsin in the stomach (133); this is usually done so thoroughly that all vitamin B_{12} from the food becomes available for absorption (388). After release from its protein link, vitamin B_{12} is bound to intrinsic factor from the stomach.

Intrinsic factor (IF) is a glycoprotein synthesized by the parietal cells of the gastric mucosa. Its release is stimulated by gastrin, histamine and insulin. A considerable excess of IF is normally formed, of which only a very small fraction is probably required for vitamin B_{12} absorption (133).

Vitamin B_{12} and IF are both substances of relatively low stability, which are readily degraded by enzymes or bacteria in the gastrointestinal tract (3, 651). By complex forming they produce a fairly stable compound, which is probably less readily consumed by bacteria (761). Once formed in the stomach or in the most proximal part of the small intestine, these vitamin B_{12}-IF complexes are carried with the food to the ileum, where they are absorbed (84).

The exact manner in which absorption takes place in the ileum is still uncertain. The enterocytes in the ileum probably have specific receptors on their microvilli for the vitamin B_{12}-IF complex (225). It is thought that these receptors are especially susceptible to IF, because free IF also attaches itself quite readily to them (2). The amount of vitamin B_{12} to be absorbed is probably determined by the number of unoccupied receptor sites in the ileum. This could explain why, of varying amounts of vitamin B_{12}, no more than 2 μg per meal is ever absorbed (133). Although the receptors in the ileum have a high affinity for the vitamin B_{12}-IF complex, they bind it only at a particular pH and in the presence of calcium or magnesium ions (125). Although coupling to the receptors is probably a rapid process (852), it nevertheless takes at least three hours for any vitamin B_{12} to appear in the circulation. The maximum concentration of vitamin B_{12} in the blood is not attained until after 8-12 hours (83). During this interval, the receptors in the ileum are blocked for further uptake of the vitamin B_{12}-IF complex (1). It is probably during this interval that vitamin B_{12} is detached from its complexes by enzymes from the brush border (539). The free IF remains attached to the receptor for some hours (394), and cannot be found in the faeces until some time later (931).

Vitamin B_{12} is found, after its absorption, in several organelles of the enterocyte, specifically in the mitochondria (674). Here, some cobalamins are incorporated if necessary in coenzyme-vitamin B_{12} complexes (675).

Transport of vitamin B_{12} from the enterocyte to the liver takes place exclusively by means of a carrier protein called transcobalamin II. Its absence leads to severe megaloblastic anaemia (351).

In addition to absorption, also some secretion of vitamin B_{12} takes place in the small intestine. The amount secreted is uncertain. Vitamin B_{12} is believed to enter the intestinal lumen with gastric juice, intestinal juice and bile (332, 650). Most of it is normally re-absorbed and thus proceeds in the enterohepatic circulation (165).

5.8.3 Folates

Folates are the compounds derived from folic acid. Food contains mainly folates (pteroylpolyglutamates), and only small quantities of folic acid (pteroylmonoglutamic acid). To cover its folate requirements, the human organism must rely on dietary folates. The requirements are estimated to amount to about 50 μg/day (383). The normal diet as a rule provides more than enough folates: an average of 600-700 μg/day, mainly in the form of green vegetables, fruit and liver (131). Yet some synthesis takes place in the organism. Certain bacteria in the colon synthesize endogenous folate, but this is scarcely absorbed (404). Without a dietary supply of folates, the organism's reserves of about 10 mg are exhausted within a few months (382). Folates are needed as coenzyme constituent in many enzymatic processes, such as the nucleic acid synthesis and amino acid metabolism.

Polyglutamates from food are probably deconjugated to monoglutamates before being absorbed (63, 718). The enzyme needed for this purpose, folate conjugase or γ-glutamyl carboxypeptidase is found in high concentrations in the lysosomes and mitochondria (401, 718). This suggests that polyglutamate deconjugation takes place intracellularly. It seems more rational, however, to assume that deconjugation precedes absorption and therefore takes place at the brush border (720) or in the intestinal lumen (718). The enzymes could be taken there by intracellular transport or they could be liberated by intraluminal degradation of exfoliated enterocytes (718). It is highly probable that this polyglutamate deconjugation is not effected by a single enzyme but by a whole series of enzymes, each of which governs one step (719). In the blood stream, only the end-product monoglutamate is encountered (63).

Some foods make less folate available for absorption than might be expected in view of their folate contents (702). This can be explained by both the presence of less readily absorbable polyglutamates (121) or by the formation of complexes with substances such as cellulose (534). It is also possible that food contains substances which interfere with the activity of folate conjugase (403).

Folate is preferably absorbed in the proximal part of the small intestine. This is also suggested by the fact that folate deficiency often follows diseases or resection of this part of the small intestine, whereas a deficiency is rarely observed in association with diseases of the ileum (170). Perfusion studies, too, have shown that monoglutamate absorption is maximal in the jejunum and negligibly small in the ileum (380). Absorption probably involves an active transport process by means of carriers (380, 381). The relevant data, however, are not entirely convincing (308, 718).

After its absorption, further conversion of monoglutamate into 5-methyl-tetrahydrofolate takes place in the enterocytes (669). The intracellular transport of all possible types of folate, like their transport from the enterocyte to the blood stream, probably takes place in the same way and with the aid of the same type of transport carrier (503, 747). The capacity of this carrier transport would seem to determine the rate at which polyglutamate as well as monoglutamate can be absorbed (878).

The entire process of deconjugation of polyglutamate and absorption with further conversion of monoglutamate is so quickly completed that an increase in serum folate concentration is observed within 15 minutes of its oral administration (380, 718). Of an oral dose of monoglutamate, 60-80% is usually absorbed even when large doses (up to 15 mg) are given (380). Of polyglutamate, a similar fraction is absorbed only of physiological doses, while less is absorbed of larger doses of polyglutamate (121, 824).

Some endogenous folate is released in the small intestine, moreover, from bile (60-90 µg/day) and exfoliated enterocytes. Normally, however, a large part of this endogenous folate is re-absorbed, and the loss is therefore limited (40).

5.9 WATER-SOLUBLE VITAMINS

5.9.1 Vitamin C

Vitamin C (ascorbic acid) has an important function in the growth process and cell metabolism. Its presence is required for formation of the ground substance of connective tissue and the matrix of bone tissue. In addition, it is probably of importance for the synthesis of some hormones and the absorption of such substances as iron (196). The vitamin C requirement is estimated to be 30 mg/day (700). Important sources are fruit, potatoes and green vegetables (196, 422). Vitamin C deficiency manifests itself by extensive capillary haemorrhages in gingiva and skin, or in muscles and joints. This syndrome is known as scurvy.

Vitamin C is absorbed in the proximal small intestine (635, 816) by diffusion and possibly also by active transport. The absorption process is undoubtedly very complicated, because vitamin C given by mouth appears in the circulation only much later (816). The capacity to absorb vitamin C is high (635). Any surplus of vitamin C is stored, but when these stores are replete, the excess of vitamin C is excreted by the kidneys.

5.9.2 Thiamine

Thiamine (vitamin B_1) plays a particular role in carbohydrate metabolism. The thiamine requirement depends on the caloric intake, and should be 0.5 mg per 1000 kilocalories (700). Sources rich in thiamine are bread, vegetables, potatoes, fruit, meat and milk (196, 422). A chronic thiamine deficiency can lead to peripheral neuropathies or to cardiac failure, a condition known as beriberi. An alternative possibility is the occurrence of an encephalopathy, which is named after Wernicke.

Thiamine is probably absorbed in the proximal part of the small intestine, for diseases of the stomach or terminal ileum do not influence its absorption (845). Thiamine is absorbed unchanged, probably by active transport (613). The organism has no thiamine reserves, any surplus of this vitamin being excreted by the kidneys (196).

5.9.3 Riboflavin

Riboflavin (vitamin B_2) is a constituent of the flavoprotein enzymes which are involved in various oxidation reactions in the human organism. The requirement for this vitamin is supposed to be 0.6 mg per 1000 kilocalories (700), which is obtained from dairy products, meat, eggs, green vegetables, fruit, potatoes and bread (196, 422). Symptoms of riboflavin deficiency are: angular stomatitis, cheilosis, glossitis (magenta tongue), seborrhoeic dermatitis, lacrimation and photophobia (196).

Riboflavin is absorbed mainly in the proximal part of the small intestine, probably by diffusion (613).

5.9.4 Niacin

Niacin (vitamin B_3), which refers to nicotinic acid as well as to nicotinamide, has a function as a constituent of certain coenzymes which are of great importance in cell respiration, glycolysis and fat synthesis. The niacin requirement is estimated to be 6.6 mg per 1000 kilocalories (700). Dietary sources are meat, vegetables, fruit, potatoes and bread (196, 422). Niacin can also be derived from tryptophan in food. Niacin deficiency causes pellagra, a condition characterized by dermatitis, diarrhoea and dementia (196).

Niacin is largely absorbed by diffusion in the proximal part of the small intestine (813).

5.9.5 Vitamin B_6

Vitamin B_6 (also called pyridoxine, but actually a collection of three pyridines) has a function in the degradation and synthesis of amino acids. The vitamin B_6 requirement is estimated to be 2 mg per day (700). Sources rich in vitamin B_6 are meat, vegetables, potatoes, rice and bread (196). Vitamin B_6 deficiency can give rise to neuropathies, dermatitis, stomatitis, glossitis, cheilosis or sideroblastic anaemia (196).

Vitamin B_6 is absorbed in the proximal part of the small intestine. Even after very extensive resections, leaving intact only about 1 metre of the proximal jejunum, vitamin B_6 absorption was found to be normal (99). Absorption probably takes place by diffusion. Virtually all vitamin B_6 in food is absorbed. Any surplus is largely excreted by the kidneys (99).

5.9.6 Pantothenic acid

Pantothenic acid is a constituent of coenzyme A, which is involved in various metabolic processes, including the citric acid cycle. It is difficult to estimate the daily requirement of pantothenic acid, which is supplied by meat, eggs, potatoes, vegetables and bread (196, 422). An intake of 5-10 mg per day is regarded as sufficient (700). There is no certainty about the question whether pantothenic acid deficiency produces any symptoms, although myospasms, general malaise and burning feet have been ascribed to such a deficiency (196).

Pantothenic acid is probably absorbed by diffusion (813).

CHAPTER 6

PATHOPHYSIOLOGY OF COELIAC SPRUE

6.0 INTRODUCTION

It is widely known that coeliac sprue is nearly always accompanied by malabsorption, and there are abundant relevant data on this subject. Far less attention has so far been paid to possible changes of the physiological processes in the small intestine in patients with coeliac sprue. There are indeed some indications that these processes take an abnormal course. This is quite conceivable, because the inflammatory lesions in the intestinal wall do involve mucosal and submucosal elements other than the enterocytes, such as the hormone or mucus producing cells, the nerve fibres and the blood vessels or lymphatics.

The following sections deal with various aspects of the pathophysiology of coeliac sprue. A survey of relevant observations so far published will be presented, with the addition of some personal observations. Before discussing the results of these observations, it would seem useful to give some information on the group of patients studied. For the methods of investigation the reader is referred to chapter 12.

6.1 COMPOSITION OF THE GROUP OF PATIENTS STUDIED

Coeliac sprue was diagnosed in 47 patients on the basis of three criteria (section 1.3). The first criterion to be fulfilled was the presence of characteristic villous abnormalities (section 3.3.2) in the first jejunal loop, 5-20 cm beyond the ligament of Treitz. A biopsy specimen was obtained from the small intestine before gluten withdrawal in each of the 47 patients with the exception of 3. In these 3 patients a biopsy specimen was not obtained until after gluten withdrawal, and in each of these cases revealed unmistakable abnormalities consistent with coeliac sprue. In view of the aim of our study – the severity of malabsorption and the effect of a gluten-free diet in coeliac sprue – the second criterion was that clinically manifest malabsorption had to be present. Coeliacs without symptoms of malabsorption, who are regularly encountered in particular among patients with dermatitis herpetiformis (section 10.2), were not included in this group. All patients, moreover, had to fulfil a third criterion, e.g. a characteristic history, or a favourable response to gluten withdrawal in clinical, biochemical or morphological respect (section 1.3).

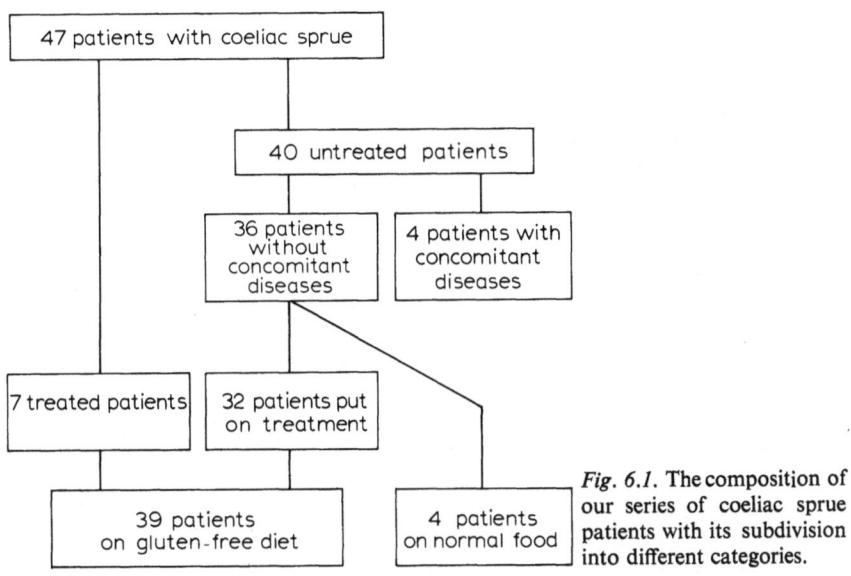

Fig. 6.1. The composition of our series of coeliac sprue patients with its subdivision into different categories.

The total number of patients who fulfilled these criteria was 47 (fig. 6.1). Of these, 7 had already been on a gluten-free diet before being referred to us. Of the 40 remaining, untreated patients, a few showed coeliac sprue as well as some other disease, such as ulcerative colitis, diverticulosis of the small intestine, or carcinoma of the pancreas. In addition, one patient had multiple stenoses on the basis of non-granulomatous duodenojejunitis (section 11.2). There remained 36 patients, therefore, who were suffering from untreated coeliac sprue without any indication of other diseases which might account for symptoms or malabsorption. Observations on clinical symptoms or biochemical abnormalities in untreated coeliac sprue were made in this group of 36 patients. The effect of gluten withdrawal could be studied in only 32 patients, because 4 patients had been on the diet only briefly, i.e. less than 6 months, or not at all. The biochemical assays during gluten depletion were made in these 32 patients. The ultimate effect of the gluten-free diet could be evaluated in a total of 39 patients, including the 7 who had been on this diet before being referred to us.

Table 6.1. Predominant symptom at presentation of 36 patients with untreated coeliac sprue.

DIARRHOEA	17 PATIENTS
ABDOMINAL PAIN	6 PATIENTS
ANAEMIA	7 PATIENTS
STOMATITIS APHTHOSA	2 PATIENTS
PETECHIAE	1 PATIENT
ANKLE OEDEMA	1 PATIENT
TETANY	1 PATIENT
NON-HEALING FRACTURE	1 PATIENT

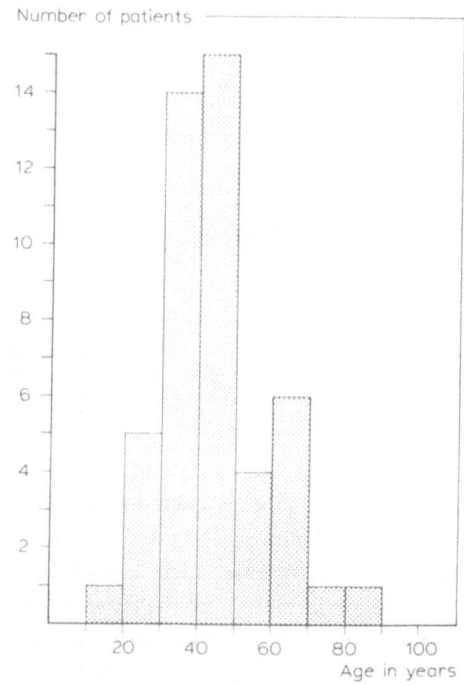

Fig. 6.2. The age distribution in our series of 47 patients with coeliac sprue at the time of diagnosis.

The total group of 47 patients included 30 women and 17 men. The age distribution at the time of diagnosis is presented in fig. 6.2. In an effort to give an impression of the severity of the clinical symptoms in these patients, table 6.1 lists the motivations for the referral of the 36 untreated patients to us. The vast majority were suffering from diarrhoea or anaemia, which in 12 patients was so severe as to necessitate immediate hospitalization. The other symptoms varied from abdominal pain or stomatitis to tetany or delayed fracture healing due to hypocalcaemia (cf chapter 8).

Little research has so far been devoted to the motility of the small intestine in coeliac sprue such as studies on the intraluminal pressure or electrical activity of the musculature of the intestinal wall. There are indications that the frequency of the basic electrical rhythm is diminished in coeliac sprue (137). Segmental contractions, moreover, are believed to diminish both in frequency and in vigour (293).

Several authors observed an abnormal passage of contrast medium in coeliac patients during fluoroscopy. The intestinal loops often impress as flaccid, atonic and collapsed, showing no reaction to filling with contrast medium, which at the same time does not provoke any peristalsis. In most cases peristalsis is slow and rather ineffective, causing an abnormally long transit time of the contrast medium (434, 563, 619, 775). In a proportion of patients, however, the small intestine is very contractile, so that passage

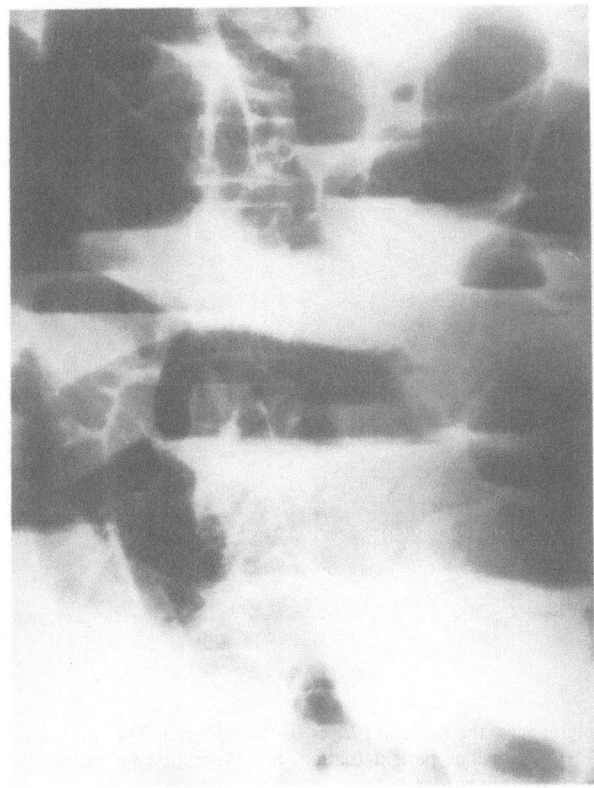

Fig. 6.3. Plain abdominal X ray in upright position, showing an ileus pattern with air-fluid levels in the small intestine. The film was obtained on a 62 – year – old untreated coeliac patient (patient no. 5, section 9.3.4) with a history of crampy abdominal pain, vomiting and abdominal distension. At the subsequent surgical exploration no mechanical obstructions were found.

of the contrast medium through the small intestine takes only a few minutes (619). It is to be borne in mind, however, that peristalsis and transit time can also vary widely in normal individuals and that, apart from the amount and composition of the contrast medium (775), psychological factors can also be of influence in this respect (118).

In some patients with coeliac sprue this atony leads to paralytic ileus (113). Features of ileus (fig. 6.3) were observed in two of our patients (no. 5 and no. 34; cf sections 9.3.4 and 9.4.3) leading to an exploratory laparotomy before coeliac sprue was diagnosed. The question arises of the aetiology of paralytic ileus in these patients. Generally speaking, paralysis can result from the influence of neurogenic, humoral or metabolic factors. A well known metabolic cause is hypopotassaemia. In retrospect, however, there was no indication of a decreased serum potassium concentration in our two patients. In one of them, who succumbed to myocardial disease shortly after, we did find an extensive accumulation of ceroid pigment in the muscular layer of the intestinal wall (fig. 6.4). In the other patient, a marked deposition of ceroid

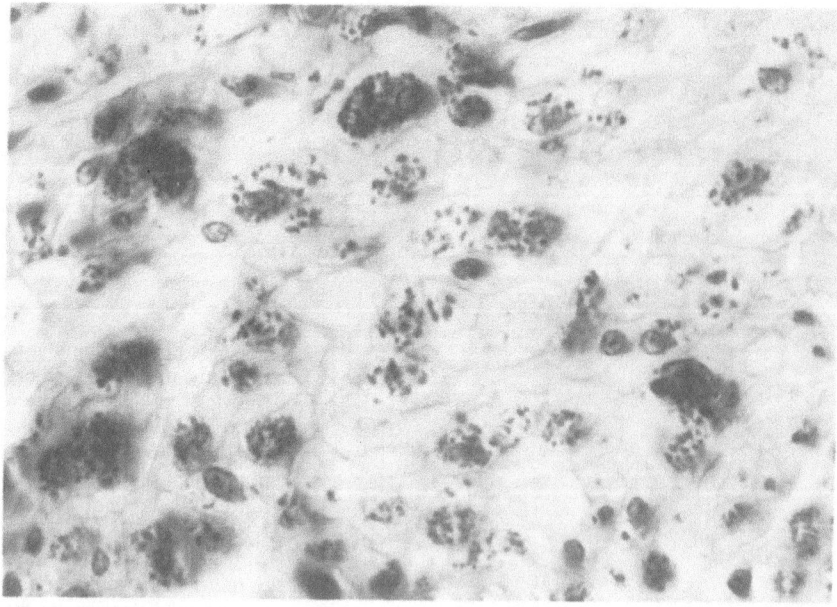

Fig. 6.4. Deposition of ceroid pigment in the muscular layer of the jejunum. This post-mortem specimen was obtained from a coeliac patient (patient no. 34, section 9.4) who presented with a paralytic ileus some months earlier.

was observed in the smooth muscle cells in a rectal biopsy specimen. The biopsy specimens from the small intestine in these patients showed a muscularis mucosae without ceroid deposition. This means that the mucosal muscle cells are not always representative of the situation in the muscular layer of the intestine. It therefore seems plausible that ceroid accumulation, resulting from vitamin E deficiency (section 7.4.6), plays a role in the aetiology of intestinal paralysis in coeliac sprue.

Another important factor may be the presence of an abnormal bacterial flora, due to which toxins and irritant degradation products (like volatile fatty acids and deconjugated bile acids) can be formed. An abnormal bacterial flora causes acceleration of transit time in most cases, but it can also give rise to ileus-like features, which disappear after medication with antibiotics (237). According to DiMagno et al. (214), the abnormal motility in coeliac sprue can be the result of a dysregulation of intestinal hormones.

Due to absence or an abnormal shape of the villi, micro-movements of the intestinal villi in the proximal small intestine are not possible in coeliac patients (771).

The sometimes pronounced disorders of motility can exert a negative influence on absorption in patients with coeliac sprue. In the event of accelerated passage, the mucosal contact time is markedly reduced. On the other hand, in cases with very slow peristalsis and dilatation of the intestinal loops, the exchange between absorbing surface and intestinal contents can be impaired as a result of the formation of a thick unstirred layer (sections 5.1.2 and 5.1.5).

6.3. INNERVATION

Regulation and coordination of intestinal motility, blood supply and secretion of digestive juices is ensured by the autonomic nervous system – probably in interaction with intestinal hormones. As already discussed in the preceding section, the motility of the small intestine is abnormal in some coeliac patients. In addition there are indications that the secretion of digestive juices, too, is not always optimal in these patients (section 6.6). It is therefore not impossible that the function of the autonomic nervous system is disturbed in these patients. In any case, abnormalities of the peripheral nerves are not uncommon in coeliac sprue (163, 611, 656). These latter are usually lesions of a degenerative nature, which are ascribed to deficiency in vitamins of the B group. Whether deficiencies in other vitamins or in certain amino acids also play a role in this context, has so far remained obscure (656). A deficiency in these nutrients could cause degenerative lesions, not only of the peripheral and the central but also of the autonomic nervous system. It is not inconceivable, moreover, that the small nerve fibers in the intestinal wall could also be damaged by the inflammatory process in the mucosa or by toxins and degradation products of an abnormal intestinal flora.

The syndrome of idiopathic intestinal pseudo-obstruction, characterized by a distended abdomen with dilatation of intestinal loops, abdominal pain, vomiting, varying diarrhoea and malabsorption, is associated with neuro-muscular dysfunction of the small intestine (549) and histological changes in the myenteric plexus (804). At first sight, this syndrome has certain similarities to coeliac sprue. However, it does not respond to gluten withdrawal but shows a response (if only transient) to broad-spectrum antibiotics (804). This suggests that an abnormal intestinal flora gives rise to the above mentioned pattern of symptoms (549). On the basis of the response to a gluten-free diet, differentiation between the two conditions is possible. By analogy to this syndrome it is not inconceivable that some abdominal symptoms such as abnormal motility could be the result of an abnormal function or structure of the autonomic nervous system. So far as we know, there are no published observations on the structure of the intestinal nervous tissue in untreated coeliac patients. Notions concerning abnormalities of the autonomic nervous system in coeliac sprue are therefore still speculative.

6.4 CIRCULATION

Hardly anything is known about the changes in the blood supply to the small intestine which can occur in coeliac sprue. Changes in vascular structure can be expected in the smaller vessels of the mucosa, specifically in that part of the small intestine in which the villi are absent or abnormal. The vascular convolutions which should be present in these villi will be either absent or deformed. An exchange between the blood vessels within the intestinal villus according to the so-called countercurrent principle, cannot take place under these circumstances.

The blood flow can be either activated or, on the contrary, impeded by the inflammatory changes in the intestinal wall, which give rise to oedema of the interstitial tissue. Distension of the wall of the small intestine due to stasis or gas formation can impair the blood supply. Also, the inflammatory process can usurp a large amount of the oxygen and nutrients supplied. It seems likely therefore that the proportion of the blood supply which is normally allocated to the absorption process, is smaller in coeliac patients. This factor can contribute to the existing malabsorption in coeliac sprue.

6.5 LYMPHATIC SYSTEM

6.5.1 Introduction

In animals subjected to experimental ligation of the efferent lymphatics from the small intestine, diarrhoea with disturbed fat absorption and increased enteric protein leakage is sometimes observed after a short time. The morphology of the intestinal mucosa in these animals can also show distinct changes, such as broadened and sometimes markedly shortened villi (275, 574, 600, 917). In human pathology, too, villous abnormalities are sometimes observed in the presence of an impaired intestinal lymph drainage, as in primary intestinal lymphangiectasia, Whipple's disease and cardiac failure (546, 678, 913).

These experimental data raise the question of the role of intestinal lymph congestion in the pathophysiology of some types of malabsorption, such as in coeliac sprue. It seems useful therefore to present some relevant observations.

6.5.2 Protein leakage and lymphocyte count

Leakage of lymph into the intestinal lumen is not infrequently associated with lymphocytopenia (431). In 8 untreated coeliac patients with a markedly increased enteric leakage, exceeding 200 ml plasma per day, the lymphocytes in the peripheral blood were counted. None of these 8 patients showed lymphocytopenia, i.e. less than 20% lymphocytes in the differential leucocyte count (242). In 4 of these patients protein leakage was again measured during a gluten-free regime. In spite of a substantial decrease of enteric leakage in all cases, the lymphocyte count increased in only one patient.

6.5.3 Influence of restriction of LCT fat on protein leakage

Absorption of long-chain triglycerides (LCT) is associated with an increased lymph flow. Restriction of these triglycerides in the diet reduces the intestinal lymph flow (340). If in coeliac sprue patients lymph congestion and leakage play a role in the aetiology of protein leakage through the intestinal wall, it should diminish during an LCT-free regime. In 3 patients who showed only a moderate response to a gluten-free diet, the protein leakage was measured both with and without supplementary LCT restriction. Two patients showed a spectacular improvement, as indicated in table 6.2. The case histories of these patients are presented in section 9.3.1 and section 11.2.2. In the third patient, fat restriction had no effect on the

93

Table 6.2. Influence of restriction of dietary long-chain triglycerides on enteric plasma protein leakage.

| PATIENT | ENTERIC PLASMA PROTEIN LEAKAGE (ml/24 hrs) | |
	On gluten-free diet	On gluten-free diet and LCT-fat restriction
# 17	430	55
# 20	260	385
# 46	200	85

extent of protein leakage. It is to be noted that in the 2 patients with an improved leakage, the peripheral lymphocyte count did not increase.

6.5.4 Abnormalities of the mesenteric lymph nodes

Of the 47 coeliac patients in our series, 24 underwent a laparotomy, usually in view of a suspected appendicitis. In 5 patients the laparotomy revealed greatly enlarged mesenteric lymph nodes. Since the presence of abdominal nodes was probably not always explicitly checked, the real number of patients with enlarged mesenteric lymph nodes may have been somewhat larger. Three patients who died from causes other than coeliac sprue (sections 9.4.3 and 9.4.4) were submitted to post-mortem examination, which in all cases disclosed enlarged lymph nodes in the mesentery. Pathological examination of these nodes revealed non-specific changes in all cases, such as follicular atrophy or hyperplasia, sinus histiocytosis, fibrosis or cavitation with fat necrosis.

6.5.5 Comment

It seems plausible that in some patients with coeliac sprue the intestinal lymph flow is indeed impaired. Due to the absence of normal initial lacteals in the damaged mucosa of the small intestine, lymph uptake can be primarily disturbed, while the 'milking' of the lacteals is also impeded (fig. 4.7). Moreover, the efferent flow of lymph can be hindered by compression of the lymphatics as a result of some oedema of the wall of the small intestine. More cranially, swollen and congested lymph nodes in the mesentery can obstruct a free lymph drainage. Laparotomy or post-mortem examination disclosed enlarged mesenteric lymph nodes in several of our coeliac patients. Histological examination of these nodes never revealed any characteristic pathology, but only non-specific changes. For that matter, many other investigators have reported enlarged lymph nodes in patients with coeliac sprue (466, 663, 912; cf chapter 11).

The impaired drainage of intestinal lymph will be the more significant because lymph production is probably increased in the damaged intestine of coeliac patients. Apart from an increased permeability of the blood capillaries, a decreased colloid osmotic pressure due to hypoalbuminaemia can also play a role in this respect.

In the case of an obstructed lymph drainage caused by abnormal mesenteric lymph nodes, only limited bypassing via collaterals is possible. The distance over which lymph can be bypassed is small, however (504, 646), and can hardly be very helpful when the drainage of a large segment of the small intestine is obstructed. In the case of severe congestion, the swollen subserous lymphatics may rupture, resulting in chylous ascites, which has in fact been described in coeliac sprue (466). On the other hand, lymph from ruptured mucosal lymphatics may also enter the intestinal lumen, as has been observed in abdominal tuberculosis (770) or primary intestinal lymphangiectasia (431, 819, 879). This entails a loss, not only of fat-like substances but also of proteins (286).

The fact that the enteric protein leakage in two of our patients with coeliac sprue showed a marked improvement after restriction of LCT fat in the diet, suggests that leakage of lymph occurs from the intestinal wall into the lumen (table 6.2). Restriction of the fat consumption reduces lymph production in the small intestine, because transport of chyle via the lymphatic system is scarcely required in that case (340). Reduced chyle production is bound to cause reduction of the congestion in the lymphatic system, and consequently less leakage occurs. In addition to chyle and tissue fluid, the intestinal lymphatics also transport lymphocytes from the lymph follicles and Peyer plaques. In the case of marked lymph leakage in the intestinal lumen, as in primary intestinal lymphangiectasia, peripheral lymphocytopenia is usually present (431, 879). In our patients with marked protein leakage, however, lymphocytopenia was never observed. Whether this may be related to a perhaps increased lymphocyte production in the intestinal wall in coeliac sprue, remains a moot question.

6.6 DIGESTIVE SECRETIONS

6.6.1 Introduction

Although patients with treated pernicious anaemia are usually in good condition and without signs of malabsorption, the view that the stomach, and specifically gastric juice, plays an essential role in digestion is still widely accepted. In patients with coeliac sprue, several investigators have observed an achlorhydria (104, 163). It therefore seemed useful to investigate the occurrence of achlorhydria in our patients. The function of the pancreas was studied in some untreated coeliac patients moreover, as some investigators have maintained that association of coeliac sprue with pancreatic insufficiency is not uncommon (60, 163, 489, 682, 937).

6.6.2 Gastric secretion

Gastric juice was collected from a total of 22 patients. In only one patient achlorhydria was found. In this patient a high acid output had been established 20 years earlier, and he was treated three times for ulcer disease. The achlorhydria now observed was associated with the presence of antibodies against parietal cells and an increased gastrin concentration of 280 pg/ml (normal value 66 ± 18 pg/ml; 496).

Tests for the presence of antibodies against parietal cells of the stomach were carried out in 16 patients, and were – apart from the above discussed patient – always negative.

6.6.3 Pancreatic secretion

A secretin test was carried out in 4 untreated patients with coeliac sprue. In all cases the amount of pancreatic juice secreted in half hourly collections increased by at least factor 2 after secretin stimulation. In 3 patients, moreover, the bicarbonate concentration was markedly increased, attaining values of 95-135 mmole/1 (31 mmole/1 in the 4th patient).

6.6.4 Comment

In our group of 22 untreated coeliacs only one case of achlorhydria was found. The association between coeliac sprue and atrophic gastritis has never been explicitly mentioned, but a relation to other types of autoimmune disease has been observed (56, 764). Other authors have likewise reported coeliac patients with achlorhydria (104). Cooke (163) even observed this phenomenon in some 15% of his patients. Our own data show, however, that achlorhydria is not a common finding in coeliac sprue. In view of the mass of experimental and clinical data it is further highly unlikely that this achlorhydria could be a factor of significance in coeliac malabsorption (cf chapter 7).

No evidence of pancreatic insufficiency was found in at least 3 of the 4 patients examined in this respect. Others, however, have reported an abnormally low response of the pancreas to parenteral administration of secretin as well as of cholecystokinin/pancreozymin, or to a test meal (60, 163, 199, 214, 489, 937). If present, this insufficiency is probably a secondary phenomenon, for after gluten withdrawal pancreatic function can show a distinct improvement (272, 899). The mechanism by which coeliac sprue causes pancreatic insufficiency, is unknown. There are some hypotheses, including one that ascribes the pancreatic abnormalities to malabsorption of proteins (384, 834). The pancreas requires a minimum of amino acids for an adequate enzyme synthesis. Without this minimal supply atrophy of the exocrine pancreatic tissue develops, which is usually reversible (45, 870). Histological abnormalities of the pancreas have indeed been found in patients with severe and even refractory sprue (682). The possibility of concomitant pancreatic insufficiency is therefore to be taken into account, particularly in coeliac patients with a high nitrogen or low (chymo)trypsin excretion with faeces, and as well in those who show a poor response to a gluten-free diet (489, 682).

Although at least 3 of our 4 untreated patients showed a normal secretin test, it is not certain that their pancreas was actually functioning normally. It is conceivable that, due to reduced endogenous production of secretin and cholecystokinin in the enterocytes, a pancreatic insufficiency did exist but failed to become manifest at vigorous exogenous stimulation. DiMagno et al. (214) have suggested that relative insensitivity of the pancreas to hormonal stimuli could also play a role in the existing pancreatic insufficiency.

It should be mentioned, finally, that the concentration of bile acids in the intestinal lumen is perhaps also decreased in coeliac sprue. Of the total pool of bile acids, which as such seems extra large (529), an abnormally small amount is released into the small intestine by gall-bladder contraction (214, 528). Together with a marked dilution of the intestinal contents due to secretion of water in the duodenum and proximal jejunum (section 7.2), this gives rise to a decreased luminal concentration of bile acids. It is believed that this concentration is sometimes lower than the critical micellar concentration (214, 578), although this is not believed to be a common phenomenon (594). The sensitivity of the gall-bladder to endogenous stimulation by cholecystokinin is probably reduced in coeliac sprue (98, 530).

6.7 INTESTINAL HORMONES

The epithelium of the stomach, duodenum and jejunum contains cells which synthesize the so-called intestinal hormones, such as gastrin, secretin and cholecystokinin as well as other hormone-like substances (666). Precisely as the proximal segment of the small intestine is most severely affected in coeliac sprue, these hormone-producing cells should also be subject to changes. One might primarily assume that the production of intestinal hormones should be reduced in coeliacs as a result of the mucosal lesions (214). The hormone-producing cells are localized mainly, however, in the crypts of the small intestine, which are largely spared from the damaging effect of gluten; they actually show a marked growth in response to the increased exfoliation of cells (587). It therefore seems probable that an increased production of intestinal hormones is to be expected in coeliac sprue.

Histological examination of biopsy specimens from the small intestine in untreated patients indicates that the number of enterochromaffin cells in the duodenum is significantly increased, and diminishes during a gluten-free regimen. The enterochromaffin cells also stain more intensively, which suggests an increased hormone production (130). Other investigators have reported an increase in the number of secretin-producing cells (687).

In view of these observations the production of intestinal hormones can be expected to be increased in coeliac sprue. Low-Beer et al. (530) did in fact find extremely high serum cholecystokinin levels in fasting coeliacs. These high levels can be caused by diminished hormone degradation as well as by increased synthesis and secretion. Moreover, the assay may have included other cholecystokinin-like substances (530). The production of amines by the APUD cells also seems to be increased in untreated patients, for the urinary excretion of 5-hydroxytryptamine (serotonin) metabolites is markedly increased, and diminishes after the institution of a diet (129, 486). DiMagno et al. (214) published observations, however, which are suggestive of a delayed and sometimes even reduced release of cholecystokinin after instillation of food or amino acids in the duodenum. A similar phenomenon was observed with regard to gastrin release after administration of a test meal to untreated coeliac patients (25). It is to be noted, however, that the above mentioned data can be interpreted in various ways (214, 215, 530, 531).

An explanation of these high serum hormone levels in coeliac sprue might be sought in reduced sensitivity of the target organs to hormonal stimuli. The less vigorous gall-bladder contraction seen in untreated patients (528) even after administration of exogenous cholecystokinin (98) would seem to suggest this. In the hands of some investigators, administration of exogenous cholecystokinin or secretin has also caused reduced secretion of enzymes, water and bicarbonate by the pancreas in coeliac sprue (384, 644, 937).

The above mentioned abnormalities in the production and release of intestinal hormones or in the sensitivity of the target organs to hormonal stimuli can result in dysregulation of gastric evacuation, intestinal peristalsis and secretion of bile and pancreatic juice in coeliac patients. This probably affords a partial explanation of the existing abnormal motility and maldigestion.

6.8 INTESTINAL MUCUS

Intestinal mucus probably protects the intestinal wall against digestive juices and bacteria which degrade and transform the ingested food. Its protective function is clearly demonstrated by the marked secretory activity of the goblet cells in the intestinal mucosa in the presence of noxious or irritant substances. The number of goblet cells also seems to increase under such conditions, to a degree which has been described as colonic metaplasia (664). In addition to the amount, the nature of mucus is one of the important determinants of its function. The composition of intestinal mucus depends on the subject's age and nutritional state, and perhaps also on genetic factors (518).

The properties of intestinal mucus may be abnormal in diseases of the small intestine (518). It is uncertain whether an abnormally large amount of mucus is formed in the small intestine in coeliac sprue. Mucus formation might be expected to be increased due to the presence of an abnormal intestinal flora and of gluten, which is toxic to coeliacs. In most cases, however, biopsy specimens from the small intestine in coeliac sprue show no increased number of goblet cells. Absence of an increase in mucus formation can be the result of a deficiency of certain necessary substances (204). The mucus production can have diminished again also, after initial hypersecretion, as if its sources were exhausted (192). If the quality of the intestinal mucus were also changed in coeliac sprue, the result would be that the mucus could no longer adequately perform its normal function. This could mean an insufficient protection of the mucosa from the influence of bacteria or proteolytic enzymes. So far, however, no factual data on the production and composition of mucus in coeliac sprue have been published.

6.9 EXFOLIATION OF ENTEROCYTES

The turnover of the small intestinal epithelium is markedly increased in patients with coeliac sprue. The number of cells exfoliated and released in the intestinal lumen is substantially increased. This increase can be readily

measured by determining the DNA content of the recovered fluid from perfused intestinal segments, for 80-95% of the cells in this fluid are exfoliated
enterocytes (683). Exfoliation in coeliac sprue is 4-6 times that in normal
subjects (178, 184). This corresponds with a 5-6 times larger cell production
observed in the mucosal crypts (929). These calculations are based on data
obtained in studies of the proximal small intestine. A less markedly increased turnover of intestinal epithelium can be expected in more distal parts of
the small intestine.

Under normal conditions the amount of enterocytes exfoliated in the
lumen is estimated to be 250 g/day (186, 507). These cells are degraded in
the intestinal lumen, and the degradation products are largely reabsorbed.
It is conceivable that the pathological mucosa of the small intestine cannot
adequately reabsorb the much larger supply of degraded exfoliated cells.

This phenomenon has been described as exfoliative enteropathy by Creamer and co-workers, analogous to the concept of exudative enteropathy
(179, 184). Exfoliative enteropathy is defined as the occurrence of deficiencies in nutrients resulting from an increased enteric loss of cell products of
exfoliated enterocytes. These deficiencies are believed to become manifest in
weight loss (184) as well as in faecal loss of iron (897), vitamin B_{12} (523),
protein (188) and lipids (169).

It is not impossible that an insufficient reabsorption of degradation products of the increased amount of exfoliated enterocytes can contribute to
the symptoms in coeliac sprue.

6.10 ENTERIC PLASMA PROTEIN LOSS

6.10.1 Introduction

Leakage of extracellular fluid from the wall of the small intestine into the
lumen is markedly increased in various conditions (431, 879). Increased
protein leakage proved to occur also in some patients with coeliac sprue
(432, 658, 685, 726). In an effort to gain an impression of the incidence and
severity of this phenomenon in coeliac sprue, the enteric protein leakage
was measured in the majority of our patients (cf chapter 12).

6.10.2 Determination of enteric protein loss

The enteric protein leakage was measured in a total of 30 untreated patients
with coeliac sprue, of whom 28 showed an increased leakage (fig. 6.5). An

Enteric plasma protein loss
(ml/24 hrs)

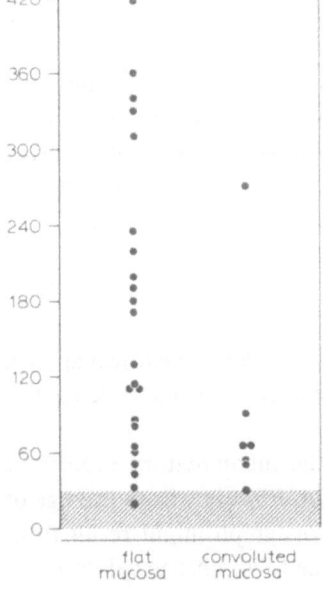

Fig. 6.5. Enteric plasma protein loss in untreated coeliac sprue. The measured amounts of enteric leakage are drawn separately for patients with a flat and with a convoluted mucosa. Statistical analysis (Mann-Whitney test) revealed no significant difference between both groups. The shaded area represents the range of normal values (cf. chapter 12).

Enteric plasma protein loss
(ml/24 hrs)

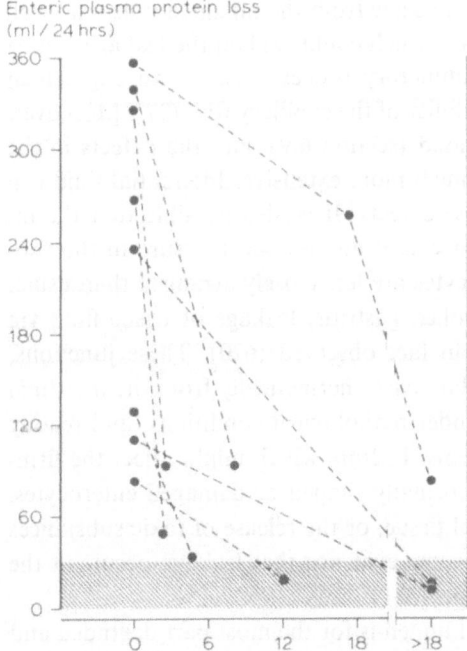

Fig. 6.6. Enteric plasma protein loss and gluten-free diet. The measured amounts of enteric leakage in corresponding patients before as well as during diet therapy are given. The shaded area represents the range of normal values (cf. chapter 12).

101

extremely high protein leakage was observed in a few cases, particularly in patients with a flat jejunal mucosa, although it was also found in the presence of apparently less severe mucosal lesions (i.e. in a biopsy specimen showing convolutions). In only 2 untreated coeliacs was the protein leakage not increased (fig. 6.5). After introduction of a gluten-free diet the majority of cases showed diminished enteric leakage (fig. 6.6). It was found to have normalized in 4 out of 8 patients. In some cases this improvement occurred within a few months (fig. 6.6), but in other patients the leakage was still high after several years on a gluten-free diet (section 9.3).

6.10.3 Comment

The above observations clearly show that an increased protein leakage via the intestinal wall existed in virtually all untreated patients with coeliac sprue.

This increased leakage is probably due to the inflammatory process in the intestinal mucosa. Protein loss can also result, however, from leakage of lymph into the intestinal lumen. This leakage of lymph might result from congestion in the intestinal lymph circulation due to an obstructed drainage (section 6.5).

The exact mechanism of protein leakage from the inflamed intestinal wall is still unknown, but some processes which could explain the leakage can be mentioned. As in any other inflammatory process there is an augmented exudation due to increased permeability of the capillary wall (27). Moreover, exfoliation of enterocytes is increased (section 6.9), and the defects in the epithelial layer are consequently much more extensive. Interstitial fluid can enter the intestinal lumen via these defects. It is also possible that the increased amount of interstitial fluid causes an elevated pressure in the subepithelial tissue so that the enterocytes are less closely arranged than usual. In dogs with experimentally provoked gastritis, leakage of tissue fluid via the so-called tight junctions was in fact observed (620). These junctions, which normally seal the intercellular spaces hermetically from the intestinal lumen, are apparently less tight under pathological conditions, and readily pass large molecules such as proteins. Factors which might affect the firmness of the tight junctions are abnormally shaped or damaged enterocytes, increased pressure in the interstitial tissue, or the release of toxic substances such as histamine (620). There is some evidence that leakage occurs at the villous tips, and is absent in the crypts (331).

Protein leaked into the intestinal lumen is for the most part degraded and reabsorbed, unless it enters the distal part of the ileum. In some coeliacs, however, it is quite possible that a considerable part of protein and protein degradation products gets lost with the faeces or urine. This may be due to the amount of protein or the site at which it is released into the small intestine, and on the other hand to decreased absorptive capacities (section 7.5).

In addition to an increased leakage of protein, coeliac patients also show an extra loss of other substances contained in the interstitial fluid. Although most of these substances are normally reabsorbed, this phenomenon may play some role in the increased faecal loss of electrolytes, iron, vitamin B_{12} or folates (179).

The structure of the intestinal mucosa shows an important degree of normalization after the institution of a gluten-free diet. The interstitial oedema in the wall of the small intestine diminishes and the integrity of the epithelial layer increases. This explains why protein leakage via the intestinal wall diminishes or returns to normal after gluten withdrawal in coeliac sprue (fig. 6.6).

6.11 INTESTINAL FLORA

6.11.1 Introduction

There are sound reasons for the assumption that the bacterial flora of the small intestine is abnormal in coeliac sprue, for there are many factors which interfere with a normal balance of micro-organisms in the small intestine. The mucosa of the small intestine is inflamed and shows lesions, and consequently the local milieu in and near the intestinal wall is changed. Another important factor is the abnormal peristalsis. Finally, due to malabsorption many food constituents are not absorbed, or only at a distal level, from which situation the micro-organisms can benefit. In view of these reasons it seemed useful to submit our patients with coeliac sprue to tests for the presence of an abnormal bacterial flora. These tests consisted of a culture of intestinal fluid, a 'breath' test with ^{14}C-glycocholic acid, and determination of urinary indican excretion (cf chapter 12).

6.11.2 Culture of intestinal fluid

In 9 untreated patients, some fluid was obtained from the jejunum by aspiration and cultured under aerobic as well as strictly anaerobic conditions. The culture results are listed in table 6.3. In 5 of the 9 cases an increased bacterial count was obtained, i.e. more than 10^3 micro-organisms per ml jejunal fluid were cultured.

Table 6.3. Results of some tests used for the demonstration of an abnormal intestinal flora in untreated coeliac patients (cf. chapter 12).

PATIENT	JEJUNAL JUICE CULTURE	^{14}C-GLYCO- CHOLIC ACID DECONJUGATION	INDICAN EXCRETION IN URINE
# 1	10^4	N.D.	142
# 5	10^4	N.D.	191
# 13	10^5	N.D.	142
# 20	5×10^5	N.D.	229
# 26	10^2	7·8	164
# 27	$< 10^2$	3·9	22
# 28	10^3	0·5	144
# 29	no growth	0·7	76
# 30	N.D.	0·4	216
# 32	10^7	0·7	57
CONTROLS	$< 10^3$ m.o./ml	$< 1,5 \times 10^{-5}$ of dose/mmole CO_2	45-120 mg/24 hrs

6.11.3 'Breath' test with ^{14}C-glycocholic acid

The so-called 'breath' test can be used to demonstrate the presence of an abnormal intestinal flora. This is possible as the degree of $^{14}CO_2$ expiration reflects the bacterial deconjugation and degradation of ^{14}C-labelled glycocholic acid in the small or large intestine (295). The test was carried out in 6 untreated patients (table 6.3), of whom 2 showed markedly increased deconjugation of glycocholic acid. There was little correlation, however, between the results of this test and the number of micro-organisms cultured or the indicanuria (table 6.3).

6.11.4 Urinary indican excretion

The urinary indican excretion was determined in 22 untreated patients, of whom 10 showed increased indicanuria. Indican excretion was as a rule normal in patients with less severe mucosal lesions in the proximal jejunum (fig. 6.7). The results obtained proved to show a fair degree of correlation with the number of micro-organisms cultured from the jejunal fluid, but the correlation with the 'breath' test results was less evident (table 6.3).

6.11.5 Effect of the gluten-free diet

In 5 patients jejunal fluid was cultured during treatment by a gluten-free diet, mostly because the clinical and biochemical effects of this treatment

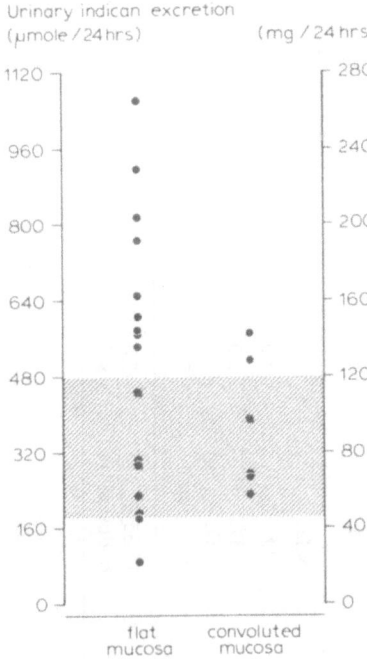

Urinary indican excretion
(μmole /24 hrs)   (mg / 24 hrs)

flat   convoluted
mucosa   mucosa

Fig. 6.7. Urinary indican excretion in untreated coeliac sprue. The amounts excreted in urine are drawn separately for patients with a flat and with a convoluted jejunal mucosa. Statistical analysis (Mann-Whitney test) revealed no significant difference between both groups. The shaded area represents the range of normal values (cf. chapter 12).

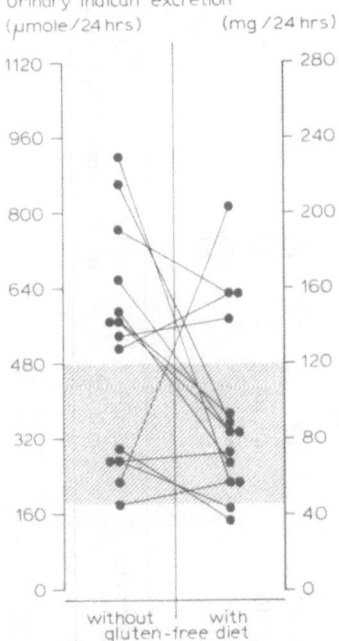

Urinary indican excretion
(μmole /24 hrs)   (mg /24 hrs)

without   with
gluten-free diet

Fig. 6.8. Urinary indican excretion and gluten-free diet. The amounts excreted by corresponding patients before as well as during diet therapy are given. Statistical analysis (Wilcoxon signed-rank test) revealed no significant improvement on diet therapy. The shaded area represents the range of normal values (cf. chapter 12).

Table 6.4. Results of some tests on an abnormal small intestinal flora in diet-treated coeliac patients (cf. chapter 12).

PATIENT	JEUNAL JUICE CULTURE	^{14}C-GLYCO-CHOLIC ACID DECONJUGATION	INDICAN EXCRETION IN URINE	^{57}Co-VIT B$_{12}$ EXCRETION IN URINE	D-XYLOSE EXCRETION IN URINE	ADDITIONAL TREATMENT
# 2	5×10^5	N.D.	160	0.6	1.8	
# 5	10^8	2.3	182	N.D.	3.1	2 g tetracycline during 4 wks
	N.D.	0.35	79	N.D.	3.8	
# 7	N.D.	2.6	130	4.4	N.D.	1 g tetracycline during 4 wks
	N.D.	3.5	N.D.	6.8	5.7	
# 21	N.D.	12.3	203	1.7	1.7	1 g miconazole during 2 wks
	2×10^5	2.95	126	11.2	N.D.	
	N.D.	16.6	N.D.	N.D.	2.2	2 g tetracycline during 12 wks
	N.D.	0.5	45	N.D.	4.8	
# 22	10^3	0.5	56	N.D.	7.5	
# 40	4×10^5	1.85	390	4.8	4.0	
# 45	N.D.	16.6	28	N.D.	2.0	1 g tetracycline during 4 wks
	N.D.	0.9	31	N.D.	4.9	
CONTROLS	$< 10^3$ m.o./ml	$< 1.5 \times 10^{-5}$ of dose/mmole CO$_2$	45-120 mg/24 hrs	15-35% of dose/48 hrs	5.0-9.3 g/5 hrs	

were disappointing. In 4 of the 5 cases culturing yielded more than 10^5 micro-organisms per ml jejunal fluid (table 6.4).

The deconjugation of ^{14}C-labelled glycocholic acid was studied in 6 patients on a gluten-free diet and found to be abnormally high in all but one patient. The indicanuria was also increased in these 6 patients (table 6.4).

In the majority of patients, however, the indicanuria normalized after gluten withdrawal (fig. 6.8).

In 3 coeliacs with persistent symptoms or biochemical changes despite several years on a gluten-free diet, tetracyclin or an oral fungistatic drug (Miconazole) were prescribed in addition to the dietary measures. In some cases the 'breath' test or the indicanuria thereupon showed improvement, as table 6.4 indicates.

6.11.6 Comment

The above observations show that the bacterial flora of the small intestine is abnormal in many patients with coeliac sprue. It was also demonstrated quite clearly that this does not apply only to untreated patients but also to some patients on a gluten-free diet.

It is somewhat difficult to establish the presence of an abnormal bacterial flora in the small intestine. Each of the various procedures commonly used for this purpose has its disadvantages and inaccuracies. For example, fluid from the small intestine is usually aspirated only from the proximal jejunum, and this is not necessarily representative of the situation elsewhere in the small intestine. One always measures the concentration of micro-organisms per ml moreover, but this is not conclusive of the total number of micro-organisms in the intestinal fluid as a whole. The technique of anaerobic culturing is very exacting, and the results are therefore often unreliable and disappointing (237).

With regard to the 'breath' test it is to be borne in mind that deconjugation of bile acids in coeliac sprue does not necessarily indicate an abnormal intestinal flora, but can also be increased for other reasons, such as structural changes in the terminal ileum or an extremely rapid passage through the small intestine. On the other hand, false-negative 'breath' test results are also possible, resulting from a delayed stomach evacuation or the presence of non-deconjugating micro-organisms (295,777).

The urinary indican excretion, finally, can be increased as a result of the fact that unabsorbed protein (and with it tryptophan) enters the colon, e.g. due to malabsorption (280). In some cases an abnormal bacterial flora is not associated with an increased indicanuria because the micro-organisms involved are apparently unable to produce indole from tryptophan (356).

Indole production can also be decreased when the luminal pH is low, due to fermentation processes (628).

It is probably due to these factors that the correlation between the various procedures used to demonstrate the presence of an abnormal intestinal flora is no more than fair (tables 6.3 and 6.4; 356).

Considering the separate procedures, we find that the culture results indicated an increased number of micro-organisms in 5 out of 9 untreated patients. This observation is in agreement with findings reported by Dellipiani (201) and Hamilton et al. (356). Brooks et al. (104), Draser et al. (236), and Neale et al. (628) never found an increased number of micro-organisms in the intestinal fluid in their patients. Modigliani et al. (601), on the other hand, found an abnormally large number of micro-organisms in nearly all untreated coeliacs.

The deconjugation of ^{14}C-labelled glycocholic acid was markedly increased in 2 of our 6 untreated patients. In a comparable number of coeliac patients Fromm et al. (295) invariably obtained a normal 'breath' test, as did Sherr et al. (777).

Indicanuria proved to be increased in about 50% of our patients, which is in agreement with the experiences reported by others (356, 525).

As a result of the presence of an abnormal bacterial flora, several metabolic disorders can develop. The great influence of the intestinal bacteria on human metabolism has been demonstrated in studies of patients with a so-called blind loop syndrome, whose symptoms are chiefly due to an abnormal intestinal flora (319, 328, 356, 630, 832). These metabolic disturbances can be roughly divided into the consumption of food constituents, the disturbance of their digestion and absorption, or the formation of (sometimes toxic) degradation products. The consumption of nutrients can amount to a few grams per hour (319), which may result in deficiencies (442, 629, 932). The increased deconjugation of bile acids can interfere with the micelle formation of lipids (831), so that steatorrhoea becomes manifest (19). The absorption of monosaccharides and D-xylose (318, 326, 471), amino acids (310), and vitamin B_{12} (309) can also be decreased due to the presence of an abnormal intestinal flora. Disturbances in the absorption of the above mentioned nutrients are interpreted by some investigators as a consequence of the consumption or degradation of these substances (201, 318), but they can equally well be the result of structural alterations of the absorptive intestinal cells (319). The deconjugated bile acids have been held responsible for these lesions (19, 328). The increased enteric leakage via the intestinal wall in the presence of an abnormal intestinal flora is perhaps also a result of this epithelial damage (435, 648).

The above considerations indicate that abnormal bacterial growth may lead to pronounced and sometimes multiple deficiencies. The question is to which extent the existing deficiencies in patients with coeliac sprue are due to the often abnormal intestinal flora in these cases. The influence of abnormal bacterial growth on malabsorption of fat, vitamin B_{12} and D-xylose in coeliac sprue has been convincingly demonstrated by the improvement of intestinal absorption after adminstration of antibiotics (table 6.4; 356, 716).

It is not quite clear why the intestinal flora is so often abnormal in coeliac sprue, but the reduced intestinal motility, malabsorption and mucosal lesions are important factors in this respect. Diminution of local immunological defence mechanisms of the small intestine is probably an additional factor. It is remarkable, however, that this abnormal intestinal flora can persist so long even after the institution of a gluten-free diet, and despite the improvement in the morphology and function of the mucosa of the small intestine. Symptoms of malabsorption in treated coeliac patients may be due to a persistent abnormal intestinal flora. It is of importance to bear this in mind because of the fact that these symptoms may be misinterpreted as indicative of the patient's carelessness in observing the prescribed dietary rules.

6.11.7 Conclusions

1. In untreated as well as in treated patients with coeliac sprue, the bacterial flora of the small intestine is often abnormal.
2. The presence of an abnormal intestinal flora is not always readily demonstrable as the procedures used for this purpose have their various disadvantages and inaccuracies.
3. Factors which permit the development of an abnormal bacterial flora in the small intestine are the reduced motility and the presence of unabsorbed food constituents in the intestinal lumen. Additional factors of importance are probably the presence of mucosal lesions and an abnormal local immunological defence.
4. The malabsorption in coeliac sprue can be due in part to the abnormal bacterial growth, either through the degradation and consumption of nutrients or through its damaging influence on the mucosa.
5. In patients with persistent malabsorption in spite of gluten withdrawal, the possibility of an abnormal flora in the small intestine has to be taken into account.

## CHAPTER 7

MALABSORPTION IN COELIAC SPRUE

7.1 INTRODUCTION

The occurrence of malabsorption in coeliac sprue is well-known for a long time. The first observations in patients with a sprue syndrome made already reference to distinct clinical symptoms of malabsorption (305, 385). The fact that this malabsorption can induce deficiencies of various nutrients, has been demonstrated by clinical surveys in the last 10-20 years. In most of these studies malabsorption was only broadly investigated, and but a few publications go into more detail.

It seemed useful therefore to publish the results of a retrospective, clinical investigation in still another group of coeliac patients. On the one hand biochemical examinations in our group of coeliac patients have been fairly extensive, with the result that the incidence of various deficiencies in the same group of patients could be reported. On the other hand insight could sometimes be gained into the mechanisms by which these deficiencies are brought about, based on our own results and data from literature. The composition of the group of patients studied has already been reported (section 6.1). For the methods of investigation the reader is referred to chapter 12.

7.2 WATER AND ELECTROLYTES

Diarrhoea is a frequent symptom in patients with coeliac sprue (table 8.1). In some cases the daily production of faeces exceeds 1000 g, but as a rule the amount of faeces is much smaller (fig. 7.1). This increase in faecal weight might be indicative of a disturbed absorption of water and electrolytes.

By means of perfusion studies, several investigators have indeed de-monstrated that absorption of water and electrolytes in the proximal jejunum is abnormal in coeliacs. As a rule, more sodium, potassium, chloride, bicarbonate and water was recovered after perfusion than had been instilled into the intestinal segment involved (78, 282, 410, 741, 759). In the majority of untreated coeliacs, therefore, there is a net secretion

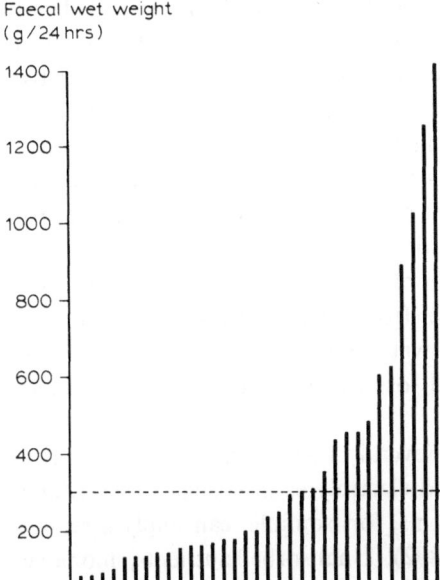

Faecal wet weight
(g/24 hrs)

Fig. 7.1. Diagram of the daily production of faeces in 33 patients with untreated coeliac sprue. The daily faecal weight was calculated from 5 day fat balance studies. The dotted line represents the upper limit of daily faeces production in controls.

of water and electrolytes in the proximal small intestine. By perfusion with labelled water, sodium or potassium, it has been demonstrated that absorption of sodium and potassium in the proximal small intestine is subnormal, whereas absorption of water is probably normal (759). Perhaps the diminished absorption results from a defect in the active transport mechanism, as is indicated by the fact that glucose is no longer able to stimulate the absorption of water and sodium chloride (282, 759). Moreover, the size of the absorptive surface has decreased due to the disappearance of villi and microvilli.

The increased secretion found in coeliac sprue patients has not yet been adequately explained. The increased permeability of the mucosa due to enlargement of the pores in the cell membrane of the enterocytes (282) can scarcely explain the increased secretion. The theory that the secretion is based on loss of extracellular fluid via the intestinal wall, which is increased due to the enhanced capillary permeability resulting from the inflammatory reaction, also seems scarcely plausible (741). A third possibility is primary stimulation of the secretory mechanism of the enterocyte. This can be effected, for example, by an increase in the cyclic AMP concentration in the enterocyte as a result of stimulation of the adenylcyclase in this cell (section

4.7). Such a phenomenon is held responsible also for the water and electrolyte secretion in other disease states, such as cholera (800). All the above mentioned hypothetical secretory mechanisms in coeliac sprue can be triggered by the effect of certain substances on the intestinal mucosa. This role has been ascribed to deconjugated bile acids (741), secretion products from undifferentiated intestinal crypt cells (378) or toxins which originate from incomplete gluten degradation, from an abnormal intestinal flora or from the inflammatory reaction in the intestinal mucosa.

In spite of a considerable secretion of water and electrolytes in the proximal jejunum, only few coeliacs suffer from severe diarrhoea (fig. 7.1). This is due to the fact that absorption of water and electrolytes in the ileum has increased (752), so that a proximal loss can still be compensated in the distal part of the small intestine (792).

It should be mentioned also that several other mechanisms can exert an influence on absorption of water and electrolytes in coeliac sprue. Malabsorption of carbohydrates and proteins, for example, can imply a reduced stimulant for sodium absorption (802). Unabsorbed nutrients, moreover, can retain an amount of water in the lumen by osmotic attraction. The aqueous diarrhoea which can occur in lactose intolerance, is thought to be partly due to this retention. Since lactase deficiency is regularly found in untreated patients with coeliac sprue (section 7.3), the malabsorption of water can perhaps be partly ascribed to osmotic retention. An abnormal bacterial flora in the small intestine can cause a reduction of intestinal transit time due to deconjugation of bile acids and to release of certain other degradation products (section 6.2). Some unabsorbed fatty acids, too, can cause accelerated peristalsis of the colon (20, 21). A decreased intestinal transit time reduces the time available for absorption (section 5.1.2). Several of the above mentioned (bacterial) degradation products cause increased secretion of water and electrolytes by the intestine as well (20, 21, 588, 742).

A remarkable finding in perfusion studies was that, despite a gluten-free diet over a period of 2-10 months, secretion in the proximal small intestine hardly diminished (78, 741, 759). Clinical experience shows, however, that the diarrhoea improves fairly soon after gluten withdrawal. This might indicate that the above described additional factors in coeliac diarrhoea improve more quickly than the primary abnormal secretion or diminished absorption of water and electrolytes.

7.3 CARBOHYDRATE

7.3.1 Introduction

A frequent symptom in patients with coeliac sprue is a distended, meteoristic abdomen, giving rise to complaints about dyspepsia, abdominal pain, borborygmi and flatulence (cf. chapter 8). The underlying increased development of gas in the small and the large intestine mainly results from carbohydrate fermentation. It can therefore be expected that digestion and absorption of carbohydrates are often disturbed in coeliac sprue. The results of pertinent studies are discussed in the following subsections.

7.3.2 Microscopic examination of faeces for starch

Faeces from 9 untreated coeliac patients were, after staining with Lugol solution, microscopically examined for the presence of starch granules. No starch was found in the faeces in 5 patients. In the remaining cases, an occasional small starch granule was found. The results, therefore, were never pathological, although all patients showed a pronounced malabsorption syndrome.

7.3.3. Glucose tolerance test

In 6 of a total of 14 untreated patients, a very slight increment of blood sugar (defined as less than 1.1 mmole/1; 639) was observed after oral administration of 100 g glucose. A low profile glucose curve was found in patients with a flat mucosa as well as in those with less severe mucosal lesions (fig. 7.2).

7.3.4 Lactose tolerance test

A lactose tolerance test was carried out in 16 untreated coeliac patients. In only 2 cases was administration of 50 g lactose followed by a normal increment of blood sugar (i.e. more than 1.2 mmole/1). In patients with a convoluted mucosa in the jejunal biopsy specimen, too, the increment was always reduced (fig. 7.3). Only 5 of the 14 patients with a low profile blood sugar curve developed symptoms as a result of the lactose administration, e.g. meteorism, abdominal cramps or diarrhoea. There was no demonstrable correlation between the development of symptoms and the increment of blood sugar.

Maximum increment blood sugar
(mmole / l)   (mg%)

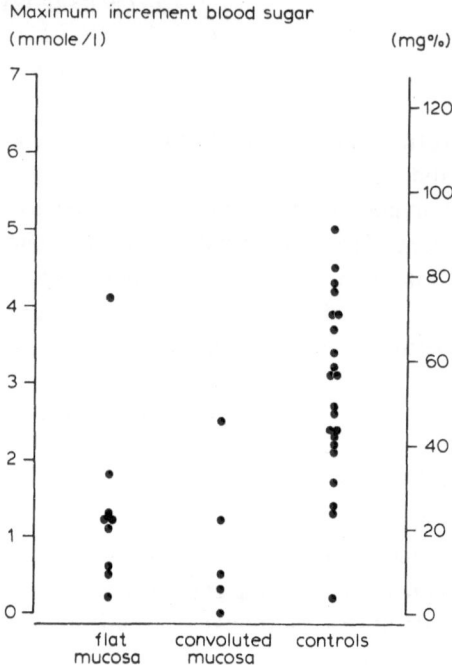

Fig. 7.2. Glucose tolerance test in untreated coeliac sprue. The increments of blood sugar are drawn separately for patients with a flat and with a convoluted jejunal mucosa. The results in 22 controls are presented for comparison. The range of normal values was not defined as a low profile curve may occur in many healthy individuals (cf. chapter 12).

Maximum increment blood sugar
(mmole / l)   (mg%)

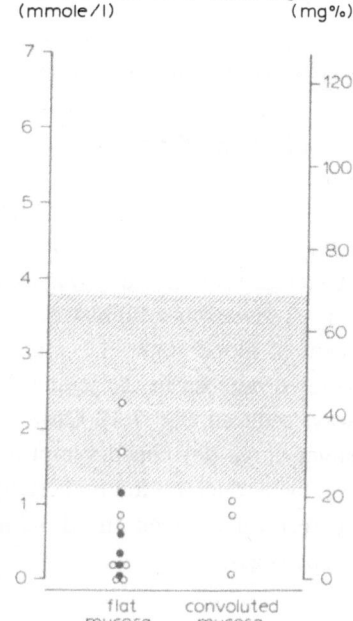

Fig. 7.3. Lactose tolerance test in untreated coeliac sprue. The increments of blood sugar are drawn separately for patients with a flat and with a convoluted jejunal mucosa. Statistical analysis (Mann-Whitney test) revealed no significant difference between both groups. Hollow dots represent patients without symptoms of intolerance, solid dots represent symptomatic cases. The shaded area represents the range of normal values (cf. chapter 12).

114

7.3.5 Lactase activity of the jejunal mucosa

The lactase content of the biopsy specimen of the first jejunal loop was determined in 5 untreated coeliacs, including patients with an abnormal as well as with a normal blood sugar increment after lactose administration. In none of the cases was any lactase activity demonstrable in the biopsy specimen.

7.3.6 Tolerance tests with other disaccharides

In 3 coeliac patients with a low profile blood sugar curve after lactose administration, a tolerance test with 50 g sucrose was carried out also. In 2 of the 3 cases a normal increment of blood sugar (3.2 and 1.5 mmole/1), was found. A tolerance test with 50 g maltose in 2 patients likewise gave normal results (blood sugar increment 1.5 and 1.25 mmole/1, respectively).

7.3.7 D-xylose test

A decreased urinary D-xylose excretion was found after oral administration of 25 g D-xylose in 88% of 33 untreated patients (fig. 7.4). Abnormal fin-

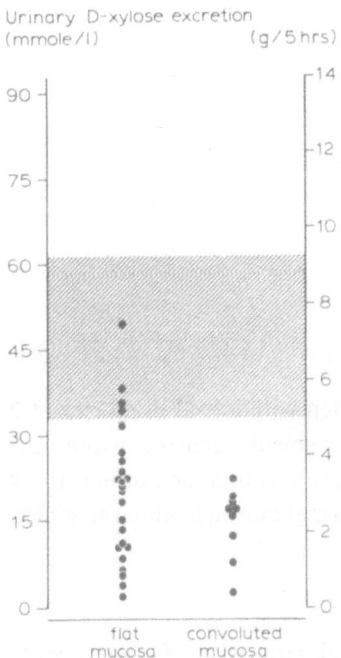

Fig. 7.4. D-xylose test in untreated coeliac sprue. The results of urinary D-xylose excretion are drawn separately for patients with a flat and with a convoluted jejunal mucosa. Statistical analysis (Mann-Whitney test) revealed no significant difference between both groups. The shaded area represents the range of normal values (cf. chapter 12).

115

dings were obtained both in patients with only slight mucosal lesions and in those with an avillous mucosa in the jejunal biopsy specimen. There was no demonstrable correlation between the degree of disturbance of the D-xylose test and the severity of the mucosal damage in the biopsy specimen.

7.3.8 Effect of the gluten-free diet

An improved and normalized increment of blood sugar after lactose administration was observed in 3 out of 8 cases after gluten withdrawal (fig. 7.5). Of the patients with a low profile blood sugar curve, only one showed clinical symptoms of lactose intolerance.

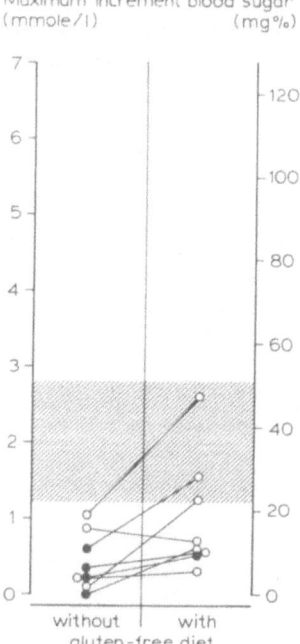

Fig. 7.5. Lactose tolerance test and gluten-free diet. The increments of blood sugar in corresponding patients before as well as during diet therapy are given. Hollow dots represent patients without symptoms of intolerance, solid dots represent symptomatic cases. Statistical analysis (Wilcoxon signed-rank test) revealed a significant improvement on diet therapy ($2\% < p < 5\%$). The shaded area represents the range of normal values (cf. chapter 12).

The D-xylose excretion improved after gluten withdrawal in all except 2 patients (fig. 7.6). In some cases the improvement occurred within 2-7 months, but in others it took longer for the result to become normal. In 18 out of 28 cases, D-xylose excretion became normal during a gluten-free diet.

7.3.9 Comment

On the basis of the results of microscopic examination of the faeces, it could

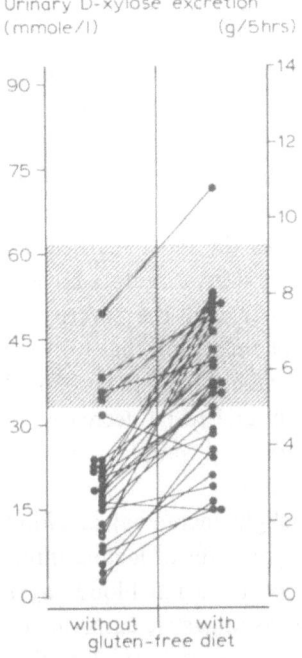

Urinary D-xylose excretion
(mmole/l)   (g/5hrs)

without | with
gluten-free diet

Fig. 7.6. D-xylose test and gluten-free diet. The results of urinary D-xylose excretion in corresponding patients before as well as during diet therapy are given. Statistical analysis (Wilcoxon signed-rank test) revealed a significant improvement on diet therapy ($p < 1\%$). The shaded area represents the range of normal values (cf. chapter 12).

be stated that digestion and absorption of starch are usually normal in coeliac patients. However, the value of microscopic examination of faeces for starch is controversial (116). Our personal experience with microscopic examination of faeces to determine digestion has been negative so far as starch is concerned. In patients with severe malabsorption we usually found no starch in the faeces; but starch was found in patients with accelerated intestinal passage (e.g. due to abuse of laxatives) (145).

Theoretically, digestion and absorption of carbohydrates can be disturbed at several different levels. In patients with coeliac sprue, deficiency of the enzyme α-amylase due to decreased secretion of this enzyme by the pancreas seems unlikely in view of the enormous functional reserve of this organ under normal conditions.

Disturbances based on abnormalities of the intestinal mucosa are more likely. For the so-called epithelial phase of carbohydrate digestion, the presence of a normal brush border is required in which, beside various disaccharidases, the transport carriers are also contained. In coeliac sprue the first morphological changes of the epithelial layer occur in the brush border. Moreover, the damage to the brush border is usually severe and fairly extensive (655, 782, 859). A decrease in the concentration of disaccharidases is bound to result.

117

Although virtually all disaccharidases are decreased in amount as a result of the above mentioned factors (553, 668), this is manifested almost exclusively in the form of lactose intolerance. This is due to the fact that, unlike the other disaccharidases, lactase activity in the intestinal mucosa is not abundant, but rather marginal under normal conditions. In coeliac patients, lactase activity can become deficient even with a relatively small decrease in the amount of lactase resulting from mucosal damage.

Lactase activity shows usually the first as well as the most marked decrease when the intestinal mucosa is damaged. Several investigators have in fact observed a correlation between lactase activity and the severity of mucosal damage (668, 686, 907). It is therefore not surprising that we were unable to demonstrate lactase activity in biopsy specimens from the proximal jejunum of untreated coeliacs. Lactase activity is bound to be decreased in every morphologically abnormal jejunal specimen, and should – in our opinion – not be quantified unless for scientific purposes.

The large majority of patients showed only a slight increment of blood sugar on lactose ingestion, but only a few showed symptoms of lactose intolerance (fig. 7.3). If no symptoms of intolerance occur, a flat blood sugar curve after lactose administration can be due to delayed gastric emptying or rapid insulin secretion. If the patient does show symptoms, on the other hand, it should be realized that lactose intolerance can also be a primary phenomenon. This may explain, for example, the lactose intolerance in

Table 7.1. Incidence of a low profile (flat) glucose tolerance curve in untreated coeliac sprue.

AUTHORS	CRITERION	NUMBER OF PATIENTS INVESTIGATED	PERCENTAGE WITH LOW PROFILE CURVE
Cooke et al. (1963)	gluc. concentration < 100 mg%	31	0
Shiner (1963)	gluc. increment < 40 mg%	7	100
Stewart et al. (1967)	gluc. increment < 40 mg%	58	84
Mann et al. (1970)	not stated	13	38
Thys et al. (1971)	gluc. concentration < 130 mg%	6	100
	< 110 mg%	6	67
Modigliani et al. (1975)	gluc. increment < 30 mg%	32	63

treated coeliacs who no longer show any other evidence of malabsorption (fig. 7.5).

In the proximal part of the small intestine absorption of monosaccharides is usually decreased in coeliac sprue. In perfusion studies virtually all untreated coeliac sprue patients are found to have a diminished absorption of glucose as well as of fructose in the proximal jejunum (62, 78, 244, 410, 752). The diminished absorption can be explained, not only by a decreased absorptive surface but also by a disturbed transport of monosaccharides through the intestinal wall. Glucose absorption does improve after gluten withdrawal, sometimes after a considerable time. In some cases glucose absorption is still abnormal while D-xylose excretion has already returned to normal (78, 410). The abnormalities of absorption found in the proximal part of the small intestine do not by any means preclude the possibility of normal glucose and fructose absorption in the distal part of the small in-

Table 7.2. Incidence of a decreased urinary D-xylose excretion in untreated coeliac sprue.

AUTHORS	CRITERION	NUMBER OF PATIENTS INVESTIGATED	PERCENTAGE WITH DECREASAD EXCRETION
Sleisenger (1961)	< 5 g/5 hrs	9	100
Cooke et al. (1963)	< 4.2 g/5 hrs	24	83
Shiner (1963)	< 5 g/5 hrs	11	100
Benson et al. (1964)	< 5 g/5 hrs	12	100
Brooks et al. (1966)	< 5 g/5 hrs	10	100
Fahrlaender et al. (1966)	not stated	14	71
Stewart et al. (1967)	< 5 g/5 hrs	57	97
Mortimer et al. (1968)	< 5 g/5 hrs	5	80
Jarnum et al. (1970)	< 5 g/24 hrs	10	90
Mann et al. (1970)	< 4.5 g/5 hrs	21	95
Thys et al. (1971)	< 3.75 g/5 hrs	8	88
Modigliani et al. (1975)	< 4 g/5 hrs	28	96
Own series	< 5 g/5 hrs	33	88

testine. All in all, therefore, there need not necessarily be carbohydrate malabsorption. The flat blood sugar curve often observed after oral glucose administration (table 7.1; fig. 7.2) does suggest that glucose absorption as a whole is decreased in untreated coeliac sprue. However, it is ill-advised to diagnose glucose malabsorption on the basis of a flat blood sugar curve or to screen for malabsorption by means of a glucose tolerance test, as is obviously frequently done (table 7.1). A low profile blood sugar curve, it should be borne in mind, may be observed in many normal individuals; according to Nolan et al. (639) even in 1 out of 4 people. In such cases the small increment of blood sugar is explained by delayed evacuation of gastric contents or abnormally rapid insulin secretion.

Although the pentose D-xylose is essentially a carbohydrate, it seems very questionable whether its absorption is a good parameter of carbohydrate absorption from food, which contains mainly hexoses. D-xylose, moreover, is an unphysiological substance, which under normal conditions is not present in food or in the human organism. In patients with untreated coeliac sprue, the absorption of this pentose is very often found to be disturbed. Our personal experience in this respect (fig. 7.4) conforms with that reported by others (table 7.2). The adequate discriminating function of the D-xylose test in coeliac sprue is probably based on the fact that this pentose is mainly absorbed in the jejunum (18). After gluten withdrawal, therefore, D-xylose absorption nearly always increases (fig. 7.6; table 7.3). The only disadvantage of this otherwise excellent test is that false low results can be ob-

Table 7.3. Incidence of a decreased urinary D-xylose excretion in treated coeliac sprue.

AUTHORS	CRITERION	NUMBER OF PATIENTS INVESTIGATED	PERCENTAGE WITH DECREASED EXCRETION
Cooke et al. (1963)	<4.2 g/5 hrs	8	38
Shiner (1963)	< 5 g/5 hrs	15	0
Benson et al. (1964)	< 5 g/5 hrs	22	41
Cerf et al. (1975)	< 5 g/5 hrs	7	86
Modigliani et al. (1975)	< 4 g/5 hrs	26	42
Own series	< 5 g/5 hrs	27	37

tained. This may be a result of delayed evacuation of gastric contents and decreased renal function, or – which is of particular importance in coeliac sprue – due to the presence of an abnormal bacterial flora (section 6.11) or greatly accelerated intestinal passage (801).

7.3.10 Conclusions

1. The clinical symptoms in coeliac sprue suggest that digestion and absorption of carbohydrates are often disturbed.
2. Microscopic examination of faeces for starch granules seems to be of no value in demonstrating disturbances in carbohydrate digestion.
3. Reduced hydrolysis of lactose is demonstrable in most coeliac sprue patients, in whom other disaccharides may be properly degraded.
4. If a patient continues to complain of dyspepsia or diarrhoea in spite of a gluten-free diet, the possibility of associated primary lactose intolerance should be considered.
5. Determination of the lactase content of the jejunal mucosa is useless in untreated coeliac sprue.
6. A flat blood sugar curve after oral glucose administration must not be used as an aid in diagnosing malabsorption.
7. D-xylose excretion is a good parameter for demonstration of malabsorption in the proximal part of the small intestine. This test is also very useful in studying the effect of a gluten-free diet in coeliac sprue.

7.4 FAT

7.4.1 Introduction

Steatorrhoea was among the first abnormalities described in patients with coeliac sprue (305). The term idiopathic steatorrhoea commonly used before gluten intolerance was discovered, also indicates the importance attached to this symptom. It was once even maintained that a decreased fat absorption was imperative to make the diagnosis (159, 289), but subsequent studies showed that not all coeliacs have steatorrhoea (table 7.4). We considered it worthwhile to study the incidence of steatorrhoea in our group of untreated coeliacs. In addition we studied the question whether there were also abnormalities in the absorption of fat-soluble vitamins or of cholesterol, on

Table 7.4. Incidence of steatorrhoea in untreated coeliac sprue.

AUTHORS	CRITERION			NUMBER OF PATIENTS INVESTIGATED	PERCENTAGE WITH STEA-TORRHOEA
Buchan et al. (1962)	>	7	g/24 hrs	36	92
Cooke et al. (1963)	>	5	g/24 hrs	49	98
Shiner (1963)	>	5	g/24 hrs	17	100
Benson et al. (1964)	>	5	g/24 hrs	7	100
Brooks et al. (1966)	>	6	g/24 hrs	10	20
Fahrlaender et al. (1966)			not stated	10	90
Stewart et al. (1967)	>	6	g/24 hrs	58	81
Gent et al. (1968)	>	7	g/24 hrs	56	75
Jarnum et al. (1970)	>	21	meq/24 hrs	10	100
Mann et al. (1970)	>	5	g/24 hrs	20	65
Thys et al. (1971)	>	8	g/24 hrs	6	83
Krondl et al. (1971)	>	2	g/24 hrs	9	100
Modigliani et al. (1975)	>	6	g/24 hrs	46	70
Own series	<	95%	absorption	32	88

the basis of the serum concentrations of these substances. Finally, we evaluated the effect of the gluten-free diet on fat absorption and on the serum concentrations of fat-soluble vitamins and cholesterol.

7.4.2 Fat absorption coefficient

The fat absorption coefficient, determined during a 5-day balance study, was found to be decreased in 91% of the 32 untreated patients with coeliac sprue. Fat absorption was disturbed in patients with severe as well as in those with less severe villous abnormalities in the proximal part of the small intestine. However, the steatorrhoea was significantly worse in the presence of a flat mucosa (fig. 7.7).

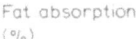

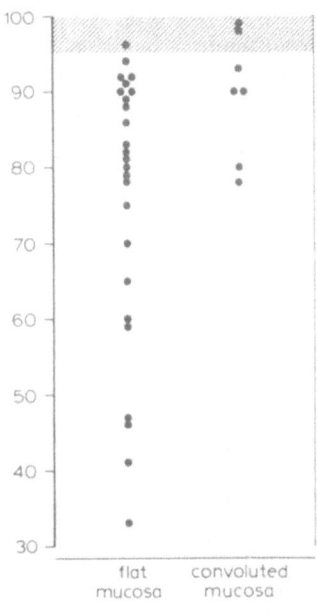

Fig. 7.7. Fat absorption in untreated coeliac sprue. The absorption coefficients are drawn separately for patients with a flat and with a convoluted mucosa. Statistical analysis (Mann-Whitney test) revealed a significant difference between both groups (p = 1%). The shaded area represents the range of normal values (cf. chapter 12).

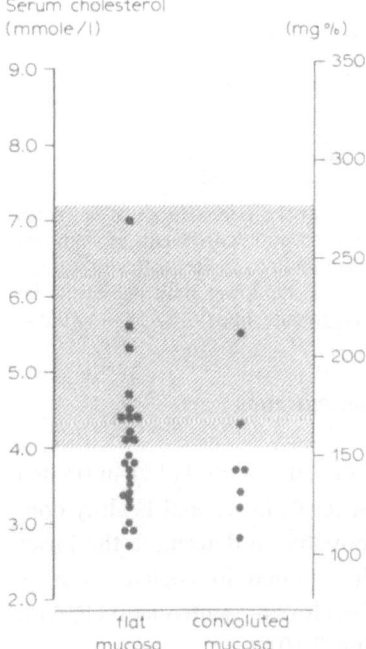

Fig. 7.8. Serum cholesterol in untreated coeliac sprue. The serum levels are drawn separately for patients with a flat and with a convoluted jejunal mucosa. Statistical analysis (Mann-Whitney test) revealed no significant difference between both groups. The shaded area represents the range of normal values (cf. chapter 12).

123

7.4.3 Serum cholesterol concentration

A decreased serum cholesterol concentration was found in 59% of the 32 untreated coeliacs. The severity of the villous abnormalities in the biopsy specimen did not seem to be a determinant of the frequency or the extent of the decreases in serum cholesterol (fig. 7.8). A rather poor correlation was found between the degree of hypocholesterolaemia and the degree of fat malabsorption (fig. 7.9).

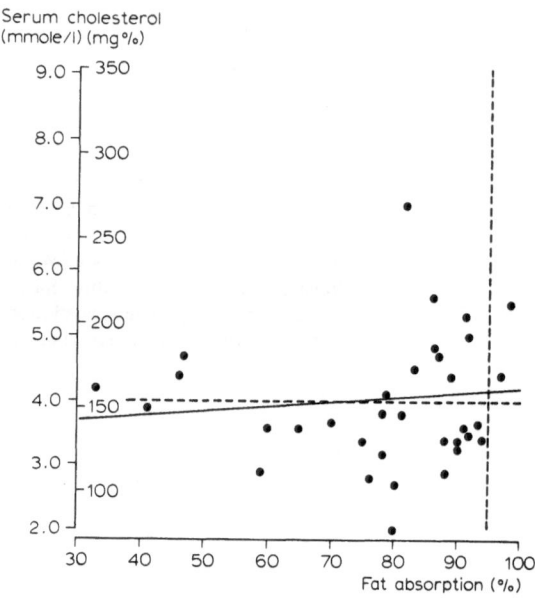

Fig. 7.9. Serum cholesterol and fat absorption. The serum cholesterol levels of untreated coeliac patients are plotted against the corresponding absorption coefficients of simultaneously conducted fat balance studies. The dotted horizontal line represents the lower limit of normal serum cholesterol, and the dotted vertical line the lower limit of normal fat absorption. The straight diagonal line is the calculated regression line ($y = 3.58 + 0.005x$; $r = 0.08$; $p > 10\%$).

7.4.4 Serum vitamin A concentration

The serum vitamin A concentration was determined in a total of 28 untreated coeliacs. Since the range of serum vitamin A levels in normal healthy controls was found to be very wide, it was impossible to determine the lower limit of normal. Interpretation of the values found in coeliac sprue is therefore difficult. The results obtained are therefore presented as such, with the values found in controls for comparison (fig. 7.10).

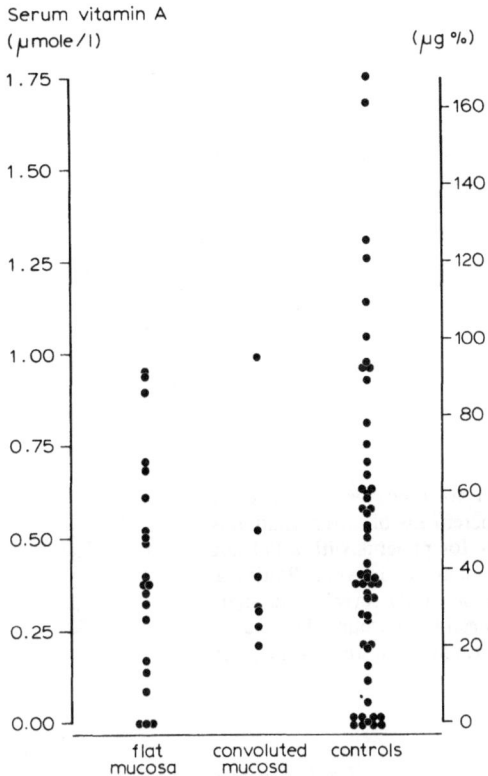

Fig. 7.10. Serum Vitamin A in untreated coeliac sprue. The serum levels are drawn separately for patients with a flat and with a convoluted jejunal mucosa. The results in 54 controls are presented for comparison.

7.4.5 Vitamin A tolerance test

A vitamin A tolerance test was carried out in a total of 26 untreated patients. This test also proved to show a wide range of normal values (fig. 7.11). Unlike the serum vitamin A concentration, the vitamin A tolerance test was found to show a fair correlation with the fat absorption coefficient (fig. 7.12).

7.4.6 Serum vitamin E concentration

The serum vitamin E concentration was decreased in 95% of 19 patients. The decrease was as marked in patients with a flat or with a convoluted mucosa (fig. 7.13). No correlation was observed between the height of the serum vitamin E level and the quality of fat absorption (fig. 7.14).

125

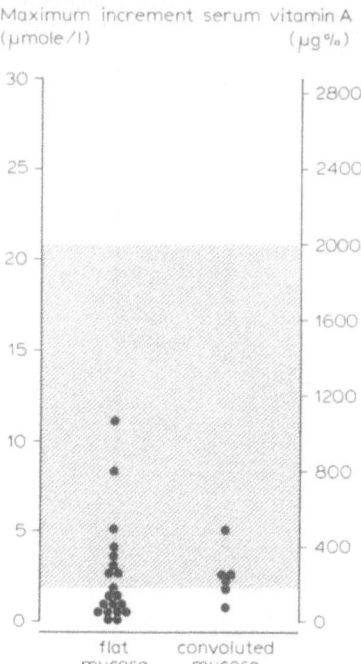

Maximum increment serum vitamin A
(μmole/l)   (μg%)

Fig. 7.11. Vitamin A tolerance test in untreated coeliac sprue. The increments of serum vitamin A are drawn separately for patients with a flat and with a convoluted jejunal mucosa. Statistical analysis (Mann-Whitney test) revealed no significant difference between both groups. The shaded area represents the range of normal values (cf. chapter 12).

7.4.7 Thrombotest

The thrombotest, with which deficiencies in vitamin K-dependent coagulation factors can be demonstrated, was decreased in 6 of the total of 20 patients. These 6 patients all showed a flat jejunal mucosa. In patients with less marked abnormalities in the jejunal biopsy specimen, the thrombotest was always normal (fig. 7.15). There was a fair correlation between the thrombotest value and the degree of steatorrhoea (fig. 7.16).

7.4.8 Effect of the gluten-free diet

Most coeliac sprue patients show improved fat absorption after gluten withdrawal. In 8 out of 9 patients with a decreased fat absorption coefficient before treatment, faecal fat excretion was less after gluten withdrawal. In 5 of these 8 coeliacs the fat absorption returned to normal (fig. 7.17).

The hypocholesterolaemia disappeared in all but one patient on the gluten-free diet. In some cases the serum cholesterol level rose within a few weeks

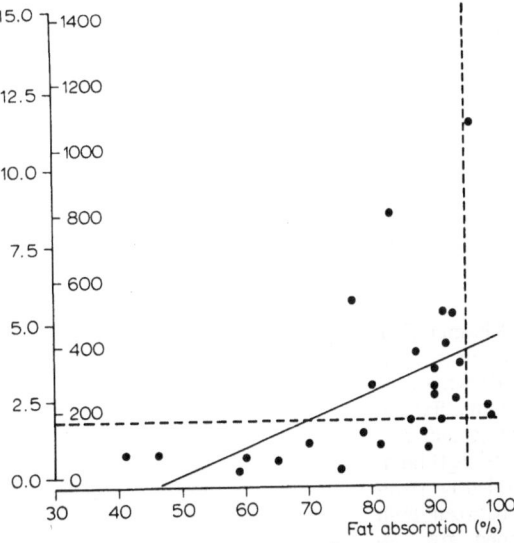

Fig. 7.12. Vitamin A tolerance test and fat absorption. The vitamin A increments of un-treated coeliac patients are plotted against the corresponding absorption coefficients of simultaneously conducted fat balance studies. The dotted horizontal line represents the lower limit of normal vitamin A increment, and the dotted vertical line the lower limit of normal fat absorption. The straight diagonal line is the calculated regression line ($y = -3.44 + 7.43x$; $r = 0.47$; $0.5\% < p < 1\%$).

(fig. 7.18). A remarkable phenomenon was that a slight decrease in serum cholesterol often followed on a substantial initial increase. This finding might indicate that the gluten-free regimen was less strictly observed after a while. Another possibility is that cholesterol synthesis, after initial maximal stimulation, gradually diminishes again after a while.

The serum vitamin A concentration showed no significant change after gluten withdrawal. It was sometimes still very low after many years.

Some effect of the diet on the vitamin A tolerance test was discernible. After gluten withdrawal the maximal increment of serum vitamin A was slightly higher in 5 out of 8 cases (fig. 7.19).

The vitamin E concentration, however, increased in response to the diet in all patients except one, although a normal vitamin E level was reached in only 3 cases (fig. 7.20).

The thrombotest (if decreased) also returned to normal on the gluten-free diet, often within a few weeks (fig. 7.21).

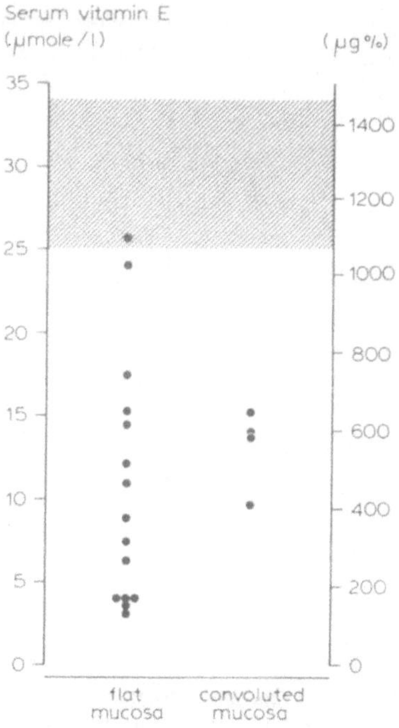

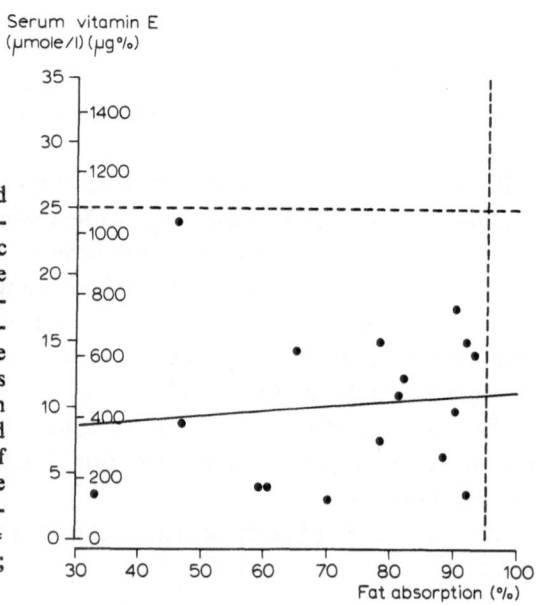

Fig. 7.13. Serum Vitamin E in untreated coeliac sprue. The serum levels are drawn separately for patients with a flat and with a convoluted jejunal mucosa. Statistical analysis (Mann-Whitney test) revealed no significant difference between both groups. The shaded area represents the range of normal values (cf. chapter 12).

Fig. 7.14. Serum vitamin E and fat absorption. The serum vitamin E levels of untreated coeliac patients are plotted against the corresponding absorption coefficients of simultaneously conducted fat balance studies. The dotted horizontal line represents the lower limit of normal serum vitamin E, and the dotted vertical line the lower limit of normal fat absorption. The straight diagonal line is the calculated regression line (y = 7.60 + 0.036 x ; r = 0.11; p > 10%).

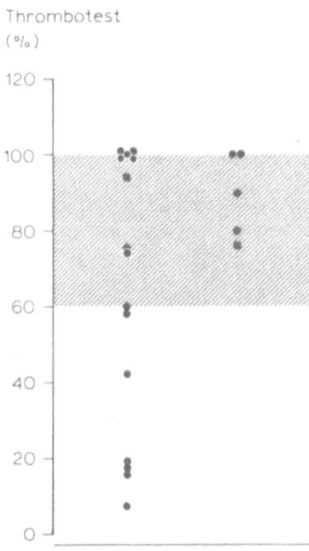

Fig. 7.15. Thrombotest in untreated coeliac sprue. The results are drawn separately for patients with a flat and with a convoluted jejunal mucosa. Statistical analysis (Mann-Whitney test) revealed no significant difference between both groups. The shaded area represents the range of normal values (cf. chapter 12).

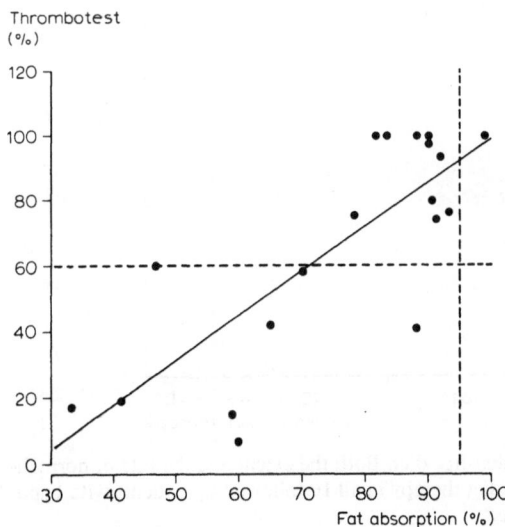

Fig. 7.16. Thrombotest and fat absorption. The results of the thrombotest of untreated coeliac patients are plotted against the corresponding absorption coefficients of simultanteously conducted fat balance studies. The dotted horizontal line represents the lower limit of normal thrombotest results, and the dotted vertical line the lower limit of normal fat absorption. The straight diagonal line is the calculated regression line ($y = -36 + 1.35x$; $r = 0.79$; $p < 0.0005$).

129

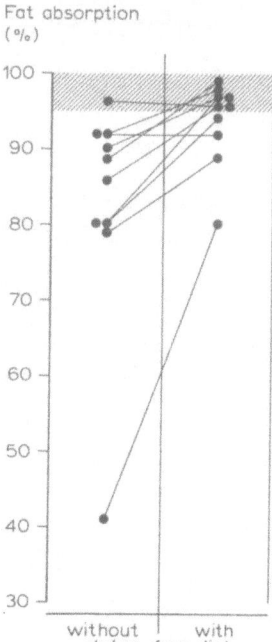

Fat absorption
(%)

Fig. 7.17. Fat absorption and gluten-free diet. The absorption coefficients in corresponding patients before as well as during diet therapy are given. Statistical analysis (Wilcoxon signed-rank test) showed a significant improvement on diet therapy ($p \leqslant 1\%$). The shaded area represents the range of normal values (cf. chapter 12).

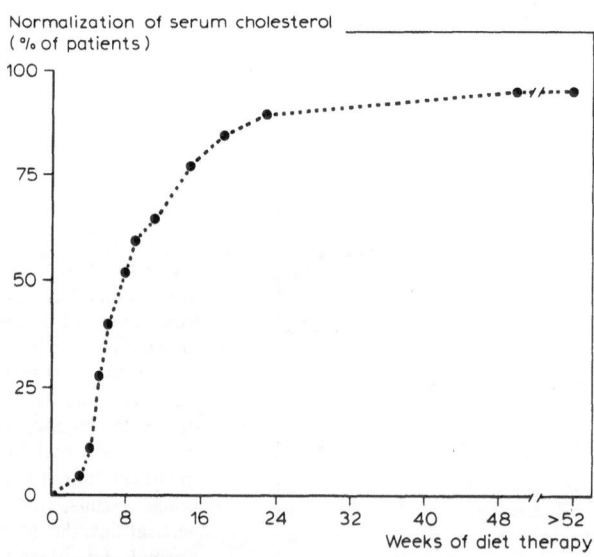

Fig. 7.18. Serum cholesterol and gluten-free diet. Both the extent and the rate of normalization of serum cholesterol levels on diet therapy in all 16 followed-up patients with hypocholesterolaemia (fig. 7.8) are recorded.

130

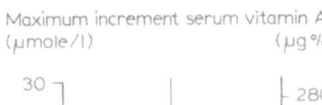

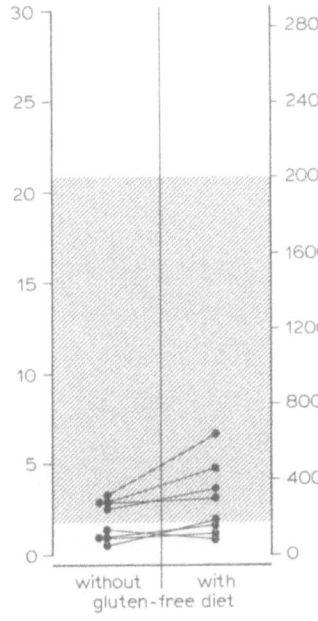

Fig. 7.19. Vitamin A tolerance test and gluten-free diet. The increments of serum vitamin A in corresponding patients before as well as during diet therapy are given. Statistical analysis (Wilcoxon signed-rank test) showed a significant improvement on diet therapy ($2\% \leqslant p \leqslant 5\%$). The shaded area represents the range of normal values (cf. chapter 12).

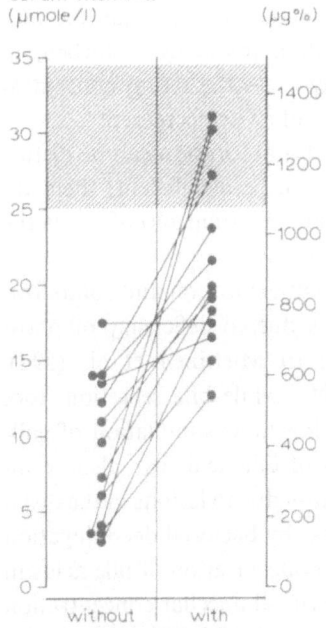

Fig. 7.20. Vitamin E and gluten-free diet. The serum levels in corresponding patients before as well as during diet therapy are given. Statistical analysis (Wilcoxon signed-rank test) showed a significant improvement on diet therapy ($p < 1\%$). The shaded area represents the range of normal values (cf. chapter 12).

131

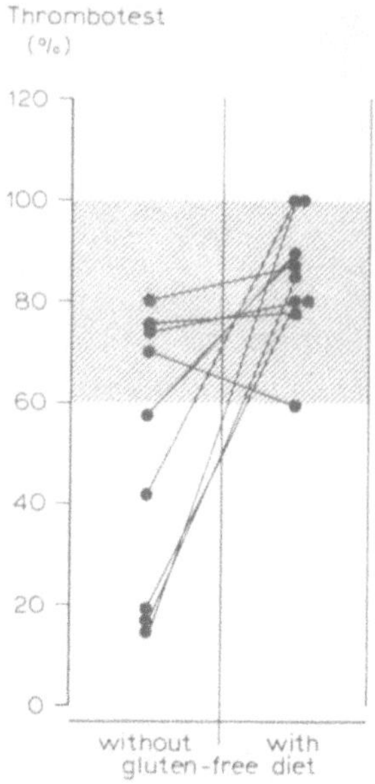

Fig. 7.21. Thrombotest and gluten-free diet. The results in corresponding patients before as well as during diet therapy are given. Statistical analysis (Wilcoxon signed-rank test) showed a significant improvement on diet therapy ($2\% < p < 5\%$). The shaded area represents the range of normal values (cf. chapter 12).

7.4.9 Comment

The results described above show clearly that uptake of fat and fat-like substances is usually disturbed, and relatively often markedly disturbed, in untreated patients with coeliac sprue. In many cases the serum concentrations of cholesterol and fat-soluble vitamins are likewise decreased.

The normal chain of events in fat digestion and absorption can be disturbed at many levels. The solubilization of fats can be insufficient; their absorption by the enterocytes can be diminished; and the transport of fat via the lymphatics can be decreased.

It is not inconceivable that such processes as emulsification and solubilization are less than optimal in coeliac patients due to deficiency of phospholipids, bile acids and lipases. According to Miettinen et al. (594), coeliacs produce less bile than normal subjects, while bile secretion, too, can be diminished as a result of decreased endogenous stimulation of gallbladder contraction (214). Moreover, the loss of bile acids can also be increased as a result of their diminished reabsorption due to lesions in the distal ileum (594), or because they are rendered useless by bacterial deconjugation (718). Due to the above mentioned factors the concentration of bile acids in the intestinal lumen can decrease to below the critical micellar concentration (578). DiMagno et al. (214) did in fact find a correlation between the micellar concentration in the intestinal fluid and the severity of steatorrhoea in coeliac patients.

According to some authors, the exocrine function of the pancreas is decreased in patients with coeliac sprue (section 6.6.3). As a rule, however, the pancreas secretes enzymes in such large amounts that a deficiency of lipases in the intestinal lumen will only occur if the pancreatic function is reduced to 10% of its original capacity (91). In coeliac patients, improvement of fat absorption was observed after administration of additional pancreatic enzymes by Cooke (163), which is in fact indicative of disturbed lipolysis. In one of our untreated coeliac patients, however, we observed no effect of high doses of pancreatic enzymes on the amount of faecal fat. Others, too, have reported negative experiences in this respect (180, 682).

Disturbance of fat absorption due to damage of the epithelium of the small intestine seems to be more important in coeliac sprue. This is also indicated by the fact that absorption of fatty acids, which require no solubilization and hydrolysis, is as markedly disturbed as absorption of triglycerides (119). The epithelial damage can involve, beside reduction of the absorptive surface, abnormal functioning of the remaining enterocytes (102). This may result in a disturbed re-esterification of absorbed monoglycerides, enabling the intracellular fatty acids to diffuse back into the intestinal lumen (880). Chylomicron formation can also be disturbed, on the one hand as a result of the already mentioned reduced re-esterification to triglycerides, and on the other hand as a result of disturbed synthesis of apolipoproteins. Such a form of secondary hypo-β-lipoproteinaemia has been described, for example, in congenital intestinal lymphangiectasia (220).

The uptake of chylomicrons in the initial lacteals may be impeded in coeliac patients, as these lymphatics are often deformed. Normal lymph drainage can be impossible due to congestion in the lymphatics (section 6.5).

It is finally to be noted that, apart from malabsorption, increased faecal loss of endogenous fat can be partly responsible for deficiency of fat and fat-like substances. These endogenous lipids originate partly from bile and from the enteric plasma loss, but most of them enter the intestinal lumen via the increased exfoliation of enterocytes (169).

Disturbances in fat absorption are likely to entail malabsorption of cholesterol and fat-soluble vitamins. In coeliac patients, the absorption of vitamin A (449), vitamin D (841), vitamin E (542) and vitamin K (774) is indeed often decreased. Consequently one might expect the serum concentrations of these vitamins to be decreased in coeliac sprue. The serum vitamin concentrations in our untreated coeliacs, however, were more often normal than could be expected on the basis of the fat absorption coefficient (figs. 7.12 and 7.16). Most other investigators, listed by Kasper et al. (461), also had unsatisfactory experiences with vitamin A as parameter of fat absorption. The serum carotene concentration is reportedly a more reliable parameter, perhaps because the human organism has no significant reserves of carotene, at it has of vitamin A (525). But on the use of carotene determination, too, opinions differ (461). The same applies to views on the value of vitamin A and carotene tolerance tests (449, 462). Our own experience with the vitamin A tolerance test was not so disappointing. In many patients the increment of vitamin A concentration was less marked then in controls (fig. 7.11), while a fair degree of correlation with the degree of fat malabsorption was also found (fig. 7.12).

The correlation between serum vitamin E concentration and fat absorption was not evident (fig. 7.14). Several other investigators reported more favourably on this correlation (469, 542). The consequences of a decreased vitamin E concentration are still questionable, moreover. In some cases vitamin E deficiency can manifest itself in ceroid accumulation in the smooth muscle cells of the intestinal wall. Because the brown colour of ceroid may be faintly visible through the serosa, this situation has been named 'brown bowel syndrome' (69, 847). Perhaps this ceroid acccumulation is related also to disturbances in the motility of the small intestine in coeliac sprue (section 6.2). A peroral biopsy of the intestinal mucosa does not seem appropriate for demonstration of ceroid. In none of our patients was ceroid demonstrable in the muscularis mucosae (not even with the aid of fluorescence), although the muscular layer of the intestine was sometimes packed with ceroid granules (fig. 6.4). A deep rectal biopsy may give more information in this respect (69).

Table 7.5. Incidence of a prolonged prothrombin time in untreated coeliac sprue.

AUTHORS	CRITERION	NUMBER OF PATIENTS INVESTIGATED	PERCENTAGE WITH PROLONGED P.T.T.
Benson et al. (1964)	> 2 secs. above control	30	47
Jarnum et al. (1970)	< 85%	10	80
Mann et al. (1970)	< 50%	14	28
Thys et al. (1971)	< 60%	8	25

The amount of circulating vitamin K can be measured only indirectly, by means of coagulation tests such as prothrombin time (PTT) and thrombotest. Neither the thrombotest (fig. 7.15) nor the prothrombin time (table 7.5) are often 'spontaneously' abnormal. This is not very surprising, for vitamin K absorption has to be markedly decreased before this becomes manifest in a prolonged PTT (773).

After gluten withdrawal usually a marked improvement or even normalization of fat absorption is seen (fig. 7.17; table 7.6). This improvement

Table 7.6. Incidence of steatorrhoea in treated coeliac sprue.

AUTHORS	CRITERION	NUMBER OF PATIENTS INVESTIGATED	PERCENTAGE WITH STEA- TORRHOEA
Buchan et al. (1962)	> 7 g/24 hrs	19	16
Cooke et al. (1963)	> 5 g/24 hrs	10	50
Shiner (1963)	> 5 g/24 hrs	17	53
Benson et al. (1964)	> 5 g/24 hrs	11	36
Bolt et al. (1964)	> 7 g/24 hrs	12	42
Brooks et al. (1966)	> 6 g/24 hrs	7	0
Cerf et al. (1975)	> 5 g/24 hrs	17	71
Modigliani et al. (1975)	> 6 g/24 hrs	28	43
Own series	< 95% absorption	10	40

was also apparent in the serum concentrations of cholesterol (fig. 7.18) and the fat-soluble vitamin E and K (fig. 7.20, fig. 7.21). The vitamin A absorption test showed only sometimes a small improvement (fig. 7.19). This indicates that the absorption of vitamin A probably differs from that of triglycerides or cholesterol and is influenced by other factors still to be identified.

7.4.10 Conclusions

1. The fat absorption coefficient was abnormal in the large majority of untreated coeliac patients. The extent of steatorrhoea seemed to depend on the severity of the mucosal lesions.
2. The serum concentration of fat-soluble vitamin A proved to be a poor

parameter of fat absorption. In this respect the serum vitamin E concentration was superior.

3. The serum cholesterol concentration – although a poor parameter of fat absorption – was found to be decreased in 59% of the untreated patients.
4. The serum vitamin E and cholesterol concentrations were found to be suitable parameters in evaluating the effect of the gluten-free diet.
5. Possible explanations of the fat malabsorption in coeliac sprue are to be found in particular in reduction of the mucosal surface area and in abnormal functioning of the remaining enterocytes.
6. Additional factors may be relative pancreatic insufficiency, deficiency of conjugated bile acids and impaired lymph transport.
7. Apart from malabsorption of exogenous fat, an increased loss of endogenous fat can contribute to the severity of steatorrhoea.

7.5 PROTEIN

7.5.1 Introduction

Many affections of the digestive tract are associated with a decreased serum albumin concentration. Hypoalbuminaemia is a common finding in coeliac sprue (table 7.7). Some coeliac patients in fact seek medical advice because

Table 7.7. Incidence of hypoalbuminaemia in untreated coeliac sprue.

AUTHORS	CRITERION	NUMBER OF PATIENTS INVESTIGATED	PERCENTAGE WITH HYPO- ALBUMINAEMIA
Buchan et al. (1962)	< 35 g/l	37	59
Cooke et al. (1963)	< 41 g/l	47	57
Benson et al. (1964)	< 38 g/l	30	73
Ross et al. (1966a)	< 35 g/l	42	55
Jarnum et al. (1970)	< 37.7 g/l	10	70
Mann et al. (1970)	< 38 g/l	19	84
Thys et al. (1971)	< 30 g/l	8	63
Modigliani et al. (1975)	< 30 g/l	46	39
Own series	< 45.8 g/l	36	86

of hypoproteinaemic oedema. For these reasons we considered it useful to study the incidence of hypoalbuminaemia in our series of coeliac patients, and to establish which mechanisms can be held responsible for this decrease in serum albumin concentration.

7.5.2 Serum albumin concentration

We determined the serum albumin concentration in each of our 36 untreated patients with coeliac sprue. Hypoalbuminaemia was found in 86% (fig. 7.22). In patients with less severe lesions in the jejunal biopsy specimen, the incidence of hypoalbuminaemia was as high as in those with a flat mucosa. Peripheral oedema was observed in all patients with a serum albumin concentration of less than 30 g/l.

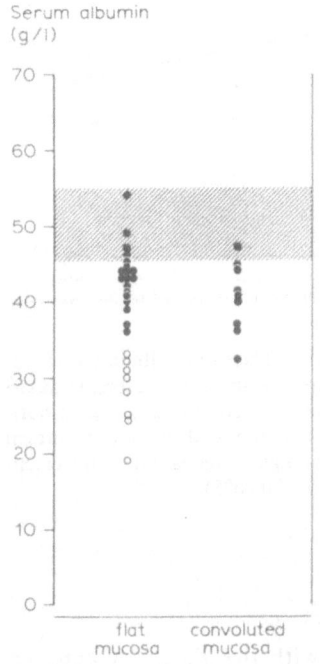

Fig. 7.22. Serum albumin in untreated coeliac sprue. The serum levels are drawn separately for patients with a flat and with a convoluted jejunal mucosa. Statistical analysis (Mann-Whitney test) revealed no significant difference between both groups. Hollow dots represent patients with peripheral oedema, and solid dots those without oedema. The shaded area represents the range of normal values (cf. chapter 12).

7.5.3 Enteric protein loss

The data obtained on the enteric protein loss were presented in section 6.10. In a summary of these data, it can be stated that increased protein loss was evident in nearly all 30 untreated patients, i.e. in 93%. Comparison of the

137

serum albumin concentration with the extent of enteric protein loss reveals a negative correlation between these two variables (fig. 7.23). The range is somewhat wide, however; at a protein loss of, for instance, 100 ml plasma per day, it was found that the serum albumin concentration could vary from 25 to 44 g/l.

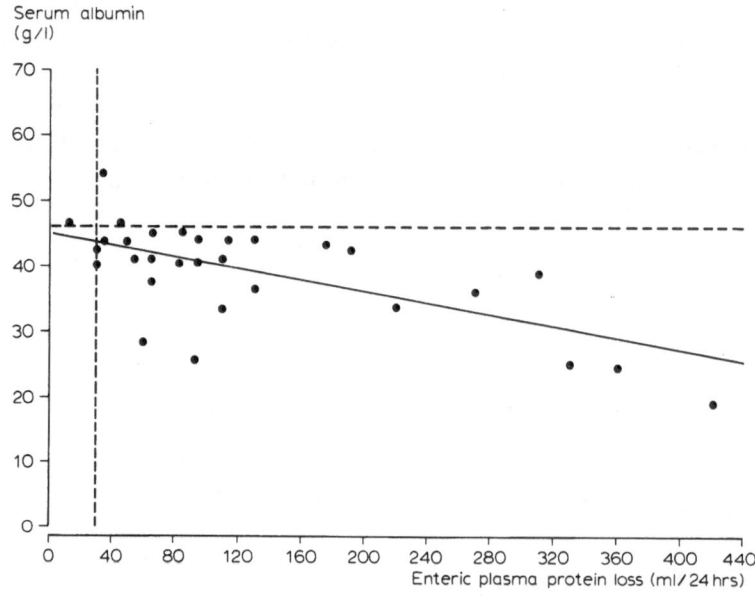

Fig. 7.23. Serum albumin and enteric plasma protein loss. The serum albumin levels of untreated coeliac patients are plotted against the corresponding amounts of protein leakage calculated from simultaneously conducted enteric protein loss studies. The dotted horizontal line represents the lower limit of normal serum albumin, and the dotted vertical line the upper limit of normal enteric protein loss. The straight diagonal line is the calculated regression line ($y = 45.2 - 0.046\,x$; $r = -0.72$; $p < 0.0005$).

7.5.4 Albumin synthesis

The rate of albumin synthesis was measured with the aid of ^{14}C-labelled carbonate, according to McFarlane (575). This was done by our colleagues Yap and Hafkenscheid, as part of their extensive studies in this field (932, 933, 934).

Synthesis was found to be normal in 5 of the 6 untreated coeliacs. Decreased albumin synthesis was observed in 1 patient (table 7.8), in whom the serum concentration of the essential amino acid tryptophan was markedly reduced. In addition, the serum concentrations of threonine, valine, leucine, and phenylalanine were moderately decreased. In 2 patients with normal albumin synthesis, however, slightly reduced serum concentrations of some essential amino acids were likewise found. The liver function tests were slightly abnormal in only 2 patients, including the one with the decreased albumin synthesis.

7.5.5 Effect of the gluten-free diet

In all patients the serum albumin concentration increased after gluten withdrawal. In about 50% of the cases the albumin concentration returned to normal within 5 months, but in some it took much longer for the hypoalbuminaemia to disappear (fig. 7.24).

Enteric protein loss diminished as a rule rapidly after gluten withdrawal, and became normal in 4 out of 8 cases (section 6.10).

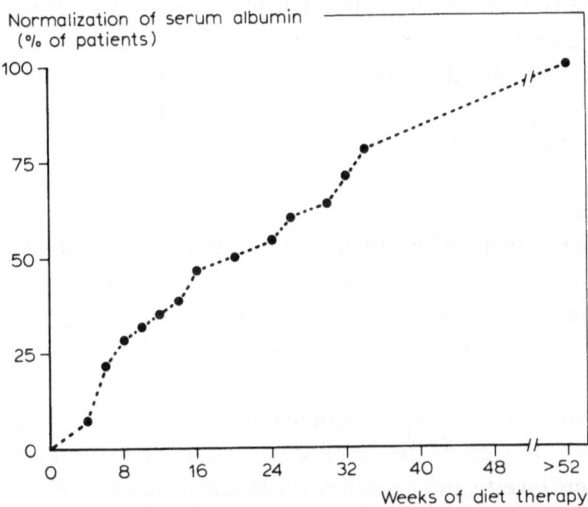

Fig. 7.24. Serum albumin and gluten-free diet. Both the extent and the rate of normalization of serum albumin levels on diet therapy in all 28 followed-up patients with hypoalbuminaemia (fig. 7.22) are recorded.

7.5.6 Comment

In view of the high incidence of hypoalbuminaemia it seems likely that digestion and absorption of dietary protein are abnormal in many cases of coeliac

Table 7.8. Serum albumin, enteric protein loss, albumin synthesis rate and serum concentration of essentia

PATIENT	SERUM ALBUMIN (g/l)	ENTERIC PROTEIN LOSS (ml plasma/ 24 hrs)	ALBUMIN SYNTHESIS RATE (g/175 cm/ 24 hrs)	FRAC-TIONAL SYNTHESIS RATE (%/24 hrs)	THREO-NINE (μmole/l)	VALINE (μmole/l)
# 1	33.0	215	20.4	16.6	167	266
# 5	34.0	110	7.0	6.7	75	145
# 20	25.4	360	26.8	45.4	165	172
# 26	44.2	82	29.2	20.2	262	274
# 27	17.7	400	20.7	34.6	28	127
# 30	26.8	330	22.8	28.0	N.D.	N.D.
Controls	45.8-55.1	< 30	22.3±6.8 (M±S.D.)	16.2±4.2 (M±S.D.)	103-172	189-350

sprue. This is also indicated by the fact that faecal nitrogen excretion is increased in some coeliac patients, although this increase can of course also be due to increased loss of endogenous protein. The faecal nitrogen excretion is less than 2 g per day under normal conditions (291, 701), but in coeliac patients can be as high as 4-7 g per day (601). In extreme cases it may even exceed the amount of nitrogen in the food (436). Several mechanisms can cause this increase of faecal nitrogen and by that a decreased serum albumin concentration.

It is conceivable that, owing to decreased endogenous stimulation, the pancreas does not always function optimally in coeliac patients. This stimulation is effected via the hormones cholecystokinin and secretin, which are both synthesized in the mucosa of the duodenum and the proximal jejunum. It is precisely in this region that mucosal lesions are most pronounced in coeliac sprue and, theoretically, the production of these hormones can therefore be decreased. In view of the diminished response to exogenous secretin observed by some investigators (section 6.6.3), the pancreas itself can also be abnormal. Another possibility is that pancreatic trypsinogen, released in the intestinal lumen, is insufficiently activated due to deficiency in enterokinase. One might presume that enterokinase deficiency develops in coeliac sprue, as this catalyser is synthesized in the duodenal mucosa, but this is not, in fact, so (506, 925). In any case it should be borne in mind that the pancreas normally secretes an enormous surplus of proteolytic enzymes (334), so that it is questionable whether decreased endogenous stimulation of pancreatic enzyme production would really have repercussions in protein digestion.

mino acids in 6 untreated coeliac patients (cf. chapter 12).

METHIONINE (μmole/l)	ISO-LEUCINE (μmole/l)	LEUCINE (μmole/l)	PHENYL-ALANINE (μmole/l)	LYSINE (μmole/l)	TRYPTO-PHAN (μmole/l)	SGOT (u/l)	SGPT (u/l)
31	101	168	84	288	40	10	21
22	58	99	49	173	9	21	10
18	53	88	38	200	28	12	3
50	75	147	91	206	64	7	11
18	60	96	60	99	79	6	11
N.D.	N.D.	N.D.	N.D.	N.D.	N.D.	12	15
20-37	49-118	110-213	53-103	150-268	34-68	< 15	< 15

The absorption of entirely or partly digested protein can also be decreased in coeliac patients. With the disappearance of villi and brush border, the size of the absorptive surface area diminishes. The importance of a sufficiently large surface area for protein absorption is demonstrated by the occurrence of an increase in faecal nitrogen excretion after extensive intestinal resections (85). The remaining enterocytes in coeliac patients have only a low enzyme activity, including peptidase activity (224, 231), so that the normal membrane digestion by peptidases may be disturbed (743). There may be also insufficient or defective transport carriers present in the brush border membrane.

Although decreased protein absorption might be theoretically expected in all cases of coeliac sprue, the various relevant observations are not unequivocal. For example, the in-vitro uptake of radioactive amino acids by duodenal biopsy specimens from coeliac patients proved to be less effective than that in normal test subjects (102). Perfusion studies of the proximal jejunum revealed decreased absorption of methionine (753) and glycine (6, 173) in untreated coeliacs. Silk et al. (790), however, observed that glycine absorption was normal in about 50% of the cases, perhaps (as the investigators themselves pointed out) because their patients were suffering from less severe forms of coeliac sprue. Absorption of dipeptides such as glycylglycine, glycylleucine and glycylalanine, too, was usually not markedly disturbed (6) or even normal (790). In view of these data it can therefore be maintained that absorption of amino acids and dipeptides is normal in a substantial number of coeliac patients. The same seems to apply to some proteins, for after consumption of casein (704) or albumin (230), a normal or even exaggerated increase of the corresponding serum amino acid levels is by no means unusual.

In addition to exogenous dietary protein, the small intestine also has to cope with an amount of endogenous protein. Normally, this endogenous supply (which consists of a small amount of extracellular protein leaked into the intestinal lumen, digestive enzymes and exfoliated enterocytes) is probably not much larger than half the amount of protein in the food (377). In patients with coeliac sprue, the amount of endogenous protein released in the intestinal lumen is usually much larger. On one hand, enteric protein loss has significantly increased (section 6.10), and on the other hand the number of exfoliated enterocytes is markedly increased in coeliac sprue (section 6.9). In view of the fact that faecal nitrogen excretion is frequently increased, the total amount of exogenous as well as endogenous protein to be digested and absorbed in the small intestine can exceed the capacity of this diseased bowel in coeliac patients.

Protein not absorbed in the small intestine can be degraded by bacteria in the large intestine and, partly, excreted in the faeces in the form of nitrogen containing degradation products. In patients with an abnormal bacterial flora in the small intestine, bacterial degradation of protein or amino acids can occur in this part of the intestine as well. A large proportion of these bacterial degradation products is absorbed in the small intestine (648). A well-known bacterial protein degradation product is indole, which is derived from tryptophan. After conversion in the liver, this substance is excreted in the urine as indican. Beside indican many other bacterial protein degradation products occur in the urine (371, 595). It is to be borne in mind, however, that increased indican excretion is not necessarily due to an abnormal bacterial flora but can also result from an excessive supply of protein to the large intestine (e.g. in the case of massive gastrointestinal haemorrhage), and perhaps also develops in association with severely disturbed protein absorption as may occur in coeliac sprue. About 50% of our untreated coeliacs showed increased urinary indican excretion as well as other symptoms of an abnormal bacterial flora in the small intestine (section 6.11). This abnormal flora can consume or degrade some of the protein in the intestinal lumen, thus precluding its absorption and further utilization.

As a result of malabsorption and increased bacterial degradation of amino acids and oligopeptides, an insufficient amount of amino acids may end up in the portal circulation. In several of our coeliac patients the serum concentrations of some essential amino acids were indeed decreased. Although this need not reflect the amino acid levels in the portal blood, it is possible that in these patients the liver was insufficiently supplied with amino acids, and that this affected protein synthesis. In one of our patients, albumin synthesis was markedly decreased (table 7.8), and in this patient the serum concentrations of several essential amino acids, specifically tryptophan, were decreased. In none of the other patients was so low a tryptophan concentration found. It therefore seems plausible that a deficiency in tryptophan – which is known to stimulate albumin synthesis (728, 934) – influenced the rate of synthesis in this case. Albumin synthesis was found to be normal in the other five coeliac patients. In view of their hypoalbuminaemia, however, a substantially increased synthesis would have been expected in these patients. For the liver as a rule adjusts albumin synthesis to its loss, which can be compensated as long as the maximal rate of synthesis, which is about twice the normal synthesis, is not exceeded (730). Perhaps the absence of a compensatory increase in albumin synthesis by the liver in the remaining patients does indicate a relative deficiency in the amino acids. This probably constitutes an important mechanism responsible for hypoalbuminaemia in coeliac sprue.

According to some authors, the supply of amino acids to the liver for protein synthesis is reduced chiefly as a result of the reduced intake of dietary protein due to anorexia (689, 790). This hypothesis does not seem very plausible, because the regularly increased faecal nitrogen excretion seems to indicate that more protein is supplied for absorption than the small intestine can cope with.

7.5.7 Conclusions

1. A decreased serum albumin concentration is found in the majority of untreated patients with coeliac sprue.
2. In absolute sense, the rate of albumin synthesis is normal in most patients, and decreased only in exceptional cases. An increase in albumin synthesis, however, expected in view of the hypoalbuminaemia, is seldom found.
3. This may be explained by a relative deficiency in necessary amino acids, as a result of malabsorption and bacterial degradation of protein in the small intestine.
4. The protein malabsorption frequently – but by no means always – observed in coeliac sprue, is probably not a result of reduced proteolysis by digestive enzymes, but more likely of a decreased absorptive surface area and enterocyte abnormalities.
5. The demands made on the absorptive capacity of the small intestine are

greater in coeliac patients as a result of the marked increase in released endogenous protein. This endogenous protein largely originates from enteric protein loss and increased exfoliation of enterocytes.

6. Some of the protein in the small intestine may be degraded by an abnormal bacterial flora and converted to products which often cannot be further utilized.

7. After gluten withdrawal the serum albumin concentration increased in all patients, and in some 50% even reached a normal level within 5 months. The serum albumin concentration therefore seems to be a simple and reliable parameter in studying the effect of diet therapy.

7.6 CALCIUM

7.6.1 Introduction

It is a well-known empirical fact that the plasma calcium concentration is decreased in many coeliac patients (table 7.9). Clinical symptoms also suggest calcium deficiency; tetany and bone pain are regularly observed (table 8.1; 60, 87, 113, 553, 723). The incidence of disorders of calcium

Table 7.9. Incidence of hypocalcaemia in untreated coeliac sprue.

AUTHORS	CRITERION	NUMBER OF PATIENTS INVESTIGATED	PERCENTAGE WITH HYPO-CALCAEMIA
Buchan et al. (1962)	< 4.5 meq/l	35	60
Cooke et al. (1963)	< 9.2 mg%	44	64
Benson et al. (1964)	< 9.0 mg%	30	67
Ross et al. (1966a)	< 9.0 mg%	35	57
Brooks et al. (1966)	not stated	11	63
Harrison et al. (1969)	< 8.9 mg%	5	80
Mann et al. (1970)	< 8.8 mg%	20	65
Melvin et al. (1970)	< 4.5 meq/l	9	44
Thys et al. (1971)	< 8 mg%	9	56
Modigliani et al. (1975)	< 8.5 mg%	46	81
Own series	< 2.35 mmole/l	35	63

metabolism was investigated in our patients. In addition to the results of these investigations, the factors which influence calcium balance in coeliac sprue are discussed.

7.6.2 Plasma calcium concentration

The plasma calcium concentration was determined in 35 untreated coeliac patients. Since the majority also showed more or less marked hypoalbuminaemia, the calcium values obtained were corrected for the existing plasma protein concentration (657). After this correction, 22 of the 35 patients (63%) proved to show a real decrease in plasma calcium concentration (fig. 7.25). Marked hypocalcaemia was observed only in patients with a

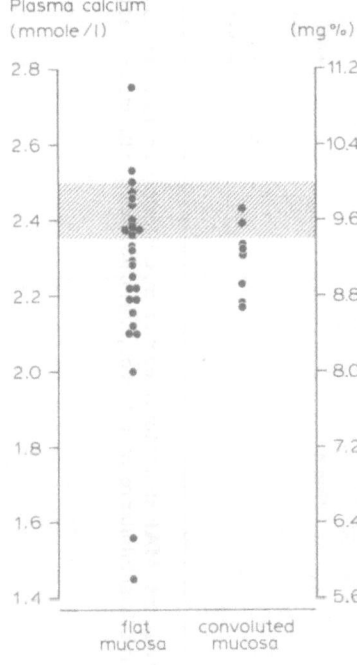

Fig. 7.25. Plasma calcium in untreated coeliac sprue. The serum levels are drawn separately for patients with a flat and with a convoluted jejunal mucosa. Statistical analysis (Mann-Whitney test) revealed no significant difference between both groups. The shaded area represents the range of normal values (cf. chapter 12).

flat mucosa in the jejunal biopsy specimen. Decreased calcium concentrations were also found, however, in patients with less severe mucosal lesions. No correlation could be established between the severity of hypocalcaemia and the degree of steatorrhoea or the volume of enteric protein leakage.

145

Table 7.10. Relevant data on calcium and bone metabolism in 11 untreated coeliac patients.

PATIENT	#1	#2	#5	#10	#13	#20	#27	#28	#29	#30	#34	CONTROLS
SERUM CALCIUM (CORR.)	1.45	2.10	2.00	2.28	2.44	2.17	1.56	2.36	2.40	2.25	2.33	2.35-2.50 mmole/l
CALCIUM ABSORPTION							AB-NORM	AB-NORM		AB-NORM		
BONE HISTOLOGY*	MAL & OP	MAL	MAL	OST FIBR	MAL	MAL	MAL	MAL	MAL	MAL & OP		
SERUM ALKALINE PHOSPHATASE	219	120	164	177	153	194	326	163	65	96	148	45-90 U/l
HYDROXYPROLINE EXCRETION	854		315	651			469	405	351		416	150-400 µmole
Tm/GFR**		1.85	0.66	0.57		1.55						0.71-1.36
X-RAY STUDIES		NORM					AB-NORM	NORM				
AMINO-ACIDURIA						NORM	AB-NORM			AB-NORM		

* Meaning of abbreviations: MAL stands for osteomalacia, OP for osteoporosis, and OST FIBR for osteitis fibrosa.
** Tm/GFR means: maximal tubular reabsorption of phosphate related to the glomerular filtration rate.

7.6.3 Calcium absorption

The absorption of a small dose (10 μCi) of ⁴⁷Ca was measured in 3 untreated patients (fig. 7.26), both by determination of plasma radioactivity during 4 hours following administration of ⁴⁷Ca and by determination of ⁴⁷Ca retention with the aid of a whole-body counter during 3 weeks. The latter method is thought to show a better correlation with the calcium balance (10, 715). Both determinations revealed low calcium absorption in each of the 3 patients. For the other findings obtained in these 3 patients we refer to table 7.10.

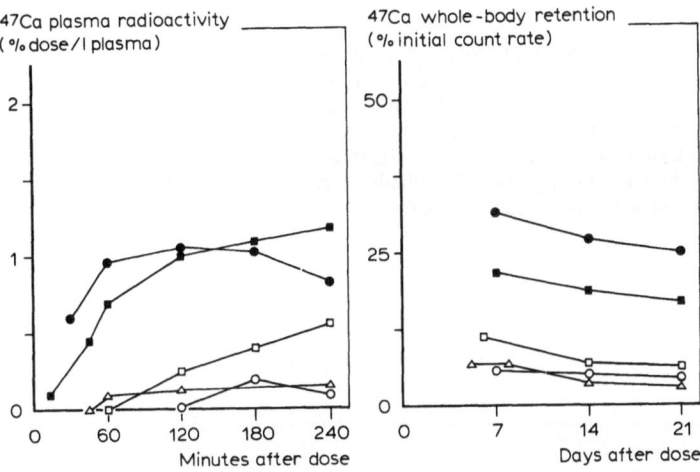

Fig. 7.26. Calcium absorption in coeliac sprue. The absorption of ⁴⁷Ca, measured by determination of both plasma radio-activity and by whole-body retention, in 3 untreated patients is given by hollow symbols. The solid symbols represent the absorption in corresponding patients during treatment with a gluten-free diet and temporary vitamin D administration (cf. chapter 12).

7.6.4 Alkaline phosphatase activity

The serum alkaline phosphatase activity was determined in 33 untreated patients and found to be increased in 19 (58%); these 19 included patients with a flat mucosa as well as with a convoluted mucosa in the jejunal biopsy specimen (fig. 7.27). The liver function tests were normal in all patients but 2. In these 2 patients the serum LAP activity (which, like the alkaline phosphatase activity, is increased in cholestasis but normal in disorders of bone metabolism) was 23 and 40 U/l, respectively (normal value < 28 U/l).

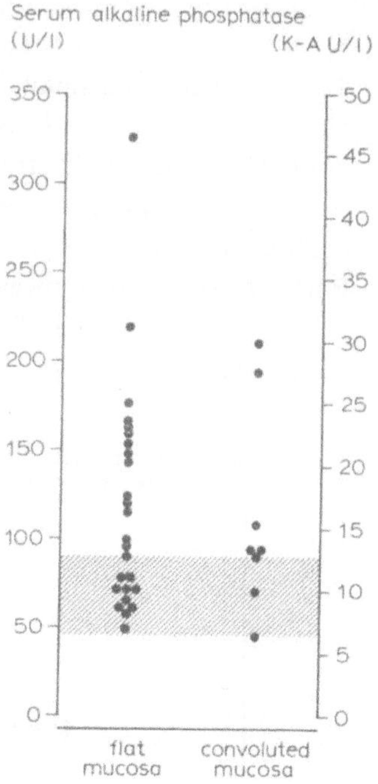

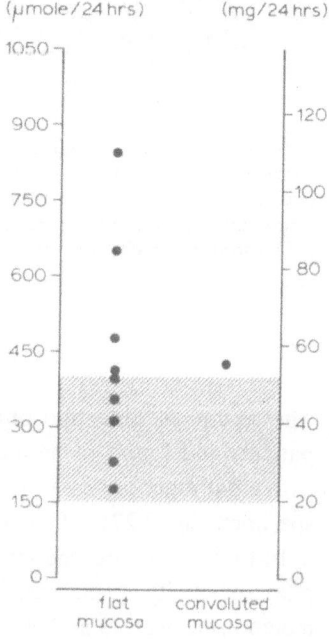

Fig. 7.27. Serum alkaline phosphatase in untreated coeliac sprue. The serum levels are drawn separately for patients with a flat and with a convoluted jejunal mucosa. Statistical analysis (Mann-Whitney test) revealed no significant difference between both groups. The shaded area represents the range of normal values (cf. chapter 12).

Fig. 7.28. Urinary hydroxyproline excretion in untreated coeliac sprue. The amounts excreted in urine are drawn separately for patients with a flat and with a convoluted jejunal mucosa. The shaded area represents the range of normal values (cf. chapter 12).

148

7.6.5 Hydroxyproline excretion

The urinary hydroxyproline excretion was determined in 10 untreated patients. Expressed as mean of excretions on 2 or 3 consecutive days, the excretion was increased in 5 (fig. 7.28).

7.6.6 Histological examination of bone tissue

In 11 untreated coeliacs a bone biopsy specimen was obtained for histological examination. Five patients showed clinical symptoms suggestive of osteomalacia, such as pain in the bones, a waddling gait or a non-healing fracture. In all cases histological evidence of disturbed mineralization was found. Osteomalacia was diagnosed in 10 patients, and osteitis fibrosa in one. The biopsy specimens from 2 patients showed distinct signs of osteoporosis. For the other observations in these cases we refer to table 7.10.

7.6.7 Two-hour phosphate clearance

In 4 patients the tubular reabsorption of phosphate was determined during a two-hour phosphate clearance test, in an effort to exclude or demonstrate hyperparathyroidism. An abnormally low phosphate clearance was found in 2 patients, one of whom also showed histological features of hyperparathyroidism in the bone biopsy specimen (table 7.10).

7.6.8 Radiographs of the hand skeleton

In one patient with marked hypocalcaemia, radiographs of the hands revealed unmistakable subperiosteal erosions. In 2 other patients, of whom only one had a slightly decreased plasma calcium concentration, no erosions were visible (table 7.10).

7.6.9 Amino-aciduria study

An abnormally high urinary excretion of some amino acids was found in 2 out of 3 patients; the amino acids in question were glycine and lysine in the one, and glycine, threonine, serine, alanine and tyrosine in the other. One of these patients also showed subperiosteal erosions in the hand skeleton (table 7.10).

7.6.10 Effect of the gluten-free diet

After gluten withdrawal, the plasma calcium concentration rose to a normal

149

level in all patients, usually within 6 months (fig. 7.29). In order to exclude the influence of persistent hypoproteinaemia, the calcium concentration was always corrected for the protein concentration (657). Administration or withholding of vitamin D caused no marked difference in the rate of normalization of the calcium concentration.

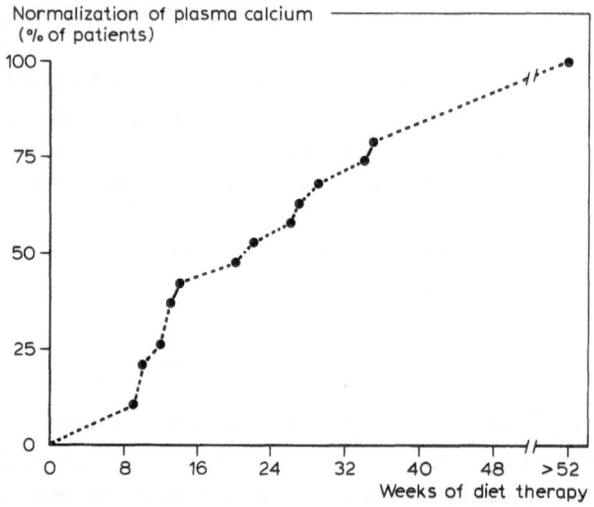

Fig. 7.29. Plasma calcium and gluten-free diet. Both the extent and the rate of normalization of plasma calcium levels on diet therapy in all 19 followed-up patients with hypocalcaemia (fig. 7.25) are recorded.

Calcium absorption and retention also improved after gluten withdrawal (fig. 7.26). In 2 patients, markedly increased calcium absorption was observed 56 and 72 weeks after gluten withdrawal, respectively. In these patients vitamin D suppletion had been discontinued more than 6 months earlier.

The serum alkaline phosphatase activity decreased to a normal value in 73% of the patients. The rate of normalization of alkaline phosphatase activity did not seem to depend on administration or withholding of vitamin D (fig. 7.30).

The urinary hydroxyproline excretion also decreased after gluten withdrawal and became normal in 3 out of 4 cases (fig. 7.31).

In 9 patients the bone biopsy was repeated after 20-80 months (mean: 36 months) on the gluten-free diet. Most of these patients had received vitamin D suppletion for a limited period. In all cases but one, histological examination of bone tissue revealed a markedly improved degree of mineralization.

150

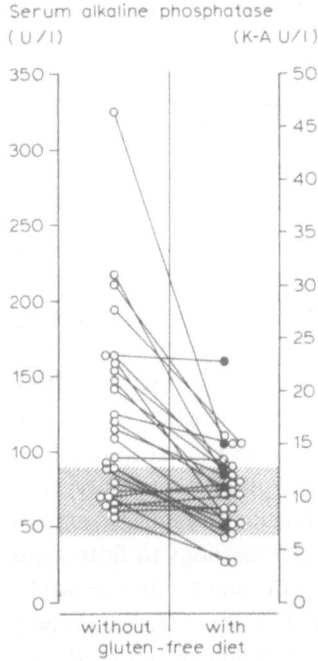

Serum alkaline phosphatase
(U/l)   (K-A U/l)

without | with
gluten-free diet

Fig. 7.30. Serum alkaline phosphatase and gluten-free diet. The serum levels in corresponding patients before as well as during diet therapy are given. Statistical analysis (Wilcoxon signed-rank test) revealed a significant improvement on diet therapy ($p < 1\%$). The solid dots represent patients who received additional vitamin D therapy. The shaded area represents the range of normal values (cf. chapter 12).

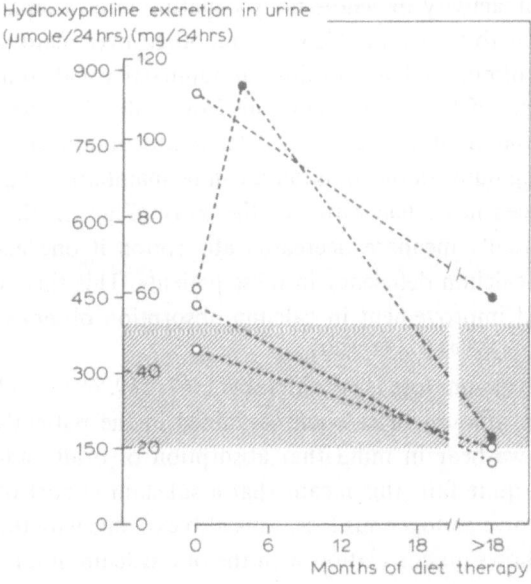

Hydroxyproline excretion in urine
(μmole/24 hrs)(mg/24 hrs)

0   6   12   18   >18
Months of diet therapy

Fig. 7.31. Urinary hydroxyproline excretion and gluten-free diet. The amounts excreted by corresponding patients before as well as during diet therapy are given. The solid dots represent patients who received additional vitamin D therapy. The shaded area represents the range of normal values (cf. chapter 12).

151

In a total of 5 patients the bone tissue had returned to complete normality, and in 4 other biopsy specimens a slight increase in osteoid was still discernible.

The amino-aciduria observed in 2 patients, disappeared 2-3 months after gluten withdrawal.

7.6.11 Comment

In nearly all untreated coeliac patients, the calcium balance proves to be negative. This is undoubtedly due to faecal calcium loss, for the urinary calcium excretion is extremely low, as can be expected in calcium deficiency (367, 589, 693).

In view of the increased faecal calcium loss, absorption of calcium from the food can be expected to be markedly disturbed in coeliac sprue. This could be a result especially of the structural abnormalities in the mucosa of the proximal small intestine, where calcium absorption is probably most important under normal conditions (906). Other phenomena can also explain calcium malabsorption, such as the binding of calcium ions to fatty acids (11) or a markedly accelerated passage through the small intestine (411). Another important factor can be the vitamin D deficiency observed in many cases (589, 841), as a result of which active transport of calcium by the intestinal mucosa is reduced.

In spite of the above mentioned disturbing factors, calcium absorption proves to be normal in some coeliacs, regardless of whether it is determined on the basis of plasma radioactivity or whole-body counting after a small (10) or a large dose of radioactive calcium (433). Several other investigators, however, regularly found diminished absorption of radioactive calcium, both from a single test dose (693), a meal (11), and from milk (71, 853). Wensel et al. (906) also found an abnormally low calcium absorption upon perfusion of the proximal jejunum. In our opinion it can be maintained that calcium absorption is reduced in coeliac sprue, as the 'normal' absorption found in some patients actually means a decreased absorption if one accounts for the pronounced calcium deficiency in these patients. This theory is supported by the marked improvement in calcium absorption observed after gluten withdrawal (fig. 7.26; 411, 433, 589).

As mentioned, the faecal calcium loss is considerable (367, 589, 693), and sometimes even exceeds the amount of calcium contained in the patient's food (589). Particularly if we bear in mind that absorption of orally administered calcium is often quite fair, this means that a substantial part of this faecal calcium must involve endogenous loss. This also explains why the amount of faecal calcium shows no correlation with the oral calcium intake

(589). Several investigators have measured this endogenous calcium loss by determination of radioactivity in the faeces after intravenous administration of calcium isotope. Endogenous calcium loss was usually markedly increased, up to 2-3 times the normal amount (367, 589, 693). Since a considerable part of the endogenous calcium is probably reabsorbed at a more distal level in the small intestine, the amount of calcium which primarily enters the intestinal lumen must be substantially higher. It is impossible to estimate even approximately the total amount of this primarily secreted, so-called digestive juice calcium (411). Moreover, it is not quite clear how and where the endogenous calcium is released. This can take place via pancreatic juice and bile (103), but also via leakage of tissue fluid from the intestinal wall into the lumen. Yet this is not sufficient to explain the enormous endogenous calcium loss found in coeliac patients. We must therefore assume that substantial secretion of calcium from the intestinal epithelium takes place (411, 589), although this has not been confirmed in perfusion studies (906).

Calcium absorption is known to adjust itself to human calcium requirements. Vitamin D is held responsible for this adjustment (section 5.6). This vitamin probably determines whether or not extra calcium is absorbed in the distal part of the small intestine, which in principle has the ability to do so. In spite of the calcium hunger due to the constantly negative balance, compensatory hyperabsorption of calcium in the distal small intestine does not seem to occur in coeliac patients. If this compensatory absorption is indeed determined by vitamin D, then there is every reason for non-absorption in the ileum, for the serum vitamin D concentration is usually decreased (589) as a result of vitamin D malabsorption (841). After parenteral administration of vitamin D, calcium absorption (11) and calcium balance (641) improve, and osteomalacia disappears (589, 693). In some cases, however, large doses of vitamin D are required to produce any effect, suggesting the existence of a partial vitamin D resistance in coeliac sprue (615). The latter may result from a decreased effect of vitamin D on the damaged intestinal mucosa (693).

As a result of the negative calcium balance, the serum calcium concentration tends to decrease. A decreased plasma calcium concentration is often found in untreated coeliac patients. We observed hypocalcaemia in 63% of our patients (fig. 7.25), which agrees with reports by other investigators (table 7.9). Secondary hyperparathyroidism can develop in response to this decreased plasma calcium concentration (117, 367, 589). In 4 patients we found evidence of hyperparathyroidism, such as osteitis fibrosa, subperiosteal erosions, decreased tubular reabsorption of phosphate or parathyreoid hyperplasia. Disorders of renal tubular function may develop as a result of this hyperparathyroidism (535, 617). We observed transient amino-aciduria in 2 coeliac patients, one of whom was suffering from proven hyperparathyroidism. Amino-aciduria in coeliac sprue has also been reported by others (355, 488).

Another consequence of the negative calcium balance is intensified mobilization of calcium from bone tissue, which in the long run leads to osteoporosis. However, osteoporosis is not very often observed in coeliac sprue. We found histological features of osteoporosis in only 2 of 11 patients in whom a bone biopsy was performed. Ross et al. (723) and Melvin et al. (589) likewise reported that osteoporosis was rare in their patients. On the basis of radiographs the incidence of osteoporosis is sometimes estimated higher (163), but proper differentiation between osteoporosis and osteomalacia is impossible on the basis of radiographs.

Osteomalacia as a result of vitamin D deficiency is a regular finding. We found signs of marked osteomalacia in virtually all biopsy specimens from untreated coeliacs; this is in agreement with findings reported by others (589). The presence of osteomalacia is usually indicated by increased serum alkaline phosphatase activity and raised urinary excretion of hydroxyprolines (table 7.10). Increased serum alkaline phosphatase activity was found in 58% of our patients, which lies in between the percentages reported by others (table 7.11). However, for correct interpretation of increased alkaline phosphatase activity, liver abnormalities always have to be excluded. In several publications exclusion of liver pathology has not been mentioned explicitly.

The iso-enzyme originating from the intestine has been found unimportant in contributing to an increase in serum alkaline phosphatase activity (366). A striking finding was that several patients with proven osteomalacia showed normal alkaline phosphatase activity (table 7.10), which was also noted by others (589). The question is whether determination of urinary hydroxyproline excretion does not supply a more sensitive parameter (table 7.10; 589).

Vitamin D absorption improves soon after gluten withdrawal (589, 841), resulting in an increased calcium absorption. The mucosal lesions in the proximal small intestine also ameliorate, as a result of which absorption increases on the one hand, and endogenous calcium loss diminishes on the other (589). In 2 patients on a gluten-free diet who were temporarily given vitamin D suppletion, we did observe increased absorption of calcium (fig. 7.26). According to other investigators (411, 433), this increase can also occur without vitamin D suppletion. The improved calcium absorption causes the calcium balance to become positive (589). As a consequence the

Table 7.11. Incidence of an increased serum alkaline phosphatase level in untreated coeliac sprue.

AUTHORS	CRITERION	NUMBER OF PATIENTS INVESTIGATED	PERCENTAGE WITH-INCREASED ALK. PHOSPH.
Cooke et al. (1963)	> 12 KAU/l*	49	67
Ross et al. (1966b)	> 4 BU/l**	25	44
Mortimer et al. (1968)	> 12 KAU/l	8	0
Harris et al. (1969)	> 13 KAU/l	111	62
Harrison et al. (1969)	> 50 U/l***	5	100
Jarnum et al. (1970)	> 39 U/l	10	80
Melvin et al. (1970)	> 13 KAU/l	9	22
Modigliani et al. (1975)	> 50 U/l	42	60
Own series	> 90 U/l	33	58

* KAU = King Armstrong Units
** BU = Bodanski Units
*** U = Bessey Units

plasma calcium concentration normalizes (fig. 7.29; 60, 104, 160), and the secondary hyperparathyroidism disappears. Newly formed bone tissue is normally mineralized again and the osteoporosis disappears once the calcium deficiency is corrected, which in some cases may take years (411). After an average of at least 2 years on a gluten-free diet, we no longer found significant abnormalities in bone biopsy specimens; this is in agreement with the findings of other investigators (589, 693). Parallel to this development, serum alkaline phosphatase activity as well as urinary hydroxy-proline excretion decreased (fig. 7.30; fig. 7.31).

7.6.12 Conclusions

1. If the existing calcium deficiency is taken into account, the absorption of a single dose of calcium tracer is usually decreased in untreated coeliac patients.
2. Active transport of calcium in the jejunum and ileum will be diminished due to vitamin D deficiency.

3. Nearly all untreated coeliac patients show a considerable faecal calcium loss, which is partly the result of an increased endogenous loss.
4. Due to a negative calcium balance, calcium from bone tissue will be mobilized, which leads to osteoporosis in the long run.
5. Secondary hyperparathyroidism with bone abnormalities and renal functional disorders can develop as a result of a decreased plasma calcium concentration.
6. The bone tissue, moreover, nearly always shows signs of insufficient mineralization as a result of the vitamin D deficiency. The true incidence of osteomalacia in coeliac sprue can only be determined by systematic bone biopsies.
7. Less complicated methods of tracing osteomalacia are determination of serum alkaline phosphatase activity and urinary hydroxyproline excretion. False negative results, however, are not uncommon.
8. After gluten withdrawal, most abnormalities quickly disappear as a result of improved absorption of vitamin D, and consequently of calcium as well, in addition to decreased endogenous calcium loss. The deficiencies and abnormalities of bone tissue, however, need more time to disappear completely.

7.7 MAGNESIUM

7.7.1 Introduction

Magnesium deficiency is thought to be regularly associated with calcium deficiency (525). Perhaps the reverse is also true. Hypocalcaemia is frequently observed in untreated coeliac patients (fig. 7.25, table 7.9), but hypomagnesaemia has not been frequently described (43). However, few investigators have systematically determined the serum magnesium concentration in their patients (601, 618, 693). We therefore considered it useful to study the incidence of hypomagnesaemia in our patients and to establish whether the plasma calcium concentration was indeed also decreased in them. The possible cause of magnesium deficiency will also be discussed in the following section.

7.7.2 Serum magnesium concentration

The serum magnesium concentration was determined in 16 untreated coeliacs, and found to be decreased in 4, all with a flat jejunal mucosa (fig. 7.32). All patients with hypomagnesaemia were in a poor clinical condition. There was a fair correlation between serum magnesium concentra-

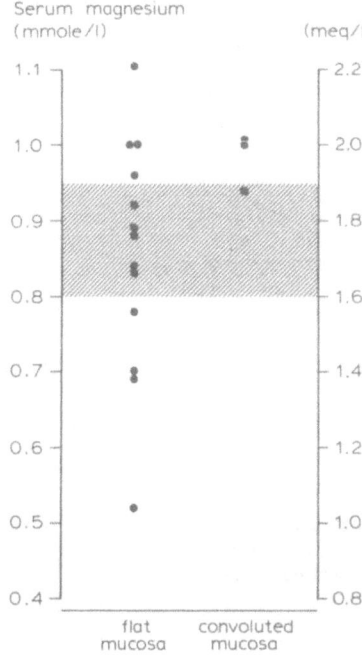

Fig. 7.32. Serum magnesium in untreated coeliac sprue. The serum levels are drawn separately for patients with a flat and with a convoluted jejunal mucosa. The shaded area represents the range of normal values (cf. chapter 12).

tion and fat absorption (fig. 7.33). In 3 of the 4 patients with hypomagnesaemia, the plasma calcium concentration was decreased. However, the calcium concentration was decreased also in 9 of the 12 patients with a normal serum magnesium concentration. None of the patients with hypomagnesaemia showed symptoms of tetany.

7.7.3 Effect of the gluten-free diet

The serum magnesium concentration always increased to a normal value after gluten withdrawal (fig. 7.34). In 2 patients with hypomagnesaemia the effect of diet therapy on serum magnesium was evaluated only after 1 year or more. In the other 2 cases the hypomagnesaemia was normalized after 2 and 9 weeks.

7.7.4 Comment

The serum magnesium concentration is decreased in a few patients with coeliac sprue (fig. 7.32; 601, 693). These are usually patients in poor condition, as has been noted before in patients with idiopathic steatorrhoea, many

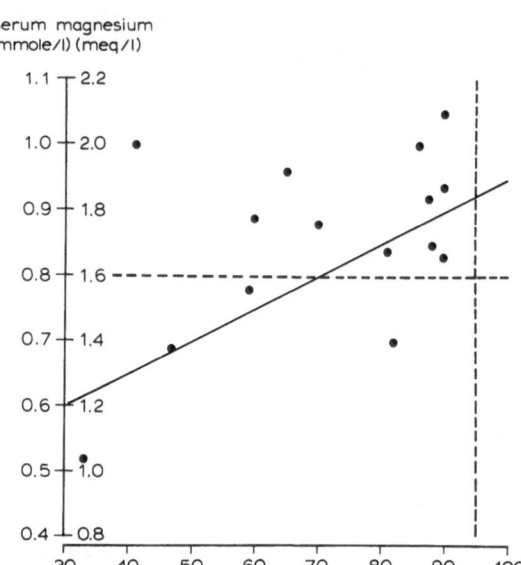

Fig. 7.33. Serum magnesium and fat absorption. The serum magnesium levels of untreated coeliac patients are plotted against the corresponding absorption coefficients of
simultaneously conducted fat balance studies. The dotted horizontal line represents the
lower limit of normal serum magnesium levels, and the dotted vertical line the lower limit
of normal fat absorption. The straight diagonal line is the calculated regression line ($y = 0.61 + 0.0034\,x$; $r = 0.48$; $2.5\% < p < 5\%$).

of whom must have suffered from coeliac sprue (87). We observed no clinical
symptoms of magnesium deficiency, such as tetany.

The hypomagnesaemia is probably partly caused by malabsorption of dietary magnesium. In this malabsorption, an important role may be played by
unabsorbed fatty acids, which bind the magnesium ions to poorly soluble
soaps. This probably explains the correlation between serum magnesium
concentration and fat absorption (fig. 7.33). It is further supported by the
observation of Booth et al. (87) who noticed an improvement of the magnesium balance in their patients with idiopathic steatorrhoea after introduction of a fat-restricted diet.

Magnesium absorption in the small intestine is supposedly very slow (330).
It is therefore readily conceivable that a shortened intestinal transit time,
present in many coeliac patients, exerts a negative influence on this absorption.

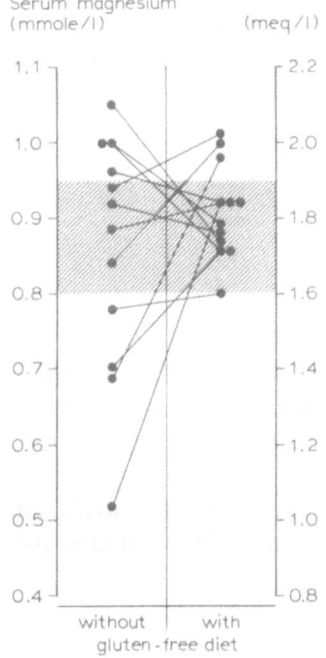

Serum magnesium
(mmole/l)   (meq/l)

Fig. 7.34. Serum magnesium and gluten-free diet. The serum levels in corresponding patients before as well as during diet therapy are given. Statistical analysis (Wilcoxon signed-rank test) did not reveal a significant improvement on diet therapy. The shaded area represents the range of normal values (cf. chapter 12).

Moreover, there is probably an increased loss of magnesium which originates from the digestive juices and the increased number of exfoliated cells. Due to this endogenous loss, the total amount of magnesium found in the faeces can be markedly increased, up to a few times the total amount of the oral intake in some cases (317).

Too little is known about magnesium absorption under normal conditions, to explain the mechanisms underlying the abnormal absorption in coeliac sprue.

The faecal magnesium loss returns to normal within a few months of gluten withdrawal (317). The serum magnesium concentration, too, increases relatively rapidly in treated patients.

7.7.5 Conclusions

1. Although there is no clinical evidence of magnesium deficiency, some patients with coeliac sprue nevertheless show hypomagnesaemia.
2. The negative magnesium balance is caused by an abnormally large faecal magnesium loss.

3. Beside poor absorption of dietary magnesium, increased loss of endogenous magnesium contributes to the large faecal magnesium loss.
4. The degree of fat malabsorption seems to influence magnesium absorption, probably because unabsorbed fatty acids bind the magnesium ions to poorly soluble soaps.

7.8 HAEMATOPOIETIC FACTORS

7.8.1 Iron

7.8.1.1 Introduction

Anaemia is a common finding in coeliac patients (table 7.12). Gee's classical description (305) already makes mention of 'cachexia, a fault of sanguification, betokened by pallor and tendency to dropsy' as a constant symptom. This anemia can be hypochromic or megaloblastic. In more than 50% of cases, the same blood smear shows evidence of iron deficiency as well as of folic acid deficiency – a so-called dimorphous picture (405). We studied the

Table 7.12. Incidence of anaemia in untreated coeliac sprue.

AUTHORS	CRITERION		NUMBER OF PATIENTS INVESTIGATED	˙ PERCENTAGE WITH ANAEMIA
Buchan et al. (1962)	< 12 g%		39	64
Cooke et al. (1963)	< 11.5 g%		50	40
Benson et al. (1964)	< 14 g%		31	55
Ross et al. (1966a)	< 12 g%		not stated	43
Mortimer et al. (1968)	< 12 g%		9	44
Jarnum et al. (1970)	< 11 g%		10	60
Thys et al. (1971)	< 12 g%		9	33
Hoffbrand (1974)	< 11.5 g% (♀) < 13.5 g% (♂)		75 47	88 90
Cerf et al. (1975)	< 12 g% (♀) < 13 g% (♂)	} 37		54
Modigliani et al. (1975)	< 12 g%		47	55
Own series	< 7.9 mmole/l (♀) < 8.7 mmole/l (♂)	} 36		75

incidence of anaemia in the untreated patients of our series and attempted to analyse the nature of this anaemia as well as the cause of the deficiency in iron, folic acid or vitamin B_{12}.

7.8.1.2 Haemoglobin concentration

Anaemia was found in 78% of the total of 36 patients with untreated coeliac sprue, of whom 14 had recently received anti-anaemic therapy (fig. 7.35). Only two of these for anaemia treated patients had a normal haemoglobin concentration. A decreased haemoglobin concentration was as frequent in patients with severe as in those with less pronounced villous abnormalities in the jejunal biopsy specimen. A striking finding was the discrepancy between men and women; anaemia was present in virtually the men, but only in two-thirds of the women. In men, moreover, the degree of anaemia depended on the severity of the mucosal lesions.

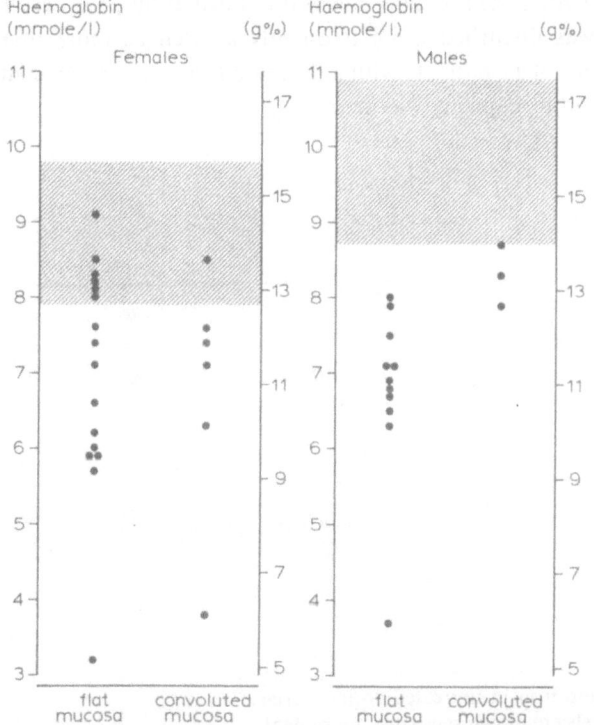

Fig. 7.35. Haemoglobin in untreated coeliac sprue. The haemoglobin concentrations are drawn separately for females and males, and for patients with a flat and with a convoluted jejunal mucosa. Statistical analysis (Mann-Whitney test) revealed no significant difference between both female groups, whereas in males a significant difference was found (p < 5%). The shaded area represents the range of normal values (cf. chapter 12).

7.8.1.3 Bone marrow study

In 21 patients, a sternal puncture was performed. In 9 cases the bone marrow showed megaloblastic characteristics, which in 5 cases were accompanied by signs of iron deficiency. In 5 of these 9 patients the serum folate concentration was determined, and found decreased in all; the serum vitamin B_{12} concentration was decreased in 2 of the 3 patients in whom it was determined. In the remaining 12 sternal punctates, evidence of iron deficiency was present in 3; 9 marrow smears were normal in all respects, although hypofolaemia was present in all patients and 2 out of 5 had a low serum vitamin B_{12}.

7.8.1.4 Serum iron concentration

The serum iron concentration was determined in 27 patients who had not previously received iron suppletion. It was found to be decreased in 41%. In patients with severe jejunal mucosal abnormalities, the serum iron concentration was disturbed more frequently as well as more markedly (fig. 7.36). In 2 out of 11 patients with a decreased serum iron concentration, the total iron-binding capacity was increased.

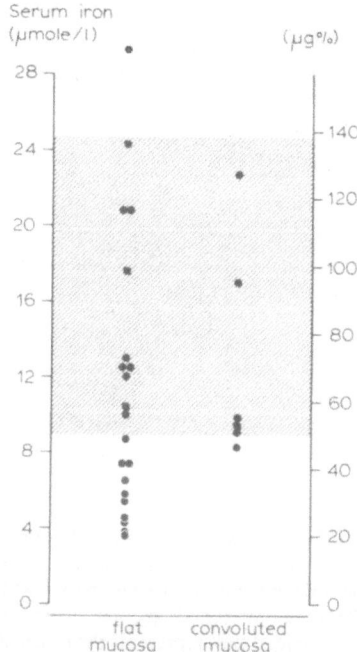

Fig. 7.36. Serum iron in untreated coeliac sprue. The serum levels are drawn separately for patients with a flat and with a convoluted jejunal mucosa. Statistical analysis (Mann-Whitney test) revealed no significant difference between both groups. The shaded area represents the range of normal values (cf. chapter 12).

7.8.1.5 Iron absorption

In 3 untreated coeliacs the iron absorption was measured with the aid of a whole-body counter after administration of a solution containing ^{59}Fe-labelled ferrous salt. The absorption was markedly decreased in 2 patients with an iron deficiency, and normal in 1 case without iron deficiency (table 7.13).

Table 7.13. Absorption of inorganic ^{59}Fe-ferrous iron in 4 coeliac patients.

PATIENT	HAEMO-GLOBIN (mmole/l)	SERUM IRON (μmole/l)	TOTAL IRON BINDING CAPACITY (μmole/l)	WHOLE BODY RETENTION OF ^{59}Fe (% of dose)	WEEKS ON GLUTEN-FREE DIET
# 9	4.9	1.4	78	N.D.	0
	6.2	5.4	69	84.0	2
# 10	7.5	1.4	79	1.4	0
	9.6	N.D.	N.D.	64.8	24
# 29	8.3	20.8	66	36.5	0
# 32	7.3	7.4	100	29.0	0
	7.0	N.D.	N.D.	94.6	6
Controls (♀) 7.9-9.8 (♂) 8.7-10.9		8.9-24.7	50-85	> 50%	

7.8.1.6 Effect of the gluten-free diet

The haemoglobin concentration increased in all patients after gluten withdrawal. Patients with severe anaemia generally also received iron, folic acid or vitamin B_{12} supplements, but even without suppletion the haemoglobin level rose (fig. 7.37).

The serum iron concentration also increased in the majority of patients. In 4 of the only 7 patients with iron deficiency, who received no iron supplements, a normal serum iron concentration was found after gluten withdrawal. In the 3 remaining cases the serum iron concentration showed no or hardly any increase, which was probably due to other causes.

In 3 patients, iron absorption was again determined after gluten withdrawal. It was found increased in all, including those whose absorption had previously impressed as being normal. As table 7.13 shows, iron absorption can sometimes improve very quickly.

7.8.1.7 Comment

Iron absorption in coeliac sprue has been studied by several investigators. The published data on this subject are rather variable, however. Badenoch

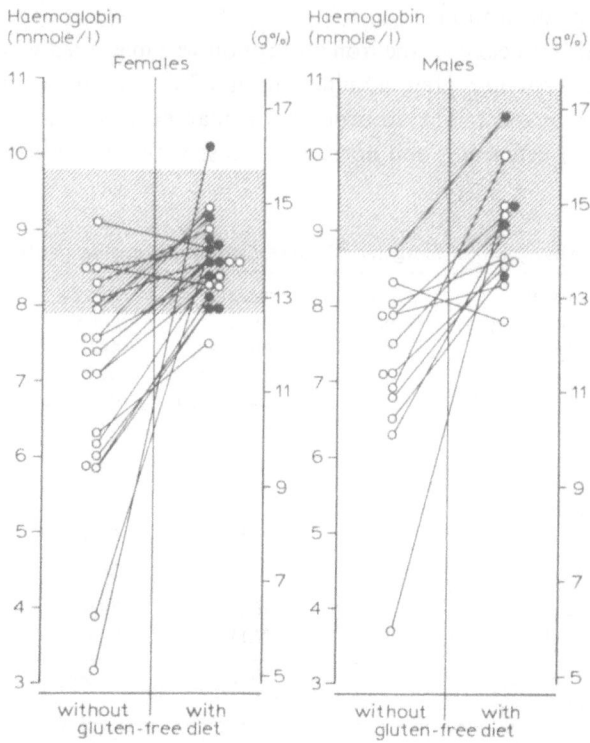

Fig. 7.37. Haemoglobin and gluten-free diet. The haemoglobin concentrations in corresponding patients before as well as during diet therapy are given. Statistical analysis (Wilcoxon signed-rank test) revealed a significant improvement on diet therapy ($p < 1\%$). The solid dots represent patients who received additional anti-anaemic therapy. The shaded area represents the range of normal values (cf. chapter 12).

et al. (34) found decreased ^{59}Fe absorption in all untreated patients with idiopathic steatorrhoea examined, regardless of whether they were or were not suffering from iron deficiency. The severity of the steatorrhoea, so far as predictable on the basis of the degree of diarrhoea, did not seem to make any difference either. According to Webb et al. (897), however, iron absorption is remarkably often normal in untreated coeliacs. Cooke (163) also regularly found normal absorption. A difficulty in the interpretation of these discrepant findings is that the presence or absence of (latent) iron deficiency is seldom explicitly mentioned, which is indispensable for correct evaluation of iron absorption (372).

It is an obvious assumption that iron absorption is disturbed specifically as a result of pathological changes in the epithelium of the proximal intestinal mucosa. The intraluminal phase of absorption is probably normal, although undegraded and unabsorbed food can influence iron solubility. These epithelial changes imply that, on the one hand, the absorptive surface is reduced (with the disappearance of villi and microvilli), while on the other hand the remaining enterocytes may be deficient in carriers for transport over the cell membrane. Intracellular iron transport as well as transfer to transferrin can be disturbed, moreover.

Coeliac patients are probably subject to an increased endogenous iron loss as well. This loss seems to be largely caused by increased exfoliation of enterocytes; a minor role can be played by increased enteric plasma leakage (179, 830).

As a result of reduced absorption and increased loss of iron, a deficiency develops. This is indicated by the decreased serum iron concentration in 41% of our patients. Other investigators have also regularly found low serum iron concentrations in coeliac sprue (table 7.14).

Table 7.14. Incidence of a low serum iron concentration in untreated coeliac sprue.

AUTHORS	CRITERION	NUMBER OF PATIENTS INVESTIGATED	PERCENTAGE WITH LOW SERUM IRON
Cooke et al. (1963)	$< 40 \ \mu g\%$	50	52
Benson et al. (1964)	$< 70 \ \mu g\%$	9	33
Ross et al. (1966a)	$< 70 \ \mu g\%$	42	24
Thys et al. (1971)	$< 60 \ \mu g\%$	9	67
Cerf et al. (1975)	$< 50 \ \mu g\%$	37	24
Modigliani et al. (1975)	$< 80 \ \mu g\%$	35	83
Own series	< 8.9 mmole/l	27	41

Iron absorption as a rule improves after gluten withdrawal, sometimes within a few weeks (table 7.13; 34, 163, 576). The rapid improvement of iron absorption is particularly impressive during corticosteroid medication (34).

As a result of improved iron absorption and decreased endogenous iron loss, the serum iron concentration increases (60) and the anaemia (if not due to other deficiencies) disappears (fig. 7.37).

7.8.1.8 Conclusions
1. The low serum iron level, present in many untreated coeliacs, is largely

due to decreased iron absorption, which fails to adjust itself to the existing iron deficiency.

2. The decreased iron absorption is presumably the result of mucosal lesions in the small intestine, which above all reduce the absorptive surface.
3. Increased endogenous iron loss via exfoliation of enterocytes and enteric leakage of extracellular fluid can aggravate the iron deficiency.
4. Iron absorption improves after gluten withdrawal and the endogenous iron loss normalizes. As a consequence the iron concentration in serum increases.

7.8.2 Vitamin B_{12}

7.8.2.1 Introduction

Megaloblastic anaemia is not uncommon in untreated coeliacs. It seemed of importance, therefore, to determine the serum vitamin B_{12} concentration. In addition the Schilling test was performed, as vitamin B_{12} absorption is reported to be often abnormal in coeliac sprue (table 7.15).

Table 7.15. Incidence of a decreased urinary *Co-vitamin B_{12} excretion in untreated coeliac sprue.

AUTHORS	CRITERION	NUMBER OF PATIENTS INVESTIGATED	PERCENTAGE WITH DECREASED *Co-VIT B_{12} EXCRETION
Cooke et al. (1963)	not stated	50	12
Benson et al. (1964)	$< 3.5\%/48$ hrs	7	43
Stewart et al. (1967)	$< 10\%/24$ hrs	11	82
Mann et al. (1970)	$< 7\%/24$ hrs	9	78
Thys et al. (1971)	not stated	6	67
Modigliani et al. (1975)	$< 8\%/24$ hrs	45	47
Own series	$< 15\%/48$ hrs	30	67

7.8.2.2 Serum vitamin B_{12} concentration

The serum vitamin B_{12} concentration was determined in a total of 10 coeliac patients who had not previously received vit B_{12} replacement. It was found to be decreased in 5 cases (fig. 7.38). Vitamin B_{12} absorption, how-

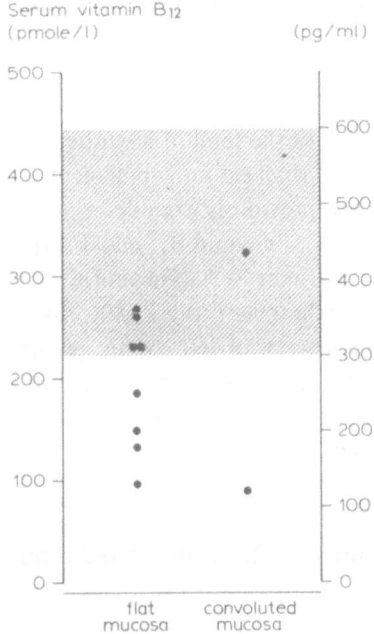

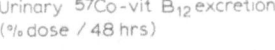

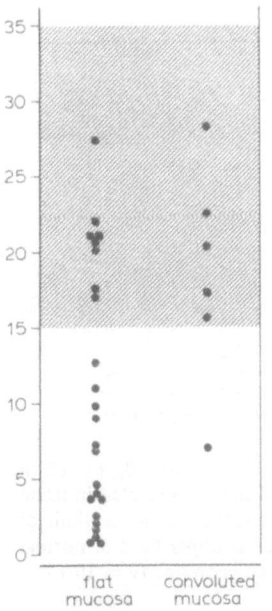

Fig. 7.38. Serum vitamin B_{12} in untreated coeliac sprue. The serum levels are drawn separately for patients with a flat and with a convoluted jejunal mucosa. The shaded area represents the range of normal values (cf. chapter 12).

Fig. 7.39. Schilling test in untreated coeliac sprue. The results of urinary ^{57}Co-vitamin B_{12} excretion are drawn separately for patients with a flat and with a convoluted jejunal mucosa. Statistical analysis (Mann-Whitney test) revealed no significant difference between both groups. The shaded area represents the range of normal values (cf. chapter 12).

167

ever, was normal in 3 of these 5 patients, which makes it difficult to explain the decreased serum vitamin B_{12} concentration.

7.8.2.3 Vitamin B_{12} absorption

Vitamin B_{12} absorption was decreased in 57% of the total of 30 untreated coeliacs (fig. 7.39). The majority of the patients received no supplement of 'intrinsic factor' because achlorhydria had been previously excluded.

No correlation was found between the severity of vitamin B_{12} malabsorption and the degree of steatorrhoea. However, increased indicanuria was more frequent in those with a disturbed Schilling test (fig. 7.40). In 2 patients the Schilling test was repeated after 1 week of tetracyclin, giving results which were not significantly different. The same applied to administration of pancreatic enzymes and bicarbonate, which likewise failed to improve vitamin B_{12} absorption in one patient.

7.8.2.4 Effect of the gluten-free diet

Vitamin B_{12} absorption nearly always improved after gluten withdrawal

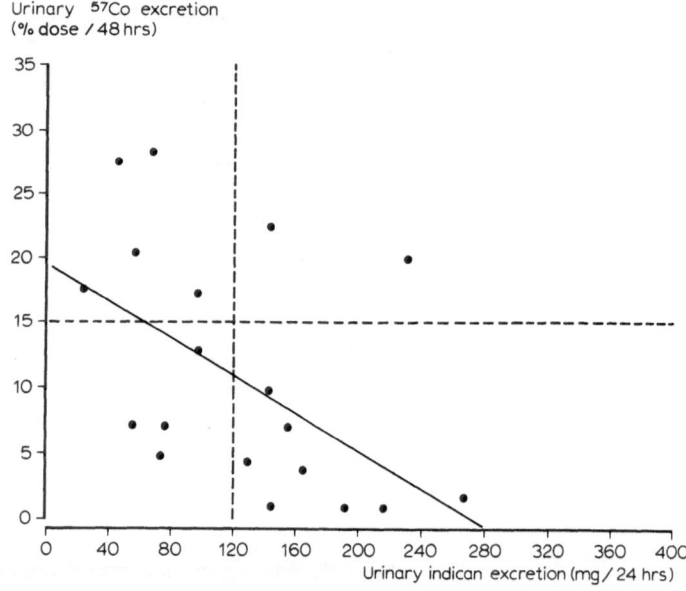

Fig. 7.40. Schilling test and indicanuria. The results of urinary ^{57}Co-vitamin B_{12} excretion of untreated coeliac patients are plotted against the amounts of indican excreted in urine of preceding or following days. The dotted horizontal line represents the lower limit of normal ^{57}Co-vitamin B_{12} excretion, and the dotted vertical line the upper limit of normal indican excretion. The straight diagonal line is the calculated regression line ($y = 19.75 - 0.07 x$; $r = -0.49$; $1\% < p < 2.5\%$).

168

(fig. 7.41). The figure does not show that the improvement occurred usually within 2-6 months; in other cases it was much more gradual and still abnormal 2 years after the institution of the diet. Marked disturbance of the Schilling test (less than 10% excretion in 48 hours) persisted in 5 patients. It was established by questioning that these patients did not properly observe the diet; this was confirmed by the finding of a flat mucosa in the jejunal biopsy specimen. In 61% of a total of 18 treated coeliacs a normal vitamin B_{12} absorption was observed (fig. 7.41).

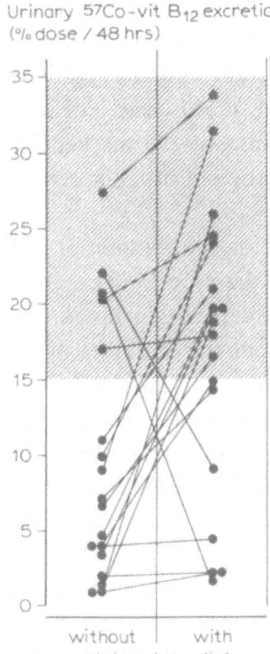

Fig. 7.41. Schilling test and gluten-free diet. The results of urinary ^{57}Co-vitamin B_{12} excretion in corresponding patients before as well as during diet therapy are given. Statistical analysis (Wilcoxon signed-rank test) revealed a significant improvement on diet therapy ($p < 1\%$). The shaded area represents the range of normal values (cf. chapter 12).

7.8.2.5 Comment

Although vitamin B_{12} deficiency which leads to megaloblastic anaemia or combined degeneration of the cord is rare in cocliac spruc (405), malabsorption of this vitamin is very frequently observed. In two-thirds of our patients we found a disturbed Schilling test, and this is in fair agreement with reports by other investigators (table 7.15). At first sight it may seem rather surprising that vitamin B_{12} absorption, which takes place in the ileum, is so often disturbed in a condition which usually involves only the proximal small intestine. In fact it is not easy to explain vitamin B_{12} malabsorption in coeliac sprue.

Gastric juice from coeliac patients contains an adequate amount of intrinsic factor (IF), as indicated also by the fact that vitamin B_{12} absorption does not improve after IF suppletion (160). Dietary vitamin B_{12} is normally attached to IF before it enters the small intestine. This complex formation with IF is thought to give the vitamin some protection from consumption or degradation by intestinal bacteria. Certain bacteria can nevertheless consume or degrade this vitamin (309, 760). The bacterial flora in the small intestine is regularly abnormal in untreated coeliacs (section 6.11), and in these patients consumption and degradation of vitamin B_{12} by bacteria can be a real problem. The correlation found between the presence of an abnormal bacterial flora and malabsorption of vitamin B_{12} is thereby explained (fig. 7.40). Bacteria which produce indole are generally found capable of binding vitamin B_{12} as well (823). Rosenberg et al. (716) clearly demonstrated the significance of an abnormal intestinal flora by the marked improvement in vitamin B_{12} absorption after administration of broad-spectrum antibiotics in an untreated coeliac patient.

There are several indications that the receptors for the vitamin B_{12}-IF complex in the ileum are readily damaged, and that the process of conjugation between receptor and complex occurs only under certain favourable circumstances. It is suspected that in various situations the receptors or the enterocytes in the ileum can be damaged so that normal vitamin B_{12} absorption is impossible (133, 457, 517, 662, 778, 852). In coeliac patients the enterocytes in the ileum may be damaged, for example, by unabsorbed food constituents, bacterial degradation products or the micro-organisms themselves. Moreover, there may be lesions in the ileal mucosa as a result of the coeliac sprue.

Stewart et al. (817) often found abnormally flat enterocytes in the distal and middle part of the ileum in coeliac patients. They found a significant correlation between the height of these cells and vitamin B_{12} absorption. Perhaps differences in enterocyte height are associated with abnormalities of the receptors or of the intracellular organelles.

Another possible explanation of vitamin B_{12} malabsorption lies in the hypothesis that the calcium and magnesium ions required for conjugation of the vitamin B_{12}-IF complex to the receptor (125), are not present in a free form because they are bound to unabsorbed fatty acids.

Although vitamin B_{12} malabsorption occurs in the majority of coeliac patients and the serum vitamin B_{12} concentration is regularly decreased (fig. 7.38; 104), megaloblastic anaemia based on vitamin B_{12} deficiency or a combined degeneration of the cord is observed only very sporadically (405, 656). This is explained by the fact that vitamin B_{12} absorption is usually less markedly disturbed and less protracted than in pernicious anaemia for example, so that vitamin B_{12} reserves remain adequate much longer (405, 525).

An abnormally high ^{57}Co-vitamin B_{12} absorption was found in none of our untreated coeliacs. This phenomenon has been observed by others, who attribute it to mucosal hyperplasia and enhanced absorption in the ileum (540).

7.8.2.6 Conclusions

1. The majority of untreated coeliac patients show moderate-to-marked vitamin B_{12} malabsorption.
2. Intrinsic factor (IF) deficiency cannot plausibly be held responsible for this finding.
3. Some of the vitamin B_{12}-IF complexes may be consumed or degraded by certain micro-organisms, as an abnormal intestinal flora is often present in coeliac sprue.
4. Unabsorbed nutrients, bacterial degradation products or the micro-organisms themselves perhaps interfere with the conjugation of the vitamin B_{12}-IF complex to the receptor in the ileum.
5. Although it is mainly in the proximal part of the small intestine that mucosal lesions occur in coeliac sprue, there may also be (usually slight) abnormalities of the enterocytes present in the distal ileum. These slight abnormalities may influence vitamin B_{12} absorption.
6. Although vitamin B_{12} malabsorption and a decreased serum vitamin B_{12} concentration are frequently observed in coeliacs, clinical symptoms of vitamin B_{12} deficiency are rare.

7.8.3 Folates

7.8.3.1 Introduction

Megaloblastic anaemia regularly develops in patients with coeliac sprue. This anaemia is usually a result of folate deficiency, and rarely due to vitamin B_{12} deficiency (section 7.8.2). Folate deficiency therefore seems to be a relatively common phenomenon in coeliac sprue. This deficiency can be manifested, not only as anaemia but also as glossitis or stomatitis aphthosa. In an effort to gain some insight into the incidence of folate deficiency, we measured the serum folate concentration in our group of untreated patients. In addition the effect of the gluten-free diet on the serum folate concentration was evaluated.

7.8.3.2 Serum folate concentration

The serum folate concentration was decreased in 91% of 22 untreated patients (fig. 7.42). In only two cases was a normal serum folate concentra-

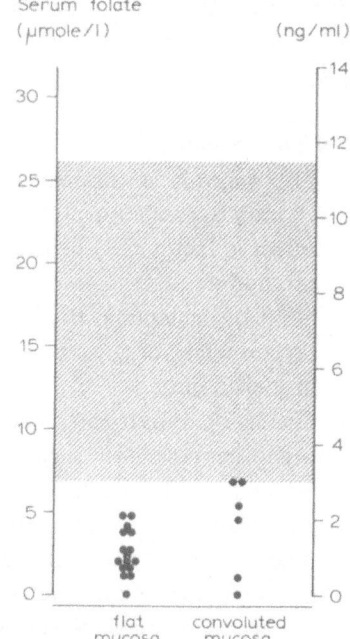

Fig. 7.42. Serum folate in untreated coeliac sprue. The serum levels are drawn separately for patients with a flat and with a convoluted jejunal mucosa. Statistical analysis (Mann-Whitney test) revealed no significant difference between both groups. The shaded area represents the range of normal values (cf. chapter 12).

tion found; both were patients with a convoluted mucosa in the jejunal biopsy specimen. The incidence or severity of hypofolaemia was not different in patients with a flat or with a convoluted jejunal mucosa. Anaemia existed in a total of 16 of the 20 patients with a decreased serum folate concentration.

7.8.3.3 Effect of the gluten-free diet

After gluten withdrawal the serum folate concentration increased in all patients, irrespective of folic acid replacement (fig. 7.43). The serum folate concentration became normal in 94% of the treated patients.

7.8.3.4 Comment

A decreased serum folate concentration was found in virtually all untreated coeliac patients (fig. 7.42). Other investigators also noticed a high incidence of hypofolaemia in coeliac sprue (table 7.16). This is not really surprising

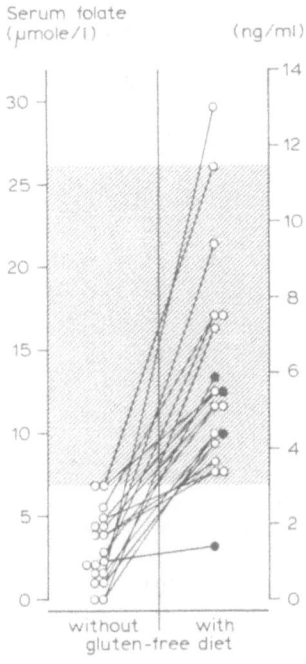

Serum folate
(µmole/l)   (ng/ml)

without   with
gluten-free diet

Fig. 7.43. Serum folate and gluten-free diet. The serum levels in corresponding patients before as well as during diet therapy are given. Statistical analysis (Wilcoxon signed-rank test) revealed a significant improvement on diet therapy (p < 1%). The solid dots represent patients who received temporarily folic acid replacement therapy. The shaded area represents the range of normal values (cf. chapter 12).

Table 7.16. Incidence of hypofolaemia in untreated coeliac sprue.

AUTHORS	CRITERION	NUMBER OF PATIENTS INVESTIGATED	PERCENTAGE WITH HYPO-FOLAEMIA
Brooks et al. (1966)	< 5 ng/ml	8	100
Cooke (1968)	not stated	51	96
Mortimer et al. (1968)	< 3 ng/ml	6	67
Hoffbrand (1974)	< 6 ng/ml	163	100
	< 3 ng/ml	163	86
Modigliani et al. (1975)	< 5 ng/ml	9	88
Own series	< 3 ng/ml	22	91

because folates can only be absorbed in the proximal part of the small intestine (380), where the mucosal lesions are most marked in coeliac sprue. The absorption of a dose of labelled or unlabelled folic acid (pteroylmonoglutamate) proves to be decreased in many coeliac patients (table 7.17).

173

Table 7.17. Incidence of an impaired folate absorption in untreated coeliac sprue.

AUTHORS	METHOD	CRITERION	NUMBER OF PATIENTS INVESTIGATED	PERCENTAGE WITH IMPAIRED ABSORPTION
Kinnear et al. (1973)	Urinary excretion of oral labelled folic acid	< mean-1 SD	8	88
		< mean-2 SD	8	50
Cooke et al. (1963)	Urinary excretion of oral versus i.m. folic acid	< 80%	33	97
	Serum folate after oral folic acid	< 40 ng/ml	15	100
Baker et al. (1964)	Serum folate after oral folic acid	< 40 ng/ml	7	100
Stewart et al. (1967)	Serum folate after oral folic acid	< 40 ng/ml	43	86
	Urinary excretion of oral labelled folic acid	< 30%/24 hrs	9	100
Modigliani et al. (1975)	Serum folate after oral folic acid	<40 ng/ml	23	100

The cause of folate malabsorption in coeliac sprue is still obscure. Perhaps the degradation of dietary polyglutamates to monoglutamate is decreased. However, a deficiency of the required enzyme conjugase (γ-glutamylcarboxy-peptidase) has never been demonstrated in jejunal biopsy specimens from coeliac patients. This is perhaps due to the fact that this enzyme is contained in the lysosomes and mitochondria, and not in the brush border of the entero-cytes (231, 402, 430). Nevertheless the observation of Hoffbrand et al. (402), who found that polyglutamate absorption can be disturbed in patients with normal monoglutamate absorption, suggests that polyglutamate degrada-tion is not always normal, and sometimes constitutes a limiting factor in folate absorption. Perhaps the enzyme is insufficiently effective due to interference with other substances in the intestinal lumen (63). Conjugase deficiency cannot be the only explanation, however, for monoglutamate ab-sorption is also disturbed in the majority of patients (table 7.17).

The reduced absorptive surface area of the jejunum due to loss of micro-villi and disappearance of villi can also play a role in folate malabsorption.

Some investigators observed a significant correlation between folate absorption and the severity of mucosal lesions (297, 480). This may be explained by a decreased attachment of folates to the epithelial surface (510), or a deficiency of transport carriers and of energy for active transport over the epithelial membrane (381). Even the transport from the enterocytes to the systemic circulation may be impaired (878). Baker et al. (35) observed that absorption of both monoglutamate and polyglutamate in coeliac patients improved after administration of an autoclaved extract of calf jejunum. This observation suggests that coeliac patients indeed have a deficiency of transport carriers or other, heat-resistant and therefore non-enzymatic substances.

The ability to convert monoglutamate in the enterocyte to a reduced and methylated form does not seem to be decreased in coeliac patients (430).

Although an abnormal bacterial flora in the small intestine usually causes increased endogenous folate synthesis and increased serum folate levels, some bacteria can in fact need folate for their metabolism. In the presence of such bacteria in the proximal jejunum, dietary folate can be consumed instead of being produced (48, 160, 404). In such cases monoglutamate absorption can improve after antibiotic medication (48).

Some other factors can conceivably also contribute to folate deficiency in coeliac patients. For example, folate requirements can be markedly increased, mainly due to an accelerated turnover of the intestinal epithelium (405). It is further not unthinkable that some coeliac patients use a diet deficient in folates because they think that raw vegetables and fruits are not readily digested by their diseased bowels.

Folate malabsorption improves after gluten withdrawal. This improvement is sometimes seen within 2 weeks, and after 6 months absorption is normal in virtually all patients (308, 478). As a result of improved absorption and disappearance of possible additional factors such as an abnormal flora in the small intestine, a deficient diet and increased folate requirements, the serum folate concentration increases (fig. 7.43).

7.8.3.5 Conclusions
1. A decreased serum folate concentration is found in nearly all untreated coeliac patients.
2. Absorption of monoglutamate as well as polyglutamate is reduced in the majority of patients.
3. Structural abnormalities of the proximal jejunum, as a result of which the absorptive surface area is decreased, seem to be an important determinant of folate malabsorption.

4. There may be a deficiency in transport carriers or energy suppliers for the active transport of folate.
5. There are no indications that conversion of monoglutamate to 5-methyl-tetrahydrofolate by the enterocytes is decreased.
6. Some dietary folate can be consumed by bacteria in the small intestine and therefore not be available for absorption.
7. The folate deficiency can be based in part on additional factors such as a deficient diet and increased requirements.
8. Folate absorption quickly improves after gluten withdrawal, and the serum folate concentration returns to normal within a few months.
9. Since the serum folate concentration is decreased in nearly all untreated coeliac patients, and practically always normalizes after gluten withdrawal, it seems to be a suitable parameter to verify both the effect and the observance of the gluten-free diet.

7.9 WATER-SOLUBLE VITAMINS

7.9.0 Introduction

Generally speaking, water-soluble vitamins are absorbed in the proximal part of the small intestine, probably by diffusion. In the case of lesions in this part of the small intestine, as for example in coeliac sprue, absorption may occur in the ileum also. Perfusion studies have shown that the capacity of only a small portion of the small intestine is sufficient to cover vitamin C requirements for example (635). Whether this also applies to vitamins of the B group, remains uncertain. Apart from malabsorption, other factors may play a role in the aetiology of a vitamin deficiency, such as the composition of the diet and the requirements for certain vitamins, which may be increased e.g. due to the accelerated turnover of the intestinal epithelium. Besides, it is possible that part of the amount of vitamin ingested does not become available for absorption due to bacterial consumption and degradation.

7.9.1 Vitamin C

The absorption of vitamin C (ascorbic acid) is normal to slightly decreased in the majority of untreated coeliac patients (816, 817). However, vitamin C deficiency is not rare, as indicated by the frequent finding of low serum concentrations, a low concentration of vitamin C in the leucocytes, and increased capillary fragility (919). In addition to low absorption, increased vitamin C requirements may play a role in this respect (919).

7.9.2 Thiamine

All untreated coeliac patients show decreased absorption of labelled thiamine (vitamin B_1). No correlation has been found between thiamine absorption and other absorption tests, or between thiamine absorption and the severity of villous abnormalities in the jejunal biopsy specimen (845). Beriberi has been observed in association with coeliac sprue (636). Thiamine absorption returns to normal after gluten withdrawal in all cases (845).

7.9.3 Riboflavin

There are no published data on the absorption of riboflavin (vitamin B_2) in patients with coeliac sprue.

7.9.4 Niacin

There are also no data on the absorption of niacin (vitamin B_3) in coeliac patients. Niacin deficiency has been described in patients with an abnormal bacterial flora in the small intestine, however (833), and is therefore not unthinkable in coeliac sprue.

7.9.5 Vitamin B_6

Decreased absorption of labelled vitamin B_6 (pyridoxine) is observed in about 50% of untreated coeliac patients (99, 817). There is no distinct correlation with other absorption tests or with the severity of villous abnormalities in the jejunal biopsy specimen (99). Most untreated coeliacs show a decreased serum vitamin B_6 concentration, but this returns to normal after gluten withdrawal (22). Sideroblastic anaemia has been described in association with coeliac sprue (198, 405).

7.9.6 Pantothenic acid

There are no data on pantothenic acid absorption in coeliac sprue. Pantothenic acid deficiency is not unthinkable in coeliac patients. According to Monro (603), some symptoms in untreated coeliac patients could be ascribed to pantothenic acid deficiency.

## CHAPTER 8

CLINICAL FEATURES

8.1 INTRODUCTION

The clinical features of coeliac sprue are hardly characteristic. Most symptoms result from the malabsorption caused by the diseased small intestine (861). The nature and severity of this malabsorption are largely determined by the extent of the intestinal lesions or, rather, by the capacity of the remaining unaffected intestine (647, 732, 817). Nevertheless, differences exist among individuals so that, given an apparently identical pathological substrate, some patients show megaloblastic anaemia whereas others suffer from osteomalacia (182).

The symptoms observed in coeliac patients are variable, and this is partly determined by the way the disease manifests itself. There are generally speaking three different types of onset. To begin with, mention should be made of the more or less acute intestinal catarrh, which usually causes the patient to report relatively quickly to his family doctor with complaints of diarrhoea, weight loss and malaise. An entirely different situation is encountered in the chronic form of the disease, in which symptoms of malabsorption are predominant. Owing to the insidious nature of the symptoms and the fact that some abnormalities are of long standing, the patient often tends to regard the symptoms as 'part of his life' or even as 'normal'. Not infrequently, the patient describes his pattern of defaecation and his stools as 'ordinary', although in fact they are far from normal. As a result, the patient sometimes postpones seeking medical advice until he is in very poor condition as a result of longstanding and marked malabsorption. In this form, the syndrome in adults differs widely from the clinical symptoms in children with coeliac sprue. It can also happen that the patient is troubled only by a single symptom – e.g. stomatitis, spontaneous fracture, increased bleeding tendency or anaemia – but at more detailed examination proves to suffer from several deficiencies. In the third category of patients attention is drawn to coeliac sprue more or less accidentally when they are examined because of dermatitis herpetiformis or in the context of a family study. In view of the above it is evident that the clinical picture and symptoms in patients with coeliac sprue can vary widely in nature and severity.

8.2 INCIDENCE OF THE VARIOUS SYMPTOMS

Before the nature of the various symptoms is discussed, it may be useful to consider their incidence. In our group of 36 untreated coeliac patients, of whom about two-thirds presented with (sub)acute intestinal symptoms and the remainder with deficiency symptoms (table 6.1), the incidence of the symptoms to be subsequently discussed was determined. The relevant data are presented in table 8.1. Our findings are largely in agreement with those reported by other investigators (53, 60, 104, 113, 160, 553, 601, 722). They can therefore be regarded as representative of the clinical syndrome of coeliac sprue as observed in a group of adult patients.

8.3 GENERAL COMPLAINTS AND SYMPTOMS

Malabsorption of nutrients and increased endogenous losses in coeliac patients lead to weight loss and in the long run even to emaciation. About one-third of our patients had a very low body weight, i.e. an obesity index according to Quetelet (476a), which was below the 2.5% limit of the Dutch population (694). In some cases the small stature of the patient – less than 164 cm for males and less than 154 cm for females (i.e. the 3% limit of the normal population (915)) – indicates that the malabsorption and losses must have existed already during the growth period. In patients under age 20 a small stature can still be based on retarded development, which can also be apparent from the bone age and the absence of secondary sex characteristics (525, 722). It is a well known fact that many coeliac patients are of small stature; in fact the condition has been jocularly described as 'jockey's disease' (33). Beside malabsorption and endogenous losses, other factors can play a role in weight loss. Anorexia, for example, is not uncommon (section 8.4), and bacterial degradation of food constituents in the small intestine can also be a factor. However, coeliac patients need not always be underweight. Some of them are in fact relatively obese (537, 553, 601). Several of our untreated patients had a Quetelet obesity index exceeding the 75% limit of the normal population (694).

When weighing these patients, one should ascertain that they are not suffering from oedema (60, 553, 723, 846) or ascites (489, 601), which could cause a flattered body weight. Oedema nearly always results from a decreased serum albumin concentration due to, among other things, an increased enteric protein loss (section 7.5). In rare cases they are an expression

179

Table 8.1. Complaints and symptoms in 36 untreated patients with coeliac sprue.

General complaints and symptoms	Number of patients
lassitude and malaise	29
weight loss	31
underweight*	9
overweight*	4
oedema	13
small stature*	4
(sub)febrile temperature*	8
nycturia	10
hypotension	0

Gastrointestinal tract

diarrhoea or frequent defaecation	27
(periodical) constipation	6
pale and pulpy stools	13
meteorism	11
borborygmi	18
flatulence	8
abdominal pain	16
anorexia	13
nausea or vomiting	8
hyperphagia	7
stomatitis aphthosa	7
glossitis	7
hepatomegaly	6

Haematopoiesis and coagulation

pallor	19
headache	10
dizziness	9
dyspnoea	11
haemorrhagic diathesis	5
Howell-Jolly bodies or target cells	8

Musculoskeletal system

skeletal deformities	9
(spontaneous) fractures	5
osseous pain	1
tetany	4

Skin, hair and nails

hyperpigmentation	13
dry and scaly skin	7
eczema	3

Table 8.1 (continued)

	Number of patients
dermatitis herpetiformis	4
loss of hair	5
psoriasis	1
watchglass nails	3
clubbing of fingertips	3
Reproductive functions	
delayed menarche	4 (out of 22 female patients)
secondary amenorrhoea	4 (out of 22 female patients)
abortion or miscarriage	6 (out of 15 pregnant patients)
infertility	5 (out of 32 married patients)
Nervous system	
gait disturbances	5
loss of reflexes	5
sensory loss	2
paraesthesiae	6

* for definition see text.

of a high output failure of the heart due to anaemia or in exceptional cases even to a thiamine deficiency (636).

In some patients the systolic blood pressure is low (i.e. lower than 100 mmHg) (60, 525, 861), for reasons which cannot be established with certainty. Some authors ascribe this to adrenocortical insufficiency (861).

We noticed that a fair number of patients had a slightly increased body temperature (i.e. a morning temperature higher than 37°C). Cooke et al. (159) noticed the same in patients with idiopathic steatorrhoea. In these patients we often also found severe anaemia, in association with which slight pyrexia is not uncommon (922).

Coeliac patients regularly suffer from nycturia, which can be so pronounced that the day-night rhythm is almost reversed. In spite of extensive investigations, this phenomenon has so far remained unexplained (389, 838, 839, 924).

8.4 GASTROINTESTINAL TRACT

As an affection of the small intestine, coeliac sprue of course causes mainly complaints about digestion. Stools are often abnormal, although some patients fail to notice this, probably because they have never passed normal stools. In the classical case, the stools are voluminous, loose, yellowish-grey, fatty and with a rancid odour. Due to the high fat content the stools do not readily wash away and have a pale colour, which is normalized after fat extraction (727). The fact that the stools float on water is largely due to the large amount of gas contained (515). This gas is partly produced by ferment-ation of undigested sugars (disaccharides). As a result, and especially be-cause of the large amounts of unabsorbed nutrients and water, the stools can be very voluminous. Nevertheless we noticed that the total weight of the daily production of faeces was usually not much increased (fig. 7.1). In the majority of our cases, moreover, the faeces did not show a typically steatorr-hoeic aspect. In no case was macroscopic blood observed. All in all, a normal appearance of the faeces is apparently compatible with the condition.

Peristalsis, sometimes visible in emaciated patients, can be either acce-lerated or retarded (section 6.2). Together with an increased amount of waste, rapid peristalsis gives rise to frequent, voluminous defaecation which can occur mostly at night (724). This acceleration of peristalsis, which may cause an explosive urge to defaecate, probably results from fermentation and the release of irritant substances such as bacterial degradation products of fat and carbohydrates, in addition to unabsorbed bile acids. The increased gas production due to this fermentation also explains other phenomena such as borborygmi, meteorism and flatulence. However, by no means all patients have accelerated peristalsis. In fact fluoroscopy often reveals de-layed passage (619). Some coeliac patients have an entirely normal pattern of defaecation or may even suffer from (periodical) constipation (256). Symptoms of paralytic ileus may be present in sporadic cases (fig. 6.3).

One can imagine that distension of loops of small and large intestine causes cramp-like abdominal pain. The complaints about abdominal pain in about 50% of patients (216, 553), however, need not always be caused by coeliac sprue. In some of our patients the pain was found to be due to other causes such as endometriosis, cholelithiasis, malrotation or abdominal angina. Palpation of the abdomen usually discloses no abnormalities. In some cases, however, the liver can be enlarged; this is often based on steatosis (233, 851).

As pointed out, weight loss is observed in many coeliac patients and anorexia, or even vomiting may be an additional factor in this respect (53, 60, 306). Perhaps some patients eat little for fear of increased ab-dominal pain or diarrhoea (338), or because they think that their bowels should be strained as little as possible. But eating can also be impeded by the presence of glossitis, stomatitis angularis (60) or stomatitis aphthosa 216, 271), which may be an expression of a deficiency in iron, folic acid, vitamin B_2 or vitamin B_{12} (53, 928). On the other hand, anorexia can be caused by an abnormal bacterial flora in the small intestine. Two of our coeliac patients with an abnormal intestinal flora continued to suffer from anorexia in spite of a gluten-free diet; the anorexia disappeared only after treatment with broad-spectrum antibiotics.

In some cases, on the other hand, patients show an excessive appetite (117, 745), although this is generally less extreme than the hyperphagia observed in patients with pancreatic insufficiency (352).

8.5 HAEMATOPOIESIS AND BLOOD COAGULATION

Anaemia is one of the most common abnormalities in coeliac sprue. Particularly clinics with a well-known interest in haematology report a high incidence of anaemia (53). Anaemia was also observed in many of our patients; it was found to be about equally often due to folic acid deficiency as to iron deficiency. Vitamin B_{12} deficiency was rarely observed, although vitamin B_{12} absorption was regularly disturbed (section 7.8.2). Symptoms of anaemia such as pallor, headache, dizziness or dyspnoea are quite common in coeliac sprue.

Due to malabsorption of the fat-soluble vitamin K, coagulation factors dependent on the presence of this vitamin may become deficient (e.g. factors II, VII, IX and X). In severe cases this may result in a haemorrhagic diathesis manifested by subcutaneous haemorrhages, epistaxis, haematuria and rectal or vaginal blood loss (265, 489, 724). A rare complication is the occurrence of retroperitoneal bleeding (33), or haemarthros (489). Purpura, which we observed on the lower legs of one of our female patients, may be a result of vitamin C deficiency. A characteristic feature in coeliac patients is a more or less marked atrophy of the spleen (405, 561). As a result of this atrophy, erythrocytes with nuclear remnants (Howell-Jolly bodies) or target cells circulate in the blood (265).

8.6 MUSCULOSKELETAL SYSTEM

The osseous abnormalities found in coeliac patients mainly result from vitamin D malabsorption. The increased calcium secretion in the proximal small intestine may play an additional role. Vitamin D deficiency in children

183

with coeliac sprue can give rise to the familiar features of rickets, e.g. frontal bossing, beading of the ribs and deformed extremities. Some adult patients still show residual symptoms. At a more advanced age, vitamin D deficiency causes osteomalacia. The patients sometimes complain of vague osseous pain low in the back or in the hips (60, 724), muscular weakness and disturbances of gait (113). The two symptoms last mentioned can also be based on a myopathy, which is not uncommon in these patients (70, 353). Physical examination sometimes reveals skeletal deformities, visible also on radiographs, along with pseudo-fractures (Looser-Milkman zones). The negative calcium balance (589) regularly leads to generalized osteoporosis which, together with osteomalacia, can give rise to compression fractures of the vertebrae or spontaneous fractures of the extremities (60). These complications as a rule do not occur unless severe disorders of mineralization have long been present; they are therefore not often observed.

Symptoms of secondary hyperparathyroidism, as a reaction to hypocalcaemia due to calcium loss, are occasionally observed (117). Probably as a result of this secondary hyperparathyroidism the plasma calcium concentration is less often decreased than might be expected, provided the calcium concentration measured is corrected for possible hypoproteinaemia (657). Nevertheless, symptoms of tetany (due either to hypocalcaemia or to a decreased serum magnesium concentration) are regularly observed in coeliac patients (60, 601, 723, 846).

8.7 SKIN, HAIR AND NAILS

Skin lesions are often observed in coeliac patients (60, 104). In such cases the skin is usually dry and rather scaly, sometimes to an extent which produces pellagra-like features. According to Wells (905) this is a false impression produced by a combination of increased desquamation and intensified pigmentation of the skin. Nicotinic acid deficiency is usually not involved (905).

Another common cutaneous abnormality in coeliac sprue is hyperpigmentation as a result of increased deposition of melanin in the skin. This hyperpigmentation can be either generalized (353, 601) or local; in the latter case the face may sometimes show the features of a so-called mask of pregnancy (127). The cause of this hyperpigmentation is still obscure. Trier (861) ascribed it to adrenocortical insufficiency, but no other investigator has so far confirmed the presence of such insufficiency. Moreover, similar hyperpigmentations are sometimes observed in cachectic or chronically undernourished patients in whom adrenal function is normal (115, 787). Increased desquamation of the skin is also observed in some cases of malnutrition, and is ascribed to deficiency in calories, proteins and essential fatty acids (905). It seems plausible that such deficiencies should also be held responsible for the skin lesions in patients with coeliac sprue (559).

Apart from eczema (294), many other skin diseases have been described in coeliac sprue, like acne rosacea (895) and psoriasis (163). The association is probably quite accidental. This does not apply, of course, to dermatitis herpetiformis which is generally known to be closely associated with coeliac sprue (section 10.2).

Complaints about loss of hair and brittle nails are not uncommon. The loss of hair can involve the scalp but also other areas such as the axillae, pubic region or extremities (745). In this respect, too, malnutrition is held responsible, while calcium deficiency cannot be excluded as a possible additional factor (905). There is no explanation for symptoms such as watch-glass nails or clubbing of fingertips (60, 216), although the latter can in some cases be due to hyperparathyroidism (698). Spooning of nails is thought to be indicative of iron deficiency (53). David et al. (193, 194) observed that, like the mucosal villi, the epidermal lines of the fingertips in untreated coeliac patients show atrophy, which is thought to improve after gluten withdrawal. The significance of their findings has been strongly doubted by others, however (572, 624).

8.8 REPRODUCTIVE FUNCTIONS

Women in poor general condition regularly show menstrual disorders. Complaints about irregular menstruation are therefore not uncommon in female coeliac patients. There may be secondary amenorrhoea which – as in the case of anorexia nervosa – disappears as the patient gains weight again. Delayed menarche or even primary amenorrhoea may also occur in coeliac patients (307); this may indicate, not only a poor general condition, but also delay of puberty due to retarded physical development (525). In addition to menstrual disorders, female coeliacs may suffer from miscarriages or infertility (447, 610), but these seem to show no correlation with the severity of malabsorption (53). The cause of this infertility is unknown, but deficiencies in vitamin B_1 or folic acid, may play a role in this respect (610).

In male coeliac patients, fertility can be reduced not only as a result of impotence but also due to abnormalities of the semen (37). That these are due to coeliac sprue is apparent from the improvement of the semen after gluten withdrawal (37).

8.9 NERVOUS SYSTEM

Several neurological abnormalities have been observed in coeliac patients (162, 611, 656). Most of these cases involve polyneuritis, but there are also reports on central system affections such as myelopathy and encephalomyelo-radiculopathy (162). The question, however, is whether the presence of these abnormalities is not often pure coincidence; particularly since the neuropathies sometimes do not develop or exacerbate until after gluten withdrawal (128, 162). As a rule the neurological lesions are ascribed to deficiency in vitamins of the B group. It is uncertain whether deficiencies in other vitamins or in certain amino acids also play a role in this respect (656). Development of a combined degeneration of the cord, however, is exceedingly rare in coeliac sprue (162, 656), although a low serum vitamin B_{12} concentration is regularly observed. The neurological symptoms are, as a rule, confined to slight reflex abnormalities and disorders of sensation. Besides, some patients complain of gait disturbances or paraesthesiae, which can in part be attributed to manifest calcium or magnesium deficiency (656). Complaints about night blindness are sometimes heard; this may result from vitamin A deficiency. Our own experience is that subjective complaints of night blindness could never be objectively confirmed.

8.10 PSYCHE

In descriptions of adult coeliac patients, notes on psychological peculiarities are regularly found (60, 104, 315). Some two-thirds of our own series of patients were described by the examining physician as excessively nervous, unstable, depressive or even hysterical. Some of them had in fact been treated by a psychiatrist before referral. The majority of these psychological disorders were probably a result of chronic fatigue, general malaise, abdominal symptoms or sterility problems. After disappearance of these symptoms as a result of gluten withdrawal, the majority of our patients proved to be quite sthenic and stable. There is a very real risk that, because a patient appears to be psychologically affected, his physical complaints are not taken seriously and interpreted as functional. In a retrospective study of all patients registered as suffering from functional abdominal disorders, Ross et al. (724) found coeliac sprue in 10% of cases!

186

CHAPTER 9

CLINICAL COURSE AND RESPONSE TO TREATMENT

9.1 SPONTANEOUS COURSE

Before dealing with the treatment of coeliac sprue, it may be useful to discuss briefly the natural history of the disease. This seems to be particularly important with a view to a more accurate assessment of the effect of the gluten-free diet.

Earlier experience has shown that children treated by a gluten-free diet during a number of years, can often later return to an unrestricted diet without suffering a relapse of symptoms. The impression was that a number of these young patients had 'outgrown' the disease, so to speak. Only a few children with coeliac sprue showed a relapse of symptoms after discontinuing the gluten-free diet, and were therefore forced to return to it (425, 776, 875).

Many patients who develop symptoms of coeliac sprue rather abruptly in adult life, are found to have already had symptoms of it in childhood. By questioning, we found that two-thirds of our group of adult patients had a

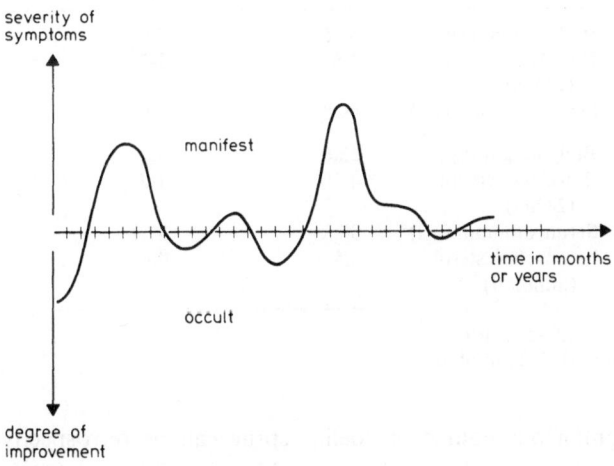

Fig. 9.1. Diagram of the variable spontaneous course of coeliac sprue, illustrating that periods with more or less severe symptoms alternate with symptom-free intervals.

187

childhood history indicative of the disease. The majority reported that they had regularly had symptoms as a child on an unrestricted diet, mostly until puberty. A symptom-free interval had usually followed – a phenomenon commonly known as 'teen-age remission' (53). This remission can persist throughout the teens. In female patients the symptoms can recur with pregnancy (776). It is also possible that coeliac sprue does not become manifest again until in late life, during the fifth or sixth decade.

It is a remarkable phenomenon that the majority of children with coeliac sprue can return to a normal diet after some time without developing symptoms. Some adult coeliacs also acquire a gluten tolerance. Several of our patients who interrupted the regimen for varying periods of time, experienced no subjective (and sometimes even no objective) untoward consequences. Untreated patients may show a very variable course of the disease, in which periods with more or less severe symptoms alternate with symptom-free intervals (fig. 9.1). This is clearly illustrated by the spontaneous improvement seen in two of our patients before a biopsy of the small intestine had confirmed the diagnosis (table 9.1).

Table 9.1. Spontaneous improvement in coeliac sprue. Observations in 2 untreated coeliac patients.

PATIENT	PARAMETER	AT FIRST EXAMINATION	JUST BEFORE DIET TREATMENT	TIME INTERVAL IN WEEKS
# 31	Body weight (kg)	59.5	62.2	27
	Bowel movements (24 hrs)	4-6	1-2	
	Serum albumin (g/l)*	44.8	50.5	
# 35	Body weight (kg)	53.6	59	14
	Bowel movements (24 hrs)	4-10	1-2	
	Serum albumin (g/l)*	37.8	47.1	
	Serum cholesterol (mmole/l)**	3.5	4.8	

* controls: 45.8 - 55.1 g/l
** controls: 4.0 - 7.2 mmole/l

The spontaneous course of coeliac sprue can be retrospectively reconstructed on the basis of data from case histories. By way of illustration we have done this for two of our patients (figs. 9.2 and 9.3). Figure 9.2 clearly shows the characteristic teen-age remission, which is almost entirely absent in

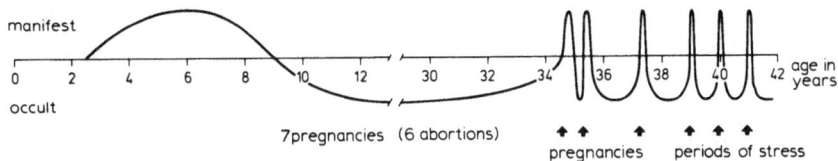

7pregnancies (6 abortions)

pregnancies   periods of stress

Fig. 9.2. Characteristic profile of coeliac sprue in a 41-year-old female patient with a history of diarrhoea and retardation of growth at the age of 26 months (reflected in her present height of 1.53m).The symptoms disappeared spontaneously at age 9, but severe diarrhoea returned when she was 34 years old, during the 8th pregnancy which led to an abortion. Of the 7 preceding pregnancies 6 had also resulted in an abortion. The next conception, after which she used a gluten-free diet, led to normal childbirth. Gluten withdrawal, prescribed on the basis of a flat jejunal biopsy, led to a normal serum concentration of albumin (54.1 g/l, from 41.1 g/l), folate (5 ng/ml, from 1.3 ng/ml) and cholesterol (5.7 mmole/l, from 3.4 mmole/l) and an improved D-xylose test (3.1 g/5 hrs, from 1.0 g/ 5 hrs). Although no longer observing dietary restrictions she is usually free of symptoms, apart from brief periods coinciding with seasonal stress in her job. She further shows normal biochemical parameters, apart from a decreased serum folate concentration (2.2 ng/ml) and a low D-xylose excretion (3.8 g/5 hrs).

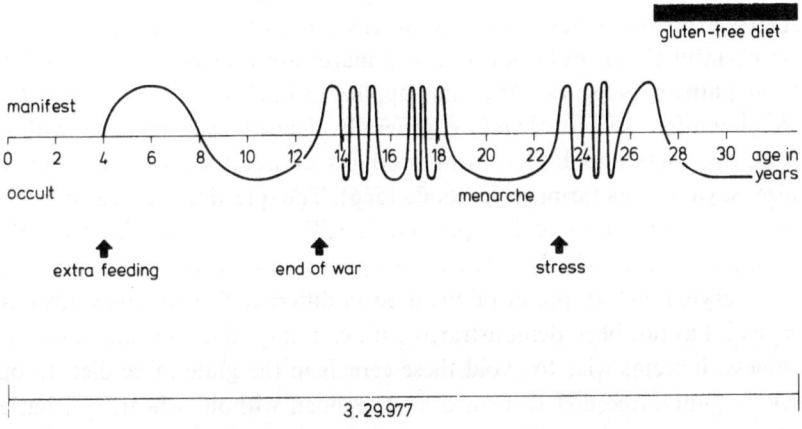

gluten-free diet

extra feeding   end of war   stress

3. 29.977

Fig. 9.3. Profile of the spontaneous course of coeliac sprue in a 44-year-old female patient, prior to gluten withdrawal. Abdominal symptoms had developed at age 4, when she had received extra feeding in view of underweight. The symptoms disappeared after a few years, and returned shortly after World War II. After a few years of varying abdominal symptoms, injections of liver extract were given at age 18, whereupon her general condition showed marked improvement and the menarche occurred. After a remission of about 5 years periodical diarrhoea recurred, but it was not until a few years later that this was interpreted as a symptom of coeliac sprue. Gluten withdrawal was prescribed on the basis of a flat mucosa in a jejunal biopsy specimen, whereupon the symptoms disappeared. The body weight increased by about 6 kg, and absorption of fat and D-xylose became normal.

189

figure 9.3. In both figures the erratic course of the disease – if untreated – is evident. The course of coeliac sprue may be different, however, varying from entirely asymptomatic to one without the slightest remission. For some patients this meant that they were in very poor health until their condition was properly diagnosed or until the gluten-free diet became known as the proper way of treatment. In the past, the prognosis for children with coeliac sprue was somewhat poor, as demonstrated by a death rate which ranged from 10% (660) to 30% (362).

9.2 TREATMENT BY THE GLUTEN-FREE DIET

9.2.1 Nature of the diet

The various diets in use before 1950 had in common that they were rather one-sided due to marked restrictions in the number of food constituents permitted (261, 346, 423, 749, 776). A turning-point in the treatment of coeliac sprue was reached in 1950, when Dicke (208, 209) published his observations on the noxious effect of gluten. Clinical experiments showed that the syndrome responded favourably to withdrawal of wheat, rye and oats from the diet. A few years later it was demonstrated that barley is likewise harmful (734). Potatoes, rice and maize are always tolerated well by coeliac patients (453), and the same applies to buckwheat and millet (586).

A gluten-free diet is therefore generally defined as a regimen without wheat, rye, oats and barley, with products of potatoes, rice, buckwheat, maize, soya, etc. as farinaceous foods (586). The question whether oats and barley are harmful to coeliac patients is still controversial, however (23, 39, 217, 453, 454, 734). Differences of opinion in this respect are apparent in the varying dietary prescriptions used in different British clinics (39). As long as it has not been demonstrated with certainty that oats and barley are harmless, it seems wise to avoid these cereals in the gluten-free diet. In our clinic, a gluten-free diet is defined as a regimen without wheat, rye, barley *and* oats.

It is to be noted – by the way – that the designation 'gluten-free' is actually a misnomer. The noxious influence of wheat and rye is based on a fraction of gluten called α-gliadin (section 2.2). The harmful protein fraction in oats and barley has a slightly different composition and a different name, e.g. avenin (oats) or hordein (barley) (38, 39). However, it seems advisable to maintain the customary designation 'gluten-free' for the time being, as long as the causative factor is not exactly known.

9.2.2 Adherence to the diet

Of the 47 coeliac patients who are under our care or have been treated by us, 43 were placed on a gluten-free diet (fig. 6.1). In a few of these patients the ultimate effect of this diet could not be evaluated, as 3 patients were simultaneously suffering from some other affection, such as ulcerative colitis, diverticulosis of the small intestine, or pancreatic carcinoma. The symptoms and lesions found in these 3 patients could not be properly interpreted, therefore. One patient was suffering from non-granulomatous duodenojejunitis (section 11.2). There remained 39 patients, in whom the effect of diet treatment could be evaluated. Within this group of patients, a distinction was made between those who stated that they had strictly adhered to the prescribed diet, those who admitted some occasional negligence, and patients who consumed regularly some gluten. The three groups thus formed consisted of:

22 patients thought to adhere strictly to the diet;

 8 patients thought to adhere well to the diet;

 9 patients thought to adhere poorly to the diet.

Comment

When dividing the patients into categories of strict, adequate or poor observance of the diet, one is forced to rely largely on the patients' statements. No reliable method has so far been developed to verify whether a patient adheres to the diet, or not. Methods recommended for this purpose, such as the D-xylose test (713), lactulose test (183), folic acid tolerance test (695) or screening for anti-gluten antibodies (837), are inadequate (36, 786). Yet the need for such verification is obvious to anyone who is evaluating the effect of treatment in coeliac sprue. It is only too often found that a patient who hardly responds to a 'gluten-free' diet at home, rapidly improves under clinical supervision. Some patients do not admit, moreover, to having partly or totally neglected dietary rules until after the occurrence of a severe relapse, a 'good' doctor-patient relationship notwithstanding. Finally there are some coeliacs who – in good faith – consume small amounts of gluten because many processed foods contain gluten which cannot be identified from the list of ingredients printed on the wrappers. It is the experience of some investigators that it is useful to have a dietician in attendance at the out-patient clinic for coeliac patients or to let her do domiciliary visits (36, 818). As long as it is uncertain which patients observe the diet strictly, and which do so only moderately well, it is impossible to evaluate the effect of gluten withdrawal on the clinical, biochemical and morphological abnormalities properly.

9.2.3 Effect on clinical symptoms

The effect of the gluten-free diet on the clinical symptoms in coeliac sprue partly depends on the clinical syndrome shown by the patient before gluten withdrawal. Those who were suffering from more or less acute intestinal catarrh, usually showed rapid improvement: the diarrhoea, abdominal cramps, nausea, flatulence and meteorism as a rule disappeared within a few days, while the appetite improved and the body weight increased. Those who had a chronic malabsorption syndrome with osteomalacia, megaloblastic anaemia or hypoproteinaemic oedema, usually showed gradual improvement, which became manifest after 1-4 months in the case of anaemia or oedema, but could take much longer in osteomalacia. Only glossitis or stomatitis aphthosa disappeared very quickly.

A difficulty in the evaluation of the effect of gluten withdrawal on the

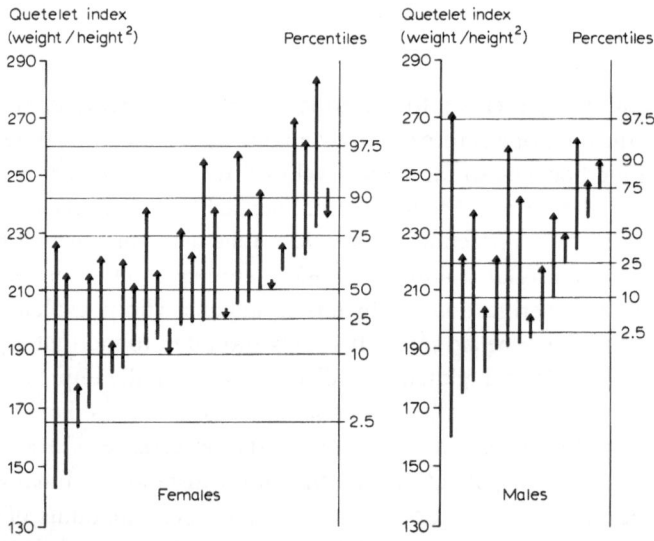

Fig. 9.4. Effect of the gluten-free diet on the body weight in coeliac sprue. The body weight is expressed by the Quetelet index (weight in hectograms, divided by height in metres; 176a, 177) as well as by the weight percentiles applying to the normal Dutch population (694). Each arrow represents one patient. A weight gain is symbolized by an arrow turned upwards, a weight loss by an inverted arrow. Statistical analysis (Wilcoxon signed-rank test) revealed a significant improvement on diet therapy ($p < 1\%$).

clinical symptoms is that it is uncertain which criteria should be applied. For patients who previously presented with symptoms of an intestinal catarrh, normalization of the defaecation or an increase in body weight, could be used as criterion. All our patients who had suffered from frequent defaecation or loose stools prior to gluten withdrawal, ultimately resumed a normal pattern of defaecation. Six patients actually developed a more or less marked form of constipation, which could usually be controlled by a cellulose-rich diet. One of these patients occasionally used a slice of ordinary bread by way of laxative. A weight gain was recorded in 35 of the 39 patients (fig. 9.4). In the majority of cases the weight gain was pronounced, and in fact 15 patients became obese. Two female patients discontinued the gluten-free diet for this reason, and 4 patients were placed on a weight-reducing diet.

The effect of gluten withdrawal was also very good and rapid in patients with symptoms resulting from anaemia, stomatitis or tetany. Many of the patients complaining of chronic fatigue or abdominal pain, however, continued to do so. On the basis of the initial symptoms, the ultimate clinical result was subjectively disappointing for 13 of the 39 patients, even though the majority of these 13 showed unmistakable improvement in biochemical parameters. In terms of the impression of the attending physician, however, the clinical effect of the gluten-free diet can be different from the patients view (table 9.2). It was a striking finding that the effect on clinical symptoms was moderate in several patients who stated a strict adherence to the

Table 9.2. Effect of diet treatment on clinical symptoms, as assessed by the attending physician.

	MARKED IMPROVE- MENT	SOME IMPROVE- MENT	NO IMPROVE- MENT
STRICT DIET	16 patients	5 patients	1 patient
RATHER STRICT DIET	7 patients	–	1 patient
NO STRICT DIET	4 patients	3 patients	2 patients

diet. There was actually little difference from the group of patients who occasionally 'sinned'. The results were evidently less good in those who neglected the dietary dictates. Some of these latter patients accounted for their carelessness because no improvement of symptoms had been experienced.

Evaluation of the clinical effect of the gluten-free diet is a subjective matter, both for the patient and for the physician. It is difficult to compare the results reported by the various investigators as a result of differences in their patients' age, condition and degree of cooperation. A study of the literature revealed that the majority of investigators found clinical improvement in 100% of their patients (60, 105, 113, 218, 803). We observed a favourable effect of gluten withdrawal in 92% of our patients which is in agreement with reports published by Cooke et al. (160), Ruffin (739), Modigliani et al. (601), and Cerf et al. (128). The only investigators to report much less favourable results were Shiner (780) and Pink et al. (682), who observed improvement in only 77% and 70% of their patients, respectively. The latter included, however, patients with associated pancreatic lesions, and refractory sprue, which explains their moderately succesful results.

9.2.4 *Effect on biochemical parameters*

It can be stated that in general biochemical abnormalities improve after gluten withdrawal. The effect of the gluten-free diet on the individual biochemical parameters was discussed in chapter 7.

In an effort to gain an impression of the ultimate and over-all effect of the gluten-free diet, we determined in the various categories of patients whether certain biochemical parameters were normalized after gluten withdrawal for a period of 6 months to 19 years (mean duration: 7 years). We focused on the parameters which in the same group of patients were most frequently disturbed prior to gluten withdrawal (fig. 10.1.c). Only the most recent biochemical findings were recorded, which in some cases differed markedly from the best results ever observed in them (fig. 9.5). A study of the data in this figure leads to the conclusion that patients who supposedly strictly observed the diet showed fewer abnormalities in vitamin B_{12} absorption, whereas all other biochemical parameters showed no differences between the 3 categories of patients on statistical analysis (Kruskal-Wall is test; 492a).

Comparison of own results with those of other investigators is not easier for the biochemical parameters than for the clinical symptoms. This is due, not to lack of suitable criteria but to the impossibility of obtaining informa-

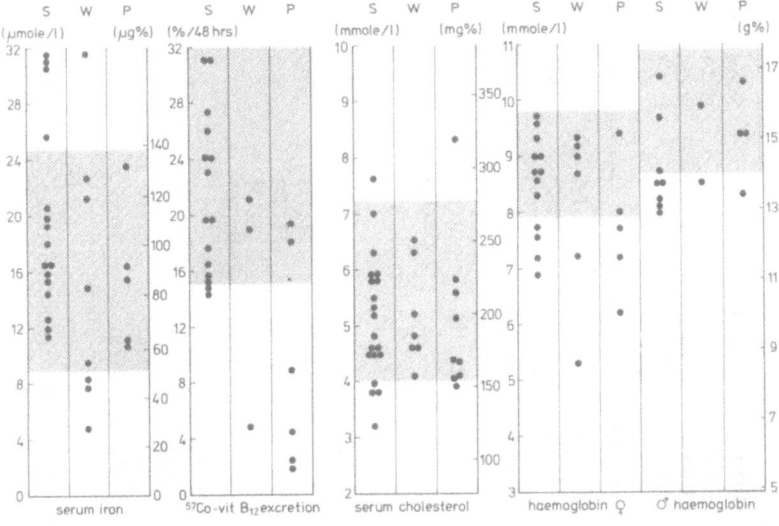

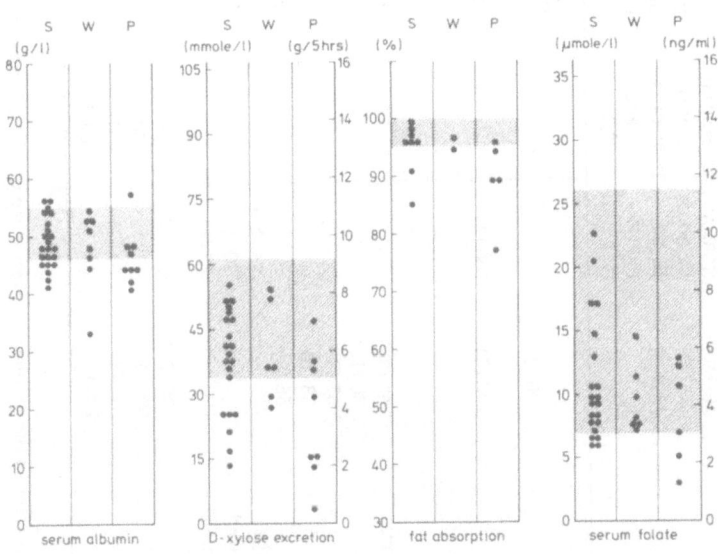

Fig. 9.5. Diagram of the effect of gluten withdrawal on biochemical parameters in coeliac sprue. As parameters were chosen the most frequently disturbed tests prior to gluten withdrawal (fig. 10.1.c). The most recent test results were recorded of patients who supposedly adhered strict (column S), well (column W) or poorly (column P) to the gluten-free diet.

195

Table 9.3. Effect of diet treatment on biochemical parameters.

AUTHORS	NORMAL SERUM IRON (%)	NORMAL ^{57}Co-VIT B_{12} EXCRETION (%)	NORMAL SERUM CHOLESTEROL (%)	NORMAL HAEMOGLOBIN (%)	NORMAL SERUM ALBUMIN (%)	NORMAL D-XYLOSE EXCRETION (%)	NORMAL FAT ABSORPTION (%)	NORMAL SERUM FOLATE (%)
Buchan et al. (1962)				100 (16)	100 (36)		84 (19)	
Cooke et al. (1963)	90 (20)			90 (20)	32 (19)	62 (8)	50 (10)	(33 12)
Shiner (1963)							47 (17)	
Benson et al. (1964)	100 (2)	100 (2)		89 (26)	100 (25)			
strict adherence						40 (15)	38 (24)	
poor adherence						48 (23)	82 (11)	
Bolt et al. (1964)						80 (10)	0 (13)	
Dissanayake et al. (1974)						23 (13)	58 (12)	
strict adherence	67 (30)			95 (37)				97 (29)
good adherence	80 (15)			100 (18)				100 (14)
poor adherence	67 (9)			92 (12)				100 (10)
Cerf et al. (1975)	33 (6)			86 (7)		14 (7)	29 (17)	80 (5)
Modigliani et al. (1975)	56 (9)	76 (21)		60 (20)		58 (26)	57 (28)	50 (6)
muc. morph. improved		80 (15)				65 (20)	72 (18)	
muc. morph. unaltered		67 (6)				33 (6)	30 (10)	
Own series	90 (29)	58 (24)	86 (36)	58 (38)	67 (39)	63 (35)	53 (15)	82 (34)
strict adherence	100 (16)	67 (15)	80 (20)	57 (21)	73 (22)	71 (21)	75 (8)	81 (21)
good adherence	63 (8)	67 (3)	100 (7)	63 (8)	75 (8)	67 (6)	50 (2)	100 (7)
poor adherence	100 (5)	33 (6)	89 (9)	56 (9)	44 (9)	38 (8)	20 (5)	67 (6)

NOTE:
The figures in brackets refer to the number of investigated patients. The various criteria for normal values are listed in tables 7.3, 7.6, 7.7, 7.12, 7.14, 7.15 and 7.16.

tion on the composition of their groups of patients and the supervision of diet observance. It hardly needs to be pointed out that patients with a long-standing severe malabsorption syndrome show a less rapid normalization of biochemical parameters than those whose condition was diagnosed soon after the onset of. symptoms. Normalization of blood chemistry is largely dependent on the suppletion of possible deficiencies. Virtually no author indicates how many patients in his series received supplements of vitamin B_{12}, folic acid, vitamin D, calcium or iron, which interferes with a correct interpretation of the great variances in published results (table 9.3).

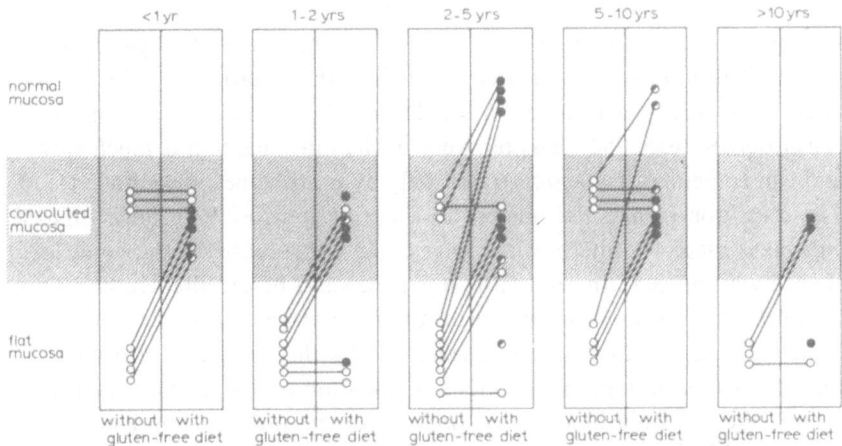

Fig. 9.6. Diagram of the effect of gluten withdrawal on the villous morphology in coeliac sprue. The stereomicroscopic aspect of mucosal biopsies from the proximal jejunum in 36 corresponding patients before as well as during diet therapy is recorded. Besides the villous morphology of 3 patients without pre-treatment biopsies is given. The different columns refer to various periods of diet treatment.

9.2.5 Effect on mucosal morphology

In all our patients, a repeat biopsy was obtained from the proximal jejunum, in between 3 months and 15 years after gluten withdrawal. In the vast majority of cases (i.e. in 24 of the 39 patients) this was performed after more than 2 years on a gluten-free diet (fig. 9.6). In a number of patients only one single biopsy specimen was obtained, while during the past 7 years multiple repeat biopsies were taken, going beyond the proximal jejunal loop. In all cases, however, the effect of the diet was evaluated on the basis of the specimen from the first jejunal loop, 10-20 cm beyond the ligament of Treitz.

As fig. 9.6 indicates, normal villi were rarely observed in the biopsy specimens, although in the majority of cases the diet had reportedly been strictly observed for over 2 years. In none of the patients who had been rebiopsied within 2 years had the mucosa resumed normal features. Another remarkable fact was that some of the patients who conceded small diet infringements showed a completely normal mucosa in the repeat biopsy specimen, whereas others showed a flat mucosa after supposedly strict observance of the diet for over 10 years.

Comment

Lesions of the intestinal mucosa gradually ameliorate after gluten withdrawal. This improvement is first apparent in the enterocytes. Within a few days, the enterocytes resume a normal intracellular structure and an intact brush border (655, 782). The recovery of the intestinal villi is much slower and can sometimes be demonstrated only by morphometric methods (135). The transition from a flat mucosa to a normal mucosa with finger-shaped villi takes place via intermediate stages, like convolutions, ridges and leaf-shaped villi (fig. 3.5). In some cases it may be years before all these stages are completed and the intestinal mucosa looks normal again (818).

Actually, it is rather incomprehensible why the complete restoration of the villous morphology takes so long. If the food no longer contained toxic agents, then it could be expected (in view of the rapid turnover of the intestinal epithelium) that the mucosa should return to normal within a few days to weeks. In-vitro culturing of flat jejunal biopsy specimens of untreated coeliac patients, showed incipient formation of villi within 48-72 hours (446, 862). According to Jos et al. (446), certain other noxious factors delay or prevent restoration of the mucosa in coeliac patients, such as incompletely degraded nutrients which as a result of the increased permeability of the epithelium enter the intestinal mucosa. It has also been suggested that local immunological factors impede rapid restoration of the mucosa (260).

It is customary to verify the effect of the gluten-free diet by taking a repeat biopsy specimen from the jejunal mucosa in all patients. As with the initial biopsy specimen on which the diagnosis was based, the secondary specimen is usually taken slightly distal to the ligament of Treitz. It is quite possible, however, that this is not the most suitable site for a control biopsy, as the mucosal abnormalities at this level disappear last of all, long after more distal intestinal loops have already become normal (734, 817). Perhaps even more important is the fact that the initial lesion can have been so severe that no restitutio ad integrum is possible (737). More exact information can be obtained by performing multiple biopsies, preferably also from more distal intestinal loops. It can thus be established whether the lesions have become less extensive (218, 737). The effect of gluten withdrawal can also be determined on the basis of a single biopsy specimen from the first jejunal loop, provided one pays special attention to the morphology of the individual enterocytes (818).

We personally observed an entirely normal villous pattern in only 6 out of 39 repeat biopsies. The majority of publications on the effect of the gluten-free diet on the mucosal morphology indicate unchanged, or still severe lesions of the proximal jejunal mucosa in a substantial number of patients (37, 60, 82, 113, 128, 160). This may well be a result of poor observance of the diet, as Dissanayake et al. (218) observed a normal jejunal mucosa in 16 of a total of 18 patients on a strict gluten-free diet.

The question whether or not complete morphological restoration always occurs after gluten withdrawal probably remains controversial as long as it is impossible to ascertain strict observance of the prescribed diet. In practice, however, it seems sufficient to require only improvement rather than normalization of the morphology for verification of the diagnosis 'coeliac sprue' (30).

9.3 ADDITIONAL MEASURES

9.3.1 Further dietary restrictions

Patients with coeliac sprue are regularly suffering from lactose intolerance. In our own series, the lactose tolerance test revealed evidence of intolerance in 4 untreated patients. As such this is not surprising, because the mucosal damage may lead to lactase deficiency (section 7.3). It is advisable to permit little or no milk in the early phase of treatment as it may cause abdominal symptoms in some patients; even long after the institution of the gluten-free diet lactose may not be tolerated (26, 152, 160, 907).

Restriction of the use of other disaccharides such as sucrose or maltose has been recommended for juvenile coeliac patients (26, 148), but seems unnecessary for adults.

Cooke's observation (163) that in exceptional cases the diarrhoea did not disappear until after abstinence from eggs, has not so far been corroborated by others.

Some investigators recommend restriction of the amount of fat in the diet, particularly for children (818). There are some theoretical arguments in favour of this. As the fat absorption is usually still disturbed in patients recently placed on a gluten-free diet, part of the non-absorbed dietary fat may enter the colon, where it is degraded by bacteria to, among other things, volatile fatty acids. These fatty acids can cause an increased frequency of defaecation. On the basis of practical experience, however, we do not believe that fat restriction is often indicated. In only one exceptional case were we forced to prescribe a low-fat diet, as the following case history shows.

Patient no. 17 (fig. 9.6) had complained of abdominal pain and lassitude throughout her childhood. At age 40 she was referred for cachexia (body weight 46 kg, height 1.73 m) and severe megaloblastic anaemia (haemoglobin 3.2 mmole/1) as a result of folate deficiency. Coeliac sprue was diagnosed on clinical grounds and an obvious improvement was seen after gluten withdrawal and folic acid suppletion. The body weight increased by 20 kg, and the serum haemoglobin, albumin and fat absorption became normal. After 8 months the diet was discontinued at the patient's request. About a year later her condition was found to have seriously deteriorated. She had lost 5 kg body weight, showed hypoalbuminaemia (28.7 g/l)

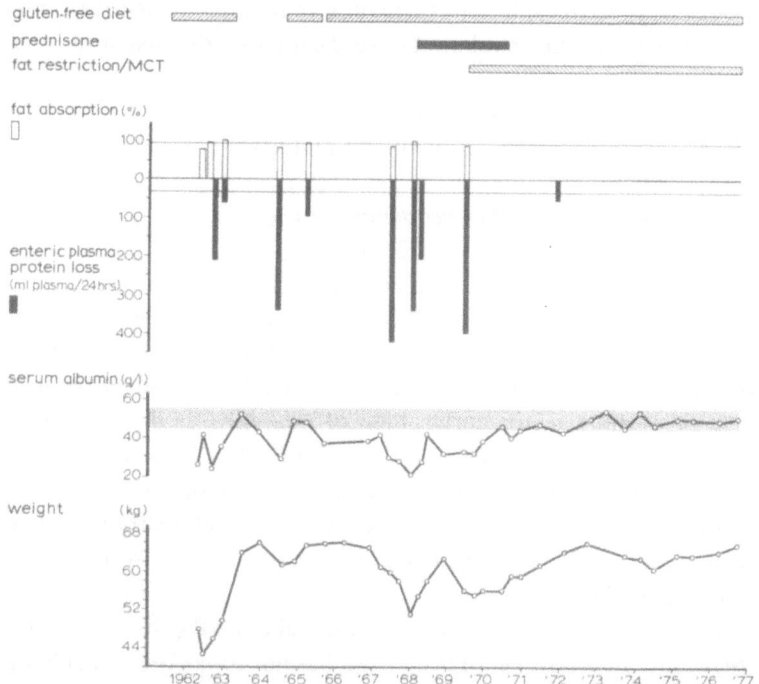

Fig. 9.7. Diagram of the effect of additional prednisone medication and L.C.T.-fat restriction in a coeliac patient on gluten-free diet (case history no. 17). As parameters are chosen the body weight, serum albumin concentration, enteric plasma protein loss and fat absorption coefficient.

and had a fat absorption coefficient of 87%. At the time the biopsy specimen from the small intestine showed a flat mucosa. After 8 months on a gluten-free diet the mucosa showed a marked improvement; body weight increased by 4 kg, fat absorption increased from 87% to 94%, and the protein loss decreased from 340 ml to 95 ml plasma per day. About 2 years after reinstitution of the diet, deterioration occurred for no apparent reason. At the time, subepithelial collagen deposition was for the first time observed in the flat jejunal biopsy. She lost 16 kg body weight, and developed extensive hypoproteinaemic oedema. During clinical observation (in order to ensure strict observance of the diet), no improvement was observed. Administration of prednisone (initially 40 mg per day, but later gradually less) caused only a partial, transient improvement. Ultimately a low-fat diet was prescribed, with suppletion of calories in the form of MCT fat. This was followed by a spectacular improvement, which persisted even after discontinuation of prednisone. The mucosal abnormalities in the proximal jejunum also improved. The biopsy specimen ultimately showed somewhat plump but otherwise virtually normal villi without subepithelial collagen deposits. The patient still keeps a fat-restricted, gluten-free diet, and has so far remained free from symptoms. Apart from a slightly decreased serum folate concentration, she shows no biochemical abnormalities.

Comment

The above case history shows that there may be reasons present for fat restriction other than the wish to prevent formation of volatile fatty acids in the colon. Our presumption in this case was that the high enteric protein loss resulted from an obstructed intestinal lymph drainage, due to abnormal mesenteric lymph nodes. Dietary fat restriction reduces the amount of chyle in the intestinal wall which has to be transported, so that the demand on the draining capacity of the intestinal lymphatic system is reduced. A reduction of lymph congestion may result in a decreased enteric protein loss (section 6.5).

9.3.2 Replacement therapy

Although absorption of food constituents improves and becomes normal soon after gluten withdrawal, it seems nevertheless sensible to prescribe temporary supplements of some lacked nutrients. Replacement therapy is probably not strictly necessary, but it does ensure a rapid disappearance of deficiencies developed in the course of time. Of our group of 39 coeliac patients, 20 received supplements of iron, folic acid, vitamin B_{12}, vitamin D or calcium in the initial phase of therapy. Vitamins A, E or K were occasionally also suppleted. When the patient is in a deplorable condition at the start of diet treatment, replacement therapy – by preference parenterally – is strongly recommended.

9.3.3 Parenteral feeding

In patients with very severe diarrhoea it may be advisable to administer all food parenterally. We ourselves were never forced to resort to total parenteral feeding except in 2 cases of refractory sprue (section 11.4). Modigliani et al (601) observed in 5 coeliac patients a spectacular improvement after parenteral feeding, such as an immediate arrest of diarrhoea, rapid weight gain and improvement of the mucosal morphology.

9.3.4 Administration of glucocorticosteroids

Four coeliac patients who had been referred to us with unexplained symptoms of malabsorption, had for some time been using glucocorticosteroids in view of a concomitant disease, such as rheumatoid arthritis, Besnier-Boeck-Schaumann disease or a suspected systemic condition. In spite of relatively large doses of prednisone (15-25 mg) or dexamethasone (1.5 mg), they continued to have or even developed severe symptoms of diarrhoea and malabsorption.

Of the total group of 47 coeliacs, 8 patients were temporarily given prednisone beside a strict gluten-free diet. Four patients had initially responded to gluten withdrawal but later showed no or hardly any response (patients no. 2, 5, 17 and 46), while the other 4 patients received corticosteroids in view of their poor general condition at the start of treatment. In the latter category of patients the effect of this medication was impressive, and the glucocorticosteroids could be gradually discontinued after 4-10 months without any untoward effect.

The following case history illustrates that no favourable response to gluten withdrawal can be forthcoming until glucocorticosteroids are given in addition.

Patient no. 5 was found to suffer from coeliac sprue at age 62. Diarrhoea had existed since early childhood, but had shown progressive exacerbation in the last 5 years. During this period the body weight decreased by about 10 kg (to 53.2 kg while 1.72 m tall), and the patient developed megaloblastic anaemia (haemoglobin concentration 6.5 mmole/l) and hypoalbuminaemia (34.4 g/l). A few months before he was referred to us, the patient had twice been hospitalized because of paralytic ileus (fig. 6.3). At that time, laparotomy had revealed no abnormalities of the abdominal organs. Since a systemic disease was suspected, the patient had received prednisone (20 mg per day) during the last 2 years. We discontinued the prednisone medication when he was admitted and prescribed a gluten-free diet because a jejunal biopsy had revealed a flat jejunal mucosa. Despite strict observance of the diet and supplements of folic acid, vitamin B_{12} and all fat-soluble vitamins, the patient showed no improvement; 2 months later, the clinical condition seemed to have deteriorated rather than improved. The clinical course took a surprising turn when 40 mg prednisone per day was prescribed in addition to the gluten-free diet (table 9.4). The prednisone was discontinued after 7 months. Today, some 5 years later, the patient is in excellent condition on a gluten-free diet. The body weight is 69.2 kg, and there are no biochemical abnormalities other than a slightly decreased D-xylose excretion (3.9 g in 5 hours). The jejunal biopsy specimen shows a convoluted pattern.

Table 9.4. Effect of additional treatment with glucocorticosteroids in a coeliac patient not responding to a gluten-free diet (patient no. 5).

PARAMETER	NO DIET PREDNISONE (20 mg)	GLUTEN-FREE DIET (8 wks) NO PREDNI- SONE	GLUTEN-FREE DIET (16 wks) PREDNISONE (40 mg, 8 wks)
Body weight (kg)	53.2	48.6	59.6
Haemoglobin (mmole/l)	6.2	4.8	7.7
Serum albumin (g/l)	34.4	34.7	49.9
Serum cholesterol (mmole/l)	2.9	3.2	4.9
Fat absorption (%)	59	N.D.	N.D.

Comment

More or less at the same time as the first publications on the results of diet treatment, reports were published on the favourable effect of glucocorticosteroids and ACTH in patients with probable coeliac sprue (8, 509, 538). Later, partial improvement of the intestinal lesions and malabsorption in patients with biopsy-proven coeliac sprue was also demonstrated during administration of prednisone (40 mg/day) (886) or dexamethasone (1.5 mg/day) (653). In-vitro organ culture studies of jejunal biopsy specimens from coeliac patients likewise proved that hydrocortisone can prevent the harmful effects of gluten (463). The mechanism of action of corticosteroids in this respect is still obscure, but various hypotheses have been advanced (463, 886).

The effect of glucocorticosteroids has been found to be decidedly inferior to that of a gluten-free diet. In 4 of our patients no effect on the intestinal symptoms or malabsorption was observed despite administration of a fair dose of prednisone (15-25 mg per day). Other investigators have also noticed that treatment with glucocorticosteroids often produced little effect in coeliac patients who subsequently responded quite well to a gluten-free diet (233).

A very evident indication for glucocorticosteroids exists in patients who show no or only an insufficient response to gluten withdrawal (128, 357, 409). This is demonstrated clearly by the case history of patient no. 5. That this effect is not based on coincidence was demonstrated by in-vitro experiments described by Klaeveman et al. (479). They demonstrated that biopsy specimens from a patient with ulcerative jejunoileitis showed no normalization during tissue culturing until glucocorticosteroids were prescribed in addition to a gluten-free diet. No explanation of this effect has so far been found.

Another indication for glucocorticosteroids exists in patients whose condition is so poor that a rapid favourable turn in the clinical course is urgently required. We personally observed an impressive improvement in 4 patients who were in very poor condition.

Whenever glucocorticosteroids are contraindicated, azathioprine medication can be tried instead (357).

9.4 COMPLICATIONS

9.4.1 Introduction

The preceding sections may have given the impression that the treatment of patients with coeliac sprue poses no problems. This will hold for the majority of cases. Once coeliac sprue is diagnosed, the average patient is likely to make a complete recovery within a few months of gluten withdrawal. Occasionally, however, the disease takes a different course. The absolute number of patients with a complicated course is probably small; yet we observed complications in a total of 8 out of 47 patients. (patients no. 2, 5, 17, 21, 27, 34, 46, 47). This large number is probably due to the fact that our patients formed a selected group due to referral from other hospitals. Brief case histories of these patients are presented in the following sections (so far as they have not been presented elsewhere in this study).

9.4.2 Abnormal bacterial flora

Patient no. 21, a woman in whom coeliac sprue was diagnosed at age 60, initially showed a good improvement after gluten withdrawal and a 3 weeks course of prednisone in view of her poor general condition. In the course of 6 months, she gained 3.5 kg body weight but showed no improvement in biochemical parameters such as serum albumin concentration (35 g/l) and D-xylose excretion (1.7 g in 5 hours). A severe relapse occurred after 6 months: the patient produced watery stools 10-20 times daily, and showed a considerable weight loss. The intestinal mucosa regressed from a convoluted pattern to a flat mucosa. The patient fervently denied negligence in observing the diet. Antigluten antibodies were not demonstrable in the serum. Laboratory findings ('breath'test for bile acid deconjugation and indican excretion) were suggestive of bacterial overgrowth, and the faeces contained numerous Candida fungi. Treatment with miconazole (250 mg q.i.d. orally) was followed by disappearance of symptoms within 48 hours, while the 'breath'test and indicanuria became almost normal. A relapse which developed a few months later, was effectively controlled with tetracycline (table 6.4).

Comment

An abnormal intestinal flora is relatively common in coeliac patients (section 6.11). In the majority of cases this abnormal bacterial flora probably causes few symptoms. The above case histories, however, demonstrate that serious effects may develop. Symptoms such as nausea, meteorism, abdominal pain and diarrhoea can in some cases be ascribed to an abnormal intestinal flora, after exclusion of other possible causes. In some cases this abnormal flora gives rise to biochemical abnormalities, such as malabsorption of D-xylose or vitamin B_{12}. It is of importance to account for this possibility in order to ensure effective therapy and, on the other hand, to avoid erroneous conclusions concerning diet observance or gluten insensitivity.

9.4.3 Other complications

At age 60, patient no. 27 was placed on a gluten-free diet in view of severe diarrhoea which she had contracted 6 months earlier during a Mediterranean trip. She had had abdominal symptoms as a child, but these had disappeared at age 12. Before institution of a gluten-free diet a jejunal biopsy was taken, which showed a flat mucosa. In view of her poor condition, expressed by anaemia (haemoglobin concentration 5.8 mmole/l), marked hypoalbuminaemia (19 g/l), fat malabsorption (47%) and hypomagnesaemia (0.63 mmole/l), glucocorticosteroids were given in addition. The patient initially showed improvement: the body weight increased by 11 kg (without oedema), the anaemia and hypoalbuminaemia disappeared, and the serum magnesium concentration also returned to normal. Scarcely 6 months later she had to be readmitted with a severe relapse of diarrhoea and marked electrolyte disturbances (plasma K^+ 2.7 mmole/l; plasma HCO_3^- 15.8 mmole/l), fat malabsorption (64%) and hypoalbuminaemia (17 g/l). Her situation was complicated by an arterial occlusion in the left lower leg, for which anticoagulants were prescribed. She admitted to having taken normal bread for several months. After an increase of the prednisone dosage and re-institution of the diet, she made another surprising recovery within a few weeks. Three months later, however, she again discontinued the regimen and severe malabsorption developed once more. Anticoagulant medication had further caused recurrent epistaxis and severe blood loss in urine and faeces. Consequently there was marked anaemia (2.3 mmole/l), and severe electrolyte disturbances (plasma K^+ 2.2 mmole/l; plasma HCO_3^- 12.4 mmole/l). Renal function, which had previously been fair, was markedly reduced (creatinine clearance 17 ml/min). In the course of a few months the renal function deteriorated further, and led eventually to a fatal issue. At post-mortem examination, both kidneys showed features of extensive interstitial fibrosis and some intra-tubulary located oxalate crystals. The glomeruli appeared completely normal.

Patient no. 34, whose defaecation pattern had been abnormal all his life, underwent a laparotomy for faecal vomiting at age 68. At this operation, markedly distended intestinal loops were found, without any sign of organic obstruction. Additional findings were enlarged mesenteric lymph nodes, which showed no specific abnormalities at histological examination. After this laparotomy the patient was transferred to our department, where studies revealed malabsorption of fat (60%), vitamin B_{12} (1.7% ^{57}Co-vit B_{12} excretion in 48 hours), and D-xylose (1.6 g in 5 hours). Additional findings were an iron deficiency anaemia (Hb 6.3 mmole/l), and decreased serum concentrations of albumin (30.7 g/l) and vitamin E (4.0 μmole/l). Since a jejunal biopsy specimen showed a flat mucosa, a gluten-free diet was prescribed. Before the effect of gluten withdrawal could be evaluated the patient died as a result of cardiac failure by recurrent arrhythmia. Post-mortem examination revealed no abnormalities of the abdominal organs other than a so-called brown bowel due to accumulation of ceroid in the muscular layer (847). A conspicuous amount of ceroid pigment was likewise found in the myocardium. It is not inconceivable that the cardiac arrhythmia in this patient resulted from myocardial degeneration caused by vitamin E deficiency, among others.

Comment

Renal failure, the direct cause of death in patient no. 27 has also been reported by other investigators (489, 724). In both publications the suspicion was expressed that this renal failure had to be ascribed to a tubulopathy, which could have resulted from a disturbed electrolyte balance due to vomiting, diarrhoea and malabsorption. The real cause of renal failure in our patient is difficult to indicate. Transient tubular necrosis could have been provoked by hypotension and potassium deficiency. This does not explain, however, her progressively deteriorating renal function. It is more likely that the interstitial fibrosis was caused by the diuretic agent furosemide (534a), prescribed in view of hypoalbuminaemic oedema. Besides hyperoxaluria, often present in coeliac sprue (574a), may have played an important role.

It need not be argued that many other complications are conceivable in the course of coeliac sprue. Some may be the result of the therapy given, such as a perforation of the stomach by glucocorticosteroid medication (patient no. 2) or sepsis caused by an in-dwelling intravascular catheter (patient A, section 11.4). Similar complications have been reported by other investigators (90, 601). The same applies to the causes of death (843) which, in view of their often accidental nature, will not be further discussed.

9.4.4 Malignant degeneration and malignancies

At age 55, patient no. 2 was diagnosed as having coeliac sprue, which had given rise to attacks of tetany over a period of 15 years. The biopsy specimens from his jejunum showed not only a flat mucosa but also a marked degree of subepithelial collagen deposition (fig. 11.3). The patient responded to gluten withdrawal by a weight gain of 12 kg (from 57 kg to 69 kg, while 1.66 m tall) and normalization of the haemoglobin concentration (from 7.1 to 8.7 mmole/l), serum calcium concentration (from 2.1 to 2.39 mmole/l) and serum cholesterol concentration (from 3.9 to 5.0 mmole/l). The serum albumin level rose from 40 to 44 g/l, D-xylose excretion from 1.3 to 3.2 g per 5 hours, and the fat absorption coefficient from 40 to 85%. Four years after the institution of the diet the patient began to complain of epigastric pain, nausea and vomiting. At that time jejunal biopsies showed the same flat mucosa as specimens obtained before gluten withdrawal. During clinical observation no effect of the gluten-free diet was observed either. Extreme dietary fat restriction also failed to give any improvement. The frequency of defaecation, 2-4 times daily in previous months, increased to 10-15 times daily. There was progressive weight loss to 52 kg, which even had to be corrected for the presence of marked hypoproteinaemic oedema (albumin 30 g/l with an enteric plasma loss of 200 ml/day). The fat absorption decreased again to 50%, associated with a decreased vitamin E concentration (7.4 mmole/l) and an abnormally low thrombotest (41%). Treatment with 40 mg prednisone daily, first by mouth and later parenterally, caused no improvement. The amount of faeces did not decrease during administration of an elementary diet or total parenteral feeding, and was eventually 1600-3300 g per day. After 2 months of treatment with large doses of prednisone, intestinal perforation symptoms suddenly occurred. Subsequent laparotomy disclosed perforation of the duodenal bulb as well as an extensive adenocarcinoma of the gallbladder with multiple metastases in the liver. The last finding was a surprise because liver function tests had not been disturbed (alkaline phosphatase activity 78 U/l; BSP retention 1.8%). The patient died from complications during the postoperative phase. Post-mortem examination revealed multiple superficial ulcers in duodenum and jejunum, and subepithelial collagen accumulation in the intestinal mucosa.

Patient no. 47 had suffered from intermittent diarrhoea and vomiting during some years in childhood. He had in addition been treated for rickets. Diarrhoea and weight loss recurred at age 42. Fatty and pale stools were produced 5 times daily. The patient's weight was reduced by about 8 kg to 45.6 kg (height 1.68 m), and he was suffering from general malaise, anorexia and vague abdominal pain. Physical examination revealed no abnormality other than a poor nutritional condition. Biochemical tests disclosed fat malabsorption (48%) as well as a markedly decreased absorption of vitamin B_{12} (3% excretion in 48 hours) and D-xylose (1.0 g excretion in 5 hours). A gluten-free diet was prescribed because a jejunal biopsy specimen showed a flat mucosa. This was followed by subjective improvement and a weight gain of 2 kg. Four weeks after gluten withdrawal progressive obstructive jaundice necessitated a laparotomy, however. This revealed an inoperable tumour in the head of the pancreas, and multiple metastases in the liver. The patient died 2 months later.

Comment

Although there had been several earlier publications on the association of steatorrhoea with malignant processes of the digestive tract and elsewhere in the organism (see 822 for a review), Gough et al. (324) were the first to suggest that neoplastic lesions could be a complication of coeliac sprue. Until that time it had often been thought that the malignancy was the primary condition, and steatorrhoea the consequence, resulting from malignant infiltration of the intestinal wall or lymph obstruction in the mesenteric lymph nodes. The coeliac patients described by Gough et al. (324) had for the most part suffered from steatorrhoea over many years before a malignant process became manifest. The jejunal mucosa in these patients, moreover, was consistent with coeliac sprue and, more specifically, showed no tumour infiltration. After Gough et al. (324), many others have described malignant processes in coeliac patients (32, 60, 104, 128, 256, 393, 413, 473, 667, 817, 843). In our own series of 47 patients we found twice a malignancy, being an adenocarcinoma of the gall-bladder and of the pancreas.

Several investigators maintain that a malignant process outside the digestive tract can as such cause mucosal abnormalities which are strongly reminiscent of those observed in coeliac sprue (176, 200, 241, 245, 508, 643, 794). If this is true, the incidence of it must be very low (200, 521). One cannot exclude the possibility, moreover, that these exceptional patients were also suffering from (previously asymptomatic) coeliac sprue.

An important fact is that the risk of malignant lymphoma or malignancy in coeliac patients far exceeds the statistical expectation. Harris et al. (365) were the first to demonstrate this statistical significance. Their conclusions were later confirmed by Stokes et al. (822) and Whorwell et al. (914). In view of this increased risk of malignancy, many 'coeliac centres' forcibly advise their patients to observe a gluten-free regime for life. The argument is usually that the harmful effect of dietary gluten on the jejunal mucosa would increase the risk of malignant degeneration. So far, however, there is no evidence to support the statement that gluten withdrawal reduces the risk of malignancies (365, 822, 914). It is strange, moreover, that most of the malignant processes observed are localized outside the jejunum (365), and that relatives of coeliacs also seem to run an increased risk (50, 822).

208

On the basis of common experience the general opinion is that development or exacerbation of abdominal pain, fever, anorexia, weight loss or skin lesions should raise a suspicion of the presence of a malignant process (112). The fact that a patient who used to respond well to gluten withdrawal suddenly deteriorates and develops features of refractory coeliac sprue, is likewise suggestive of the presence of a malignant process (patient no. 2; 112, 324).

9.5 CONCLUSIONS

1. The spontaneous course of coeliac sprue is somewhat variable, due to abrupt exacerbations and symptom-free intervals.
2. The evaluation of the effect of gluten withdrawal is seriously hindered by the impossibility of assessment of the adherence to the diet.
3. The effect of diet treatment on clinical symptoms depends on the clinical presentation before gluten withdrawal. Rapid improvement is seen in patients suffering from diarrhoea, glossitis or stomatitis. Symptoms resulting from chronic malabsorption take longer to ameliorate, while complaints of lassitude or abdominal pain often persist.
4. Biochemical abnormalities improve in general after gluten withdrawal. Patients who admit to adhere poorly to the diet show, apart from the Schilling test, no more abnormal biochemical tests than those who supposedly observe the prescribed diet more faithfully.
5. The effect of gluten withdrawal on the mucosal morphology of the proximal jejunum is often disappointing. A normal villous pattern was seldom found, and never observed within 2 years of diet therapy.
6. It is advisable to take additional measures in the early phase of treatment, such as restriction of milk (lactose) or fat, and replacement of lacked nutrients.
7. Patients in a poor general condition do benefit from additional glucocorticosteroid medication. In exceptional cases gluten withdrawal is insufficient to cause any improvement until glucocorticosteroids are given temporarily in addition.
8. An abnormal intestinal flora may be partly responsible for the malabsorption syndrome in coeliac sprue, necessitating in some patients the prescription of antibiotics.
9. Malignancies are relatively often seen in coeliac patients. Exacerbation of symptoms and the occurrence of therapy-resistance should raise a suspicion on the presence of a malignant process.

## CHAPTER 10

ASSOCIATION WITH OTHER DISEASES

10.1 INTRODUCTION

Reports on the association of coeliac sprue with other diseases have regularly been published (56, 764). The fact that some coeliacs suffer from concomitant diseases is as such not strange. The incidence of some conditions, however, exceeds that in the remainder of the population. A well-known example of this is the association of coeliac sprue with dermatitis herpetiformis (DH) (57, 106, 287, 296, 557, 560, 849). The association between coeliac sprue and other diseases is much less pronounced, but the possibility of a certain relation between these diseases and coeliac sprue is still open for the time being.

10.2 DERMATITIS HERPETIFORMIS

10.2.1 Personal observations

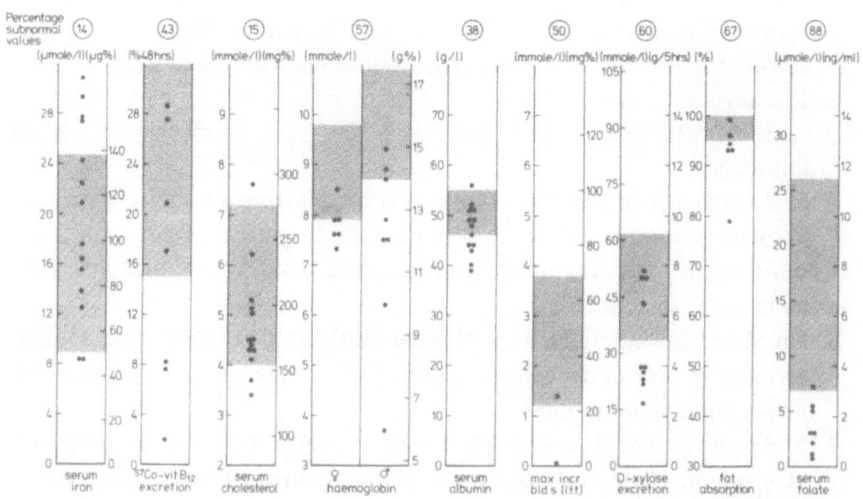

Fig. 10.1.a. Diagram of various biochemical investigations in dermatitis herpetiformis patients with villous abnormalities.

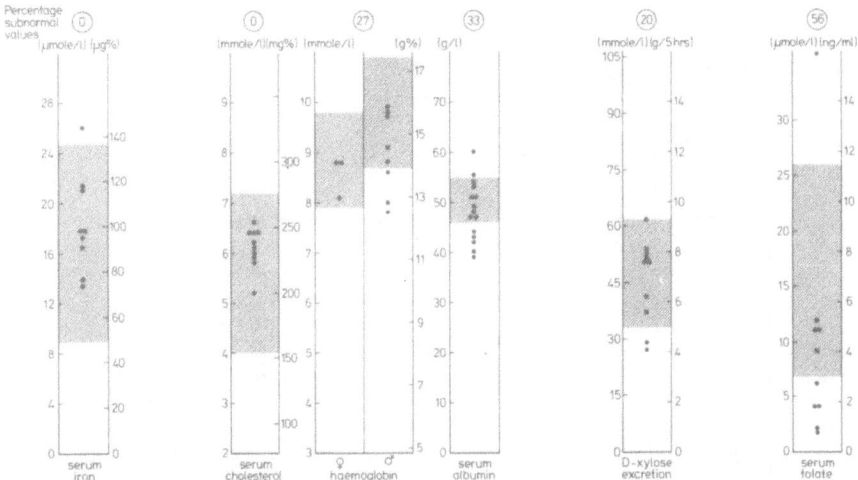

Fig. 10.1.b. Diagram of various biochemical investigations in dermatitis herpetiformis patients without villous abnormalities.

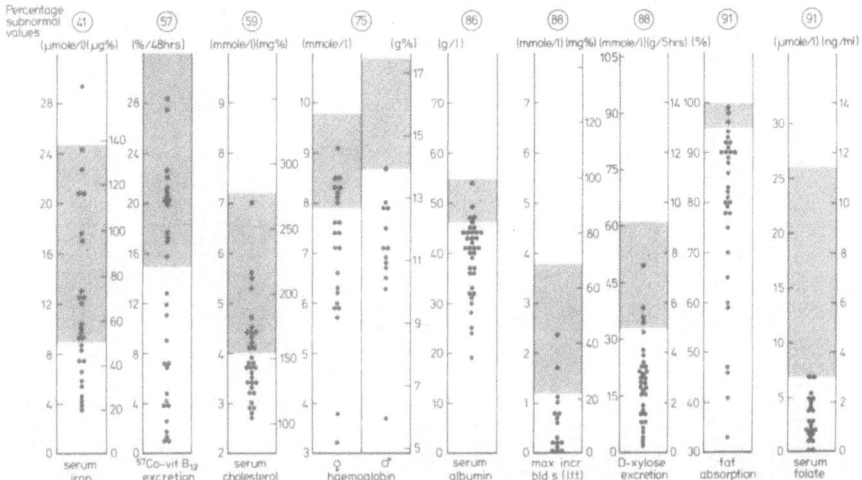

Fig. 10.1.c. Diagram of various biochemical investigations in untreated coeliac patients.

We examined a total of 34 patients with DH, which had been diagnosed on the basis of the morphological aspect and localization of the lesions, and verified by histological examination of a skin biopsy specimen. Another necessary criterion was the favourable effect of dapsone on the skin lesions and symptoms.

On the basis of preferably multiple biopsy specimens from the proximal jejunum, abnormalities of the intestinal mucosa were determined in exactly

211

Table 10.1. Abnormal biochemical results in dermatitis herpetiformis patients.

AUTHORS	SERUM IRON	SERUM VIT B_{12}	^{57}Co-VIT B_{12} EXCRETION	SERUM CHOLESTEROL	HAEMOGLOBIN	SERUM ALBUMIN	D-XYLOSE EXCRETION	FAT ABSORPTION	SERUM FOLATE
Fraser et al. (1967)					2/12	0/12	4/11	5/11	
Fry et al. (1967)	4/13	1/13	0/13		5/13			7/13	11/13
Marks et al. (1968)		14/27	3/17			1/28	15/28	7/25	18/27
Shuster et al. (1968)	4/16	0/10	3/13				3/13	6/18	
Brow et al. (1971)	0/14	0/10	0/5		18/22		2/21	2/21	16/18
Sönnichsen et al. (1971)			3/5				2/7	2/7	
Ruppin et al. (1975)						6/15			
Own series	2/23		4/7	2/23	12/25	10/28	8/20	4/6	5/18

212

50% of these 34 DH patients. The biopsy specimen showed an entirely flat mucosa in 6, a so-called convoluted pattern in 7, and only minor changes such as ridges or leaf-shaped villi in 4 of these patients. Of the 17 patients with mucosal abnormalities, 4 showed a clinically and biochemically manifest malabsorption syndrome, so that they were considered as coeliac patients.

As mentioned, 50% of our DH patients showed no abnormalities of the intestinal villi. Since in 14 cases only a single biopsy specimen had been obtained from the jejunal mucosa, all patients were invited for secondary multiple biopsies. In 5 cases no repeat biopsy was obtained owing to intercurrent death (1), very advanced age (2) or refusal to cooperate (2). Secondary multiple biopsies never necessitated revision of the previous classification. The multiple biopsy specimens, usually 6 per patient, revealed mucosal abnormalities in none of these cases.

Biochemical tests were carried out both in the DH patients with villous abnormalities (including the above mentioned 4 coeliacs) and in those with a normal villous pattern. The results are presented in fig. 10.1 (a and b). For comparison, the results of our group of 36 coeliac patients are also listed (fig. 10.1.c). Statistical analysis (Wilcoxon signed-rank test) of the biochemical test results revealed a significantly higher concentration of haemoglobin, folate and cholesterol in blood or serum of DH patients without mucosal lesions, compared to those with an abnormal jejunal mucosa. The D-xylose test differed also significantly.

Analysis of the biochemical results shows that decreased serum iron or cholesterol concentrations were rarely found in our DH patients. Malabsorption of D-xylose and vitamin B_{12}, however, was relatively common, and the same applies to a decreased serum folate level, hypoalbuminaemia and steatorrhoea. A striking feature was that a decreased serum albumin level was found as often in DH patients with as in those without villous abnormalities. However, the former showed a significantly higher incidence of anaemia and D-xylose malabsorption.

10.2.2 Comment

The association between DH and coeliac sprue was quite evident in our observations. Four patients with coeliac sprue were suffering also from DH. The biochemical findings showed that a subclinical form of malabsorption was present in many more DH patients. This was quite evident in the group of DH patients with an abnormal villous pattern: biochemical abnormalities were found in 14-67% of the cases. Malabsorption seemed to be less common in the group of patients with a normal jejunal mucosa, but it was still present in a substantial number of patients.

Similar absorption studies in patients with DH have been published (table 10.1). Comparison reveals a number of discrepancies. Some authors found a high incidence of an abnormal haemoglobin concentration (106), serum iron (296), folate (106), vitamin B_{12} (560), or albumin concentration (740). Absorption studies also yielded different results; some reports listed a high incidence of malabsorption of vitamin B_{12} (811), fat (296) or D-xylose (560). Our own observations also differ in some respects from those reported by others as regards serum folate and albumin levels (table 10.1). Differences in the composition of the various investigated groups are most likely to account for this. Only some of the biochemical abnormalities, such as anaemia or abnormal D-xylose test, were found to depend on the presence or absence of morphological mucosal lesions (fig. 10.1.a and b). Others have confirmed this with regard to anaemia, steatorrhoea or decreased D-xylose excretion (296, 560).

We found an abnormal villous morphology in exactly 50% of our DH patients. Most other investigators found a decidedly higher incidence (table 10.2). Since mucosal lesions may be patchy in DH patients (106), multiple biopsies are advised. In all DH patients with a normal mucosa in a single specimen, however, the multiple secondary biopsies also failed to reveal villous abnormalities.

Some investigators hold that all DH patients have an abnormal intestinal mucosa, even if it looks apparently normal. Fry et al. (298), for example, found an increased number of lymphocytes among the enterocytes in the jejunal biopsy specimen in virtually all their cases. In perfusion studies, Kumar et al. (494, 495) demonstrated that absorption in the jejunum of DH patients was usually abnormal, even when the mucosal morphology appeared normal. The high incidence of hypoalbuminaemia in our DH patients without villous abnormalities, supports this observation. An important argument in this context can be found in the observations of Weinstein et al. (901). These investigators found that the morphologically normal jejunal mucosa in 2 DH patients became pathological within a few months on a high-gluten diet. This phenomenon was not observed in two healthy volunteers tiven the same high-gluten diet. Taken together, these observations indicate that the jejunal mucosa is essentially abnormal in every DH patient, and sensitive to gluten if sometimes only in large doses.

The association between DH and coeliac sprue has not so far been fully explained. Several observations, often not more than fragments of the aetiological puzzle, indicate an immunological pathogenesis (299). It has

Table 10.2. Villous morphology in dermatitis herpetiformis patients.

AUTHORS	NUMBER OF PATIENTS INVESTIGATED	FLAT MUCOSA	CON-VOLUTED MUCOSA	SLIGHTLY AB-NORMAL MUCOSA	NORMAL MUCOSA
Fraser et al. (1967)	12	3	4	2	3
Bendl et al. (1968)	10	3	—	2	5
Marks et al. (1968)	26	5	13		8
Marks et al. (1970)	28	10	8	10	—
Brow et al. (1971)	22	15	—	6	1
Graber et al. (1971)	9	3	3	3	—
Gebhard et al. (1973)	28	—	15	4	9
White et al. (1973)	31	—	23		8
Fry et al. (1974a)	42	9	8	6	19
Ruppin et al. (1975)	16				16
Own series	34	6	7	4	17

been established, for example, that immune complexes circulate in the blood of all DH patients (602). IgG and IgM antibodies against nuclear substance or reticulin are also regularly present in the blood (765). Several observations indicate moreover, that IgA deposits are to be found in the skin of DH patients, both at the sites of lesions and in apparently unaffected parts of the skin (167, 585, 767). Apart from IgA, complement is also found in the lesions (768). A combination of the above mentioned findings would seem to suggest that the skin lesions in DH patients result from deposition of circulating immune complexes, involving IgA and complement (299).

For the moment this hypothesis raises more questions than it answers. The circulating immune complexes prove to be of a varying nature and are as frequent in DH patients with as in those without a gluten-free diet. Such complexes are also often found in the circulation of coeliac patients without DH (602). It is further not readily understandable why DH patients should often have an abnormal intestinal mucosa, whereas only a few patients with coeliac sprue develop DH. Until these questions can be answered, dermatitis herpetiformis has to be regarded as a separate, if associated, entity rather than as a complication of coeliac sprue.

215

10.3 CONCOMITANT DISEASES

10.3.1 Personal observations

Several patients in our series had a concomitant disease or stated they had been suffering from other diseases as well. Table 10.3 lists these diseases and the number of cases observed.

Table 10.3. Concomitant diseases in coeliac sprue.
– Observations in 47 patients. – verg. Table 10.4

DISEASE	NUMBER OF PATIENTS
Diabetes	2
Hyperthyroidism	1*
Idiopathic thrombopenia	1
Achlorhydria	1
Rheumatoid arthritis	1
Chronic bronchitis	6
Fibrosing alveolitis	1
Idiopathic pulmonary haemosiderosis	1
Sarcoidosis	1*
Peptic ulcer	4*
Intestinal diverticulosis	1
Ulcerative colitis	1
Renal tubular disease	1
Endometriosis	1
Stein Leventhal's syndrome	1
XO-XY mosaicism	1
Anorexia nervosa	1
Vascular occlusive disease	5

* Diagnosed and treated before referral.

10.3.2 Comment

The list of concomitant diseases in our patients shows that coeliac sprue can be associated with a wide variety of other diseases. Several publications have drawn attention to possible disease relationships (table 10.4). In view of personal observations as well as data from the literature, it seems questionable whether the incidence of these diseases in coeliac patients is higher than that in non-coeliacs. It would therefore seem rather premature to call these diseases associative, let alone to philosophise about possible explanations of this relationship (764).

Table 10.4. Concomitant diseases in patients with proven or possible coeliac sprue.
— cases collected from literature —

DISEASE	NUMBER OF PATIENTS	REFERENCES
Diabetes	30	57, 72, 128, 163, 338, 358, 393, 417, 418, 484, 489, 499, 553, 601, 846, 871, 873
Thyroid disease	17	163, 338, 493, 496, 499, 541, 601, 796, 875
Addison's disease	2	142, 323
Haemolytic anaemia	1	337
Achlorhydria	7	104, 160, 405
Acromegaly	1	601
Rheumatoid arthritis	3	104, 256, 337
Lupus erythematodes	2	795
Sjögren's disease	3	498, 685
Vasculitis-arteritis	8	221, 372, 601, 795, 843
Polymyositis	4	372
Epilepsy	4	601, 611
Neurological disorders	24	128, 162, 601
Chronic bronchitis	12	163, 187, 256, 601
Fibrosing alveolitis	10	415, 497, 711, 750
Idiopathic pulm. haemosiderosis	1	502
Birdfancier's lung	5	64
Hay fever	5	399
Sarcoidosis	2	393, 458
Atopic eczema	4	399
Chronic hepatitis	13	46, 142, 163, 256, 338, 476, 499, 744
α 1-antitrypsin deficiency	—	884
Cystic fibrosis	6	320, 464, 836
Pancreatic insufficiency	11	59, 60, 272, 489, 601, 682, 899
Eosinophilic gastroenteritis	1	59
Ulcerative colitis	4	160, 257, 744
Renal disease	2	489, 724
Cystinuria	2	355, 358

CHAPTER 11

SPECIAL FORMS OF SPRUE

11.1 INTRODUCTION

Patients with coeliac sprue show per definition both a distinct clinical and biochemical improvement after gluten withdrawal. In addition the lesions of the small intestine in these patients should improve. In the characteristic case this improvement – particularly that in clinical symptoms – ensues rapidly and ultimately becomes a complete remission. Rubin et al. (736) maintain that complete remission occurs per definition in every coeliac patient on a strict gluten-free diet.

One is regularly confronted nevertheless with patients who show a slow and incomplete improvement upon gluten withdrawal, and who sometimes require other measures in addition, such as administration of glucocorticosteroids (section 9.3). One generally tends to regard these patients as coeliacs (90), although some authors do not agree (736). This point of view is difficult to hold in the rare cases of patients who, like many other coeliacs, present with a malabsorption syndrome and a flat jejunal mucosa but, despite strict observance of a gluten-free diet and a variety of other measures, show progressive deterioration and ultimately die as a direct or indirect result of their malabsorption. Adequate classification of these cases is not yet possible. Terms such as 'unclassified sprue', 'intestinal atrophy' or 'fatal malabsorption syndrome' are used in this situation. Some investigators suspect a relation to coeliac sprue, and express this in terms such as 'malignant coeliac syndrome' or 'unresponsive coeliac disease'. Their suspicion is usually based on the fact that the patient had previously shown a complete or incomplete remission in response to gluten withdrawal.

In some patients with such an unresponsive malabsorption syndrome, ulcerations of the small intestine are found (56). We consider it useful to discuss this group of patients in a separate section. The same applies to patients in whom increased deposition of collagen is found in the jejunal mucosa. In the final section personal observations on 2 patients with refractory sprue will be presented.

218

11.2 ULCERATIVE DUODENOJEJUNOILEITIS

11.2.1 Introduction

Although the first reports on the presence of ulcers of the small intestine in patients with malabsorption date back at least 50 years (721), Bayless et al. (55) were the first to point out the more than accidental nature of this complication in patients with coeliac sprue. From the literature and from personal communications up to 1974, they collected some 30 cases of ulcers in coeliac patients (56). A small number of cases can be added to this series, e.g. those reported by Krondl et al. (492), Haex (348), Marche et al. (555) and Connon et al. (154), as well as some of our own patients.

11.2.2 Personal observations

We encountered once a case of ulcerative duodenojejunitis, while in another patient a complication was seen, which may have been a result of a jejunal ulcer. Their case histories will be presented. In addition we saw a female patient (no. 17, section 9.3), whose jejunal biopsy specimens showed extensive erosions, with marked infiltration of the mucosa by micro-organisms and granulocytes. The post-mortem on patient no. 2 (section 9.4) moreover, who died of a metastatised adenocarcinoma of the gall-bladder, revealed multiple superficial ulcers in duodenum, jejunum and ileum which consisted of granulation tissue.

Patient no. 46 had suffered from rickets in childhood but reportedly had never had abdominal symptoms. At age 33 she had been treated for tuberculous cervical lymphadenitis. She was further under medical care in view of chronic bronchitis. At age 51 she was referred to our department with complaints of nausea, postprandial vomiting, borborygmi and frequent passage of pulpy stools, symptoms which had been present over the past 7 years. An exploratory laparotomy had been performed prior to her referral, as a gastric carcinoma was suspected. No lesions of the stomach and other abdominal organs had been found on that occasion. In the course of these 7 years the patient's body weight had decreased from 82 to 50 kg (height 1.62 m). In view of extensive strictures in the duodenum and jejunum (fig. 11.1), another laparotomy was performed shortly after her referral. This revealed a markedly distended duodenum with severe stenoses in the duodenum and proximal 70 cm of the jejunum. The wall of the proximal jejunum was swollen and several large lymph nodes were palpable in the mesentery. After resection of the proximal jejunum, a gastrojejunostomy was established in view of the non-resectable lesions in the duodenum. Pathological examination of the resected intestine disclosed many ulcers of varying width and depth. Their floors and surroundings consisted of a cellular inflammatory infiltrate containing numerous granulocytes,

219

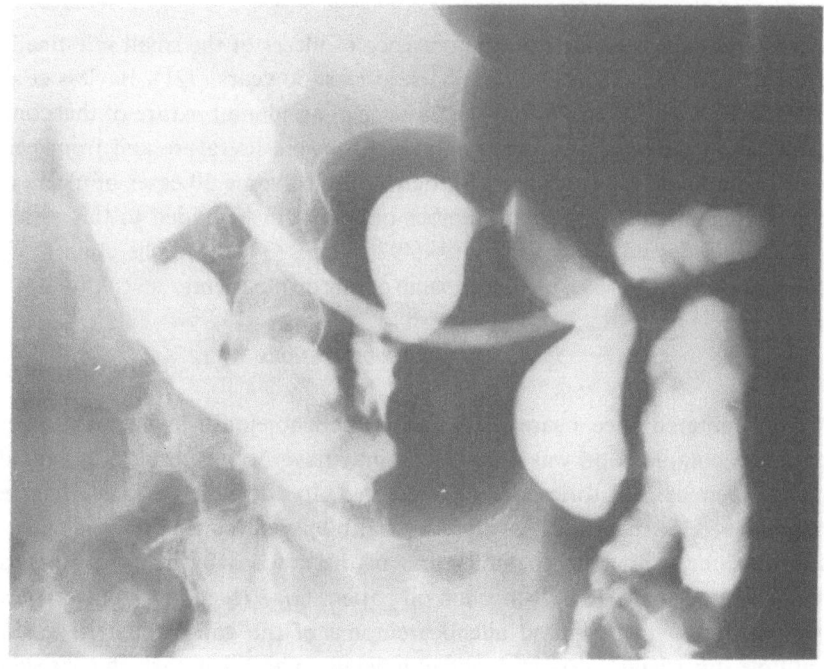

Fig. 11.1. X-ray film of a barium-meal in a patient with ulcerative duodenojejunitis (patient no. 46; for case history see text).

lymphocytes, plasma cells and eosinophils. The submucosa showed extensive oedema and proliferation of connective tissue, but there were no signs of granuloma formation or transmural inflammatory reaction. The muscularis mucosae was intact throughout. The mucosa of the resected specimen showed short to absent villi in the proximal part, which seemed less abnormal at more distal levels. The enlarged mesenteric nodes showed a marked increase in plasma cells and eosinophils, again without granuloma formation. There were no signs of malignancy, moreover. Severe diarrhoea developed after the operation, and a few months later the patient showed symptoms of tetany and stridor. The corrected serum calcium level was only 1.59 mmole/1. A biopsy specimen from the iliac crest showed marked osteomalacia. For other biochemical data we refer to table 11.1. In view of a flat mucosa in the biopsy specimen from the proximal jejunum, 40 cm past the gastro-enterostomy, a gluten-free diet was prescribed. About a year later the patient felt subjectively improved, but no significant objective improvement was observed (table 11.1). Her massive enteric protein leakage showed a favourable reaction on fat

Table 11.1. Effect of additional treatment with glucocorticosteroids (25 mg prednisone) in a patient with ulcerative duodenojejunitis, poorly responding to a gluten-free diet (patient no. 46).

PARAMETER	NO DIET	ON DIET (15 mths)	ON DIET (18 mths) & PREDNISONE (30 mg; 3 mths)
Body weight (kg)	60.5	61.2	67.9
Fat absorption (%)	83	82	85
Serum cholesterol (mmole/l)	4.2	4.2	5.0
Serum albumin (g/l)	39.6	35.8	39.0
Enteric plasma leakage (ml/24 hrs)	140	200	30
D-xylose excretion (g/5 hrs)	0.7	7.0	6.8
Haemoglobin (mmole/l)	6.9	5.3	8.2
Plasma calcium (corr) (mmole/l)	1.62	2.23	2.38

restriction of the diet, which might indicate an obstructed intestinal lymph drainage (table 6.2). After prescription of glucocorticosteroids in combination with the gluten-free diet marked improvement of the body weight and enteric protein loss was observed within a few months (table 11.1).

Patient no. 48 (who, as the number indicates, presented after completion of our series) had two children long identified as coeliac patients. He had been in good health all his life, but at age 69 experienced an acute attack of abdominal pain with restlessness and vomiting, necessitating analgesic injections. After a symptom-free period of about 6 months, the patient again developed symptoms of upper abdominal pain with vomiting of bile-coloured fluid, and watery diarrhoea, 4 times daily. Physical examination of the emaciated patient (50.5 kg while 1.76 m tall) revealed no abnormalities other than a slightly atrophic tongue. The abdomen was not distended and no masses were palpable. Laboratory findings included anaemia (haemoglobin 6.0 mmole/l), marked hypoalbuminaemia (serum albumin 26.7 g/l), a decreased D-xylose test (2.3 g in 5 hours) and increased indicanuria (daily average 300 mg). Radiographs of the small intestine revealed a fistula between the proximal jejunum and the transverse colon. At about the same site there was a fistula between the first and the second jejunal loop (fig. 11.2). At operation the fistular process proved to be readily resectable and the normal continuity of jejunal loops and transverse colon was restored. Pathological examination of the resected specimen revealed no specific inflammatory lesions or any indication of a malignant process. The same applied to the enlarged mesenteric lymph nodes. However, a flat jejunal mucosa was found in the proximal as well as in the distal resection area. Severe diarrhoea developed in the post-operative phase and the patient was given a gluten-free diet. The diarrhoea then disappeared and the body weight increased by 13 kg in 4 months. His jejunal biopsy specimen showed at that moment a convoluted mucosa, which became flat again after 3 months on a normal diet.

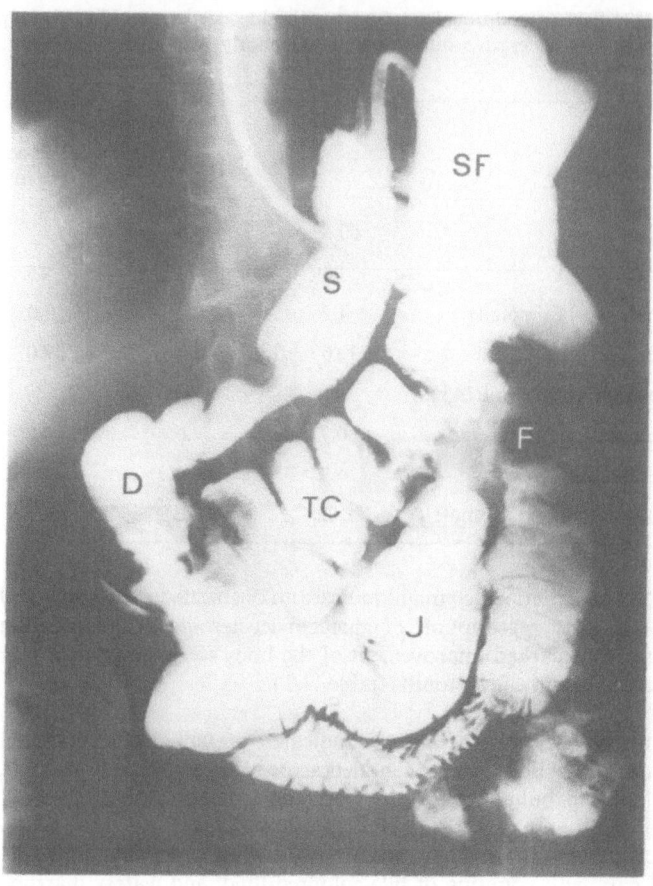

Fig. 11.2. X-ray film of a barium-meal in a coeliac patient with a jejunocolic fistula (patient no. 48; for case history see text). The fistula (F) between jejunum (J) and transverse colon (TC) is well visible (S stands for stomach, D for duodenum, and SF for splenic flexure).

11.2.3 Comment

Analysis of the various published case histories of patients with malabsorption and ulcers of the small intestine, leads to the impression that these patients form a very heterogeneous group. In part this is also expressed in the various names used by authors to decribe this condition, for example: 'intestinal ulcerations', 'recurrent benign ulcers', 'severe mucosal damage' 'chronic ulcerative jejunoileitis' and 'non-granulomatous jejunoileitis'.

In about half of the cases there were anamnestic indications that the patients were suffering from coeliac sprue (55, 141, 142, 143, 195, 769). Several patients showed no or only an insufficient response to gluten withdrawal, but improved after additional glucocorticosteroid medication (444, 479). In a substantial number of cases there were no more criteria of coeliac sprue present other than a flat mucosa in the proximal jejunum (49, 153, 438, 780). In some cases, the localization of the villous abnormalities was not typical of coeliac sprue (143, 555). There was also considerable variation in the localization and morphology of the intestinal ulcers. In some cases they were found mostly in the ileum or even in the colon (49, 142, 143, 827), being either superficial (49, 141, 143, 555) or very deep (55, 143). The cellular infiltrate in the floor or wall of the ulcers also varied, consisting of lymphoid cells (55, 143, 555), plasma cells or even polymorphonuclear cells (55, 143). In some cases there was a minimal cellular reaction (49) or only dense fibrinous tissue (142, 555) at the ulcer sites.

There are many known causes of ulceration in the small intestine (143, 896). It is difficult to exclude that in some published cases ulcers have been due to one of these causes. The high frequency of intestinal ulceration in coeliac patients suggests, however, a relationship with coeliac sprue (55, 56). In view of the differences in localization and nature of the ulcers, the aetiology may have been different also. As long as there is no clear understanding of the underlying cause or mechanisms, it seems hardly sensible to regard all these patients with intestinal ulcers as a single separate group. It must be stated on the other hand, that coeliacs whose damaged mucosa shows ulceration, differ from other coeliacs in that they often do not respond to gluten withdrawal until after additional glucocorticosteroid medication (patient no. 46). Another striking characteristic of these patients is the high rate of complications such as perforations, haemorrhages and obstruction, which are often fatal (56). The development of the fistula between jejunum and colon in our patient no. 48 may well have resulted from perforation of a jejunal ulcer. This complication seems rather unique. In view of the high rate of complications and the regular necessity of additional glucocorticosteroid medication, it does seem justifiable to regard coeliac patients with ulcers of the small intestine as a separate category.

11.3 'COLLAGENOUS' SPRUE

11.3.1 Introduction

Some patients with coeliac sprue show a marked increase in the amount of subepithelial collagen in the lamina propria. In view of this phenomenon, Weinstein et al. (900) decided to distinguish, within the group of patients with atypical coeliac sprue or 'unclassified sprue', a subgroup of patients suffering from 'collagenous' sprue. They introduced this entity with reference to the case history of a female patient with a severe malabsorption syndrome who failed to respond to gluten withdrawal prescribed on the basis of a flat jejunal mucosa. A wide variety of other therapeutic measures likewise failed to influence the downhill course of her condition. A striking feature in this case was the progressive deposition of collagen in the subepithelial tissue of the small intestine. The aetiology of this unusual form of progressive malabsorption, which led to the patient's death, remained unexplained. Collagen deposition has been demonstrated in jejunal biopsy specimens from coeliac patients by several other investigators, and was also found in the jejunal biopsies of some of our patients.

11.3.2 Personal observations

Our series of 47 patients included 3 cases in whom unmistakable collagen deposition in the subepithelial tissue was noticed (fig. 11.3). The width of the collagen band in these cases ranged from 10 μm to 40 μm. The case histories of these patients were presented in section 9.3 and 9.4, as the course of their disease was complicated (patients no. 2, 17 and 34). Apart from one patient who died shortly after the institution of the diet (patient no. 34) multiple repeat biopsy specimens were later obtained in the other cases. In one patient the subepithelial collagen deposits had completely disappeared at the repeat biopsy after 4 years on a gluten-free diet. The remaining patient still showed a distinct collagen band 5 years after gluten withdrawal, although the width of the band had diminished somewhat.

Post-mortem examination of two patients with refractory sprue (section 11.4) revealed no sign of subepithelial collagen deposition anywhere in the small intestine.

11.3.3 Comment

Collagen deposition in the lamina propria is regularly observed in coeliac patients. Gluten provocation in a treated coeliac patient is followed within 48 hours by the appearance of minute amounts of collagen beneath the basement membrane (784). A distinctly recognizable amount of collagen may be found in no fewer than one third of the intestinal biopsies of untreated coeliac patients (96, 160, 420). A wide subepithelial collagen band is fairly rare, although Bossart et al. (96) observed it in 8% of their untreated coeliacs. Other investigators have also reported the presence of subepithelial collagen deposits (49, 143, 409). It is to be noted, however, that the very large

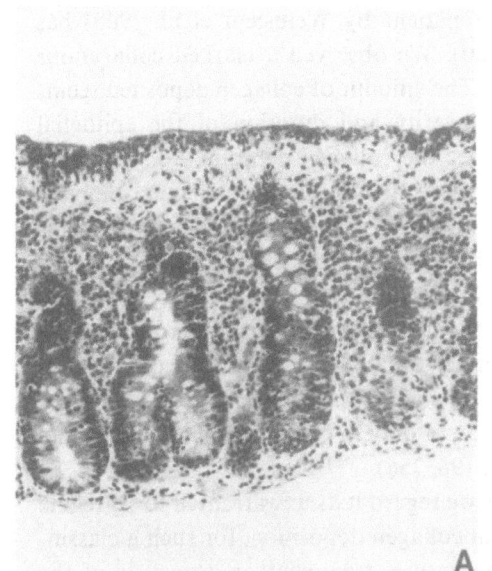

Fig. 11.3. Subepithelial collagen deposition in 3 coeliac patients (patients no. 2, 34 and 17 respectively).

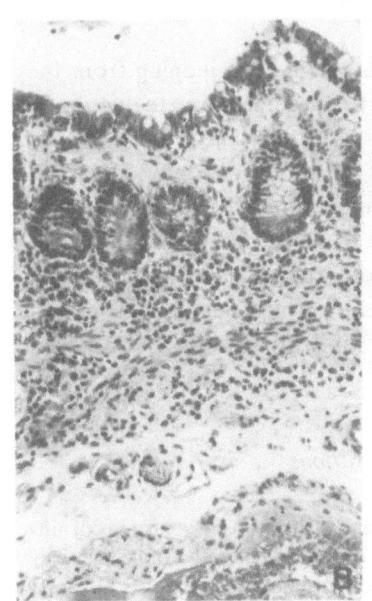

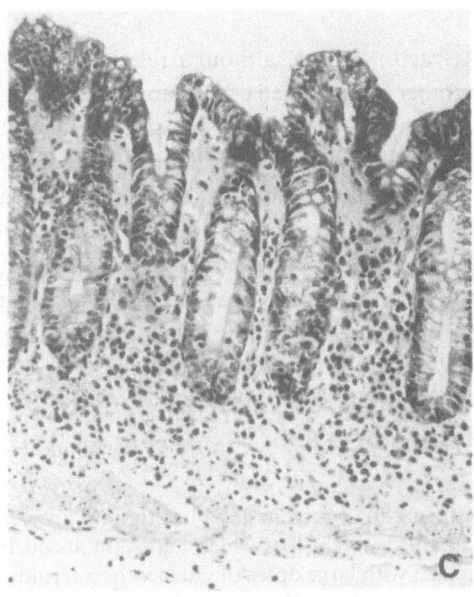

amount of collagen found in their patient by Weinstein et al. (900) has rarely been described (141, 221, 420). We observed a marked collagenous band in 3 of our patients (fig. 11.3). The amount of collagen deposited seems to be determined in part by the severity and duration of the epithelial damage, for in therapy-resistent cases the collagen deposits are sometimes seen to increase (96, 141, 900). Studies involving frequent jejunal biopsies show that the collagen can disappear within 2-6 months after gluten withdrawal. The presence of collagen beneath the epithelium of the small intestine seems of little prognostic value. Several patients respond well to gluten withdrawal, with or without temporary glucocorticosteroid medication (52, 409, 444). Patients who prefer to continue without dietary restriction can also prove to be doing quite well (96). For the rest, subepithelial collagen deposits are by no means found only in coeliac patients. It is sometimes also observed in tropical sprue (96, 756).

For the above mentioned reasons we regard it as unwarranted to segregate patients on the basis of subepithelial collagen deposition, for such a classification gives no information on the nature, treatment or prognosis of the intestinal lesions.

11.4 REFRACTORY SPRUE

11.4.1 Introduction

Refractory sprue, although relatively rare, is not unique judging from the number of published case histories (table 11.2). The names given to this condition range from 'unresponsive coeliac disease', 'collagenous sprue' or 'unclassified sprue' to 'ulcerative jejunoileitis', 'intestinal atrophy' and 'fatal malabsorption syndrome'. We prefer the name refractory sprue, which is non-committal about a possible relationship to coeliac sprue and does not emphasize the occurrence of certain morphological phenomena. The patients in question may well belong to a heterogeneous group, having as common denominator the failure to respond to any kind of treatment, clearly expressed by the adjective 'refractory'.

11.4.2 Personal observations

Patient A had been in good health until age 42, apart from several episodes of unexplained weight loss which had spontaneously ceased. At the age of 42 she was treated with large doses of glucocorticosteroids for complaints of malaise, anaemia and weight loss. These complaints were thought to be caused by adrenocortical hypofunction. She responded well to this therapy, and gained 18 kg body weight. Two years later she was treated by local irradiation for suspected reticulumcell

AUTHORS	PREVIOUS HISTORY OF COELIAC SPRUE	REPORTED NUMBER OF CASES
Himes et al. (1957)	doubtful	1
Kelley et al. (1958)	doubtful	1
Hourihane (1963)	no details	1
Shiner (1963)	no details	1
Smitskamp et al. (1965)	present	1
Pink et al. (1967)	no details	2
Stewart et al. (1967)	no details	1
Cooke (1968)	no details	2
C.P.C. (1968)	present	1
Jeffries et al. (1968)	absent	1
Barry et al. (1970)	doubtful	1
C.P.C. (1970)	absent	1
Weinstein et al. (1970)	doubtful	1
Krondl et al. (1971)	no details	1
C.P.C. (1972)	doubtful	1
Doe et al. (1972)	doubtful	1
Marche et al. (1974)	doubtful	1
Modigliani et al. (1975)	no details	1
Own series	doubtful	2

sarcoma near the left sacro-iliac joint. Only a year later, at age 45, she complained of watery diarrhoea (20 times per day) and regular vomiting, resulting in a weight loss of 12 kg. She was referred to our department for more extensive investigations. Examination revealed a severe hypoalbuminaemia (30 g/l) and marked steatorrhoea (fat absorption coefficient 55 %). Serum calcium and magnesium concentrations were decreased (1.51 mmole/l after correction, and 0.30 mmole/l, respectively). Since after ACTH stimulation the plasma cortisol level of 250 μg/l increased by factor 4, hypoadrenocorticism was excluded. A gluten-free diet was prescribed as the biopsy specimen from the proximal jejunum showed a flat mucosa. The diarrhoea, however, did not cease. Continuous intravenous administration of glucose solution, plasma, minerals and vitamins during some weeks was complicated by sepsis. Subsequent parenteral glucocorticosteroid administration during the course of several weeks failed to prevent the patient's death, only 5 months after the diarrhoea started. The post-mortem was performed within 2 hours of death. The small intestine, which felt thin over its entire length, was resected. Neither the mesenteric blood vessels nor the abdominal lymph nodes were abnormal. The liver showed extreme fatty degeneration but no tumour metastases; the pancreas was entirely normal. No signs of malignancy were observed in and around the left sacro-iliac joint. The very thin mucosa of the small intestine showed no villi from the pylorus to the ileocaecal valve. The enterocytes were cubical. A striking finding was the small number of crypts, in which little mitotic activity was discernible (fig. 11.4.a). Nowhere in the mucosa of the small intestine were ulcerations or subepithelial collagen found.

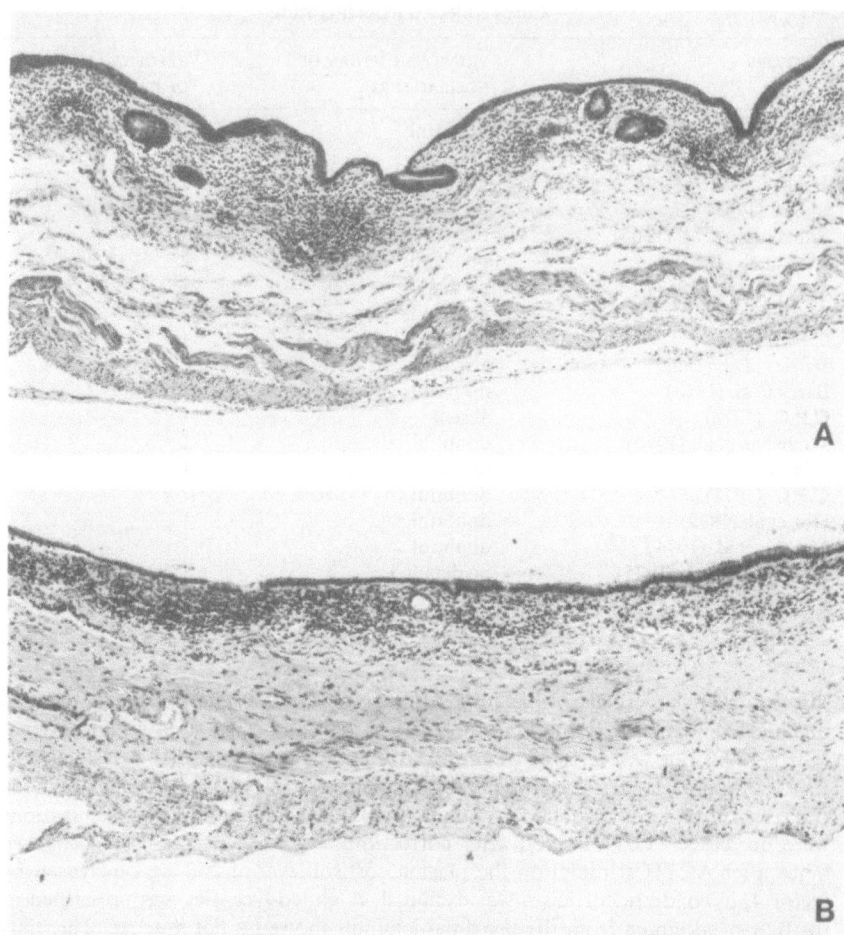

Fig. 11.4. Post-mortem specimen of the small intestine from 2 patients with refractory sprue (patients A and B; for case histories see text). The thinness of the intestinal wall and paucity of mucosal crypts are apparent.

Patient B began to pass frequent pulpy stools at age 54 and lost 6 kg body weight. He also felt tired and listless. When questioned he stated that as a child he had sometimes suffered from meteorism, diarrhoea, anaemia, and retardation of growth. The abdominal symptoms which had now developed were so severe that hospitalization was necessary. The patient was vomiting and produced large amounts of watery faeces (1-5 kg per day). The body weight had decreased to 50 kg (height 1.68 m). Biochemical tests revealed a normal haemoglobin concentration but a markedly decreased serum folate level (less than 1 ng/ml). The serum albumin concentration was markedly decreased (19 g/l), due to an increased enteric protein loss (500 ml plasma per day). There was moderate steatorrhoea (absorption coefficient 68%), decreased excretion of D-xylose (2 g in 5 hours) and vitamin B_{12} (0.6% in 48 hours). The number of micro-organisms in the proximal jejunum was not increased, while urinary indican excretion was normal. The 'breath'test for bile acid deconjugation showed an increased peak value (5.25×10^{-5} of the administered dose), probably due to reduced reabsorption of bile acids in the ileum. Cholestyramine had no effect on the diarrhoea. Gluten withdrawal prescribed in view of a flat jejunal mucosa with marked inflammatory changes and superficial erosions, had no effect, no more than 3 weeks of an elementary diet or parenteral administration of fluids, plasma, minerals and vitamins. The progressive deterioration of the patient's condition was accelerated by disturbed liver function and sepsis. The patient died cachectic, 7 months after the onset of diarrhoea. At the post-mortem, performed within 2 hours of death, a palpably thin small intestine was resected. A small amount of serous fluid was found in the abdominal cavity. The liver showed extensive steatosis and signs of cholangitis. The pancreas was normal, apart from slight atrophy of the exocrine glands. The spleen was atrophic. The mesenteric blood vessels seemed normal. The abdominal lymph nodes were markedly enlarged; microscopy revealed a chronic inflammatory infiltrate with an increase of connective tissue. No signs of a specific inflammatory or malignant process were found. The mucosa of the small intestine was flat over its entire length, and lined by cubical to high-cylindrical enterocytes. The lamina propria contained a dense inflammatory infiltrate consisting of granulocytes as well as plasma cells and lymphocytes. In this patient the number of mucosal crypts was also extremely reduced with a minimal mitotic activity (fig. 11.4.b).

11.4.3 Comment

The confrontation with patients suffering from refractory sprue comes usually as a surprise. As a rule there are hardly any indications that one is dealing with refractory sprue, and the non-responsiveness of the patient to a gluten-free diet is usually unexpected. The symptomatology of refractory sprue, after all, is virtually identical to that of coeliac sprue. Only a few symptoms stand out in patients with refractory sprue, such as abdominal pain and signs of intestinal obstruction (55, 141, 221), although these are sometimes also observed in cases with uncomplicated coeliac sprue. Some patients show variable skin lesions (141, 221, 555) or fingerclubbing (142), but these symptoms are hardly characteristic (table 8.1). The severe hypoalbuminaemia observed in nearly all patients also does not differ significantly from that in gluten-sensitive sprue (52). According to Creamer (182), radiographs of the small intestine in refractory sprue are characteristic in that they show a tubular intestine without mucosal plication. This phenomenon, known as moulage, can also occur in other intestinal diseases, including coeliac sprue (434, 563).

As the designation indicates, patients with refractory sprue fail to respond to all therapeutic measures. Efforts to influence the downhill course by even unconventional measures such as administration of pancreatic enzymes (682, 900), salazosulphapyridine (141, 900), tuberculostatics (49), broad-spectrum antibiotics (233, 555, 900) or cytostatics (555), proved to be quite unsuccessful. The patients ultimately die from complications, or from cachexia due to extensive malabsorption.

In nearly all published cases with refractory sprue a post-mortem was performed, which sometimes revealed an extremely thin-walled and atrophic small intestine (682, 900), as it was found in our two patients. Enlarged mesenteric lymph nodes were regularly observed (52), consisting of fibrotic tissue (142, 143), or cavities containing accumulated chyle or other lipid material (555). In a few cases the post-mortem did reveal other pathological abnormalities, such as a malignant process (section 9.4.4), evidence of abdominal tuberculosis (253), pancreatic lesions (682) or signs of malignant lymphoma formation in the small intestine (421), well-known causes to bring on a therapy-resistant malabsorption syndrome. The significance of extraintestinal vasculitis, cryoglobulinaemia, discrete thrombosis or obstructed lymph flow found in some patients, has remained obscure (143, 221, 555). The same applies to the mycelia or bacteria found in some intestinal ulcers (49, 55).

There are several hypotheses on the pathogenesis of refractory sprue. Some authors hold that these patients are hypersensitive to several antigens or allergens other than gluten, which originate from the food, intestinal bacteria, or result from degradation of the mucosa of the small intestine (233, 444). The increased permeability of the intestinal mucosa found in all untreated coeliac patients (267, 590) could play a role in this respect, although this fails to explain why only a few coeliac patients are affected. According to another theory are the longstanding mucosal lesions too extensive and severe to permit any recovery (141, 182). There are several other, purely speculative hypotheses (141, 142, 143, 603, 809).

In our own two cases we were struck by the extreme atrophy of the intestinal wall over the entire length. Histological examination of the intestinal mucosa revealed the features of an exhausted regeneration: a small number of crypts in which little mitotic activity was discernible (fig. 11.4). Others have reported similar findings (49, 420, 601, 682, 900), or published illustrations showing an intestinal mucosa with similar features (141, 143, 555). That a decreased production of enterocytes is present in such patients was demonstrated by Barry et al. (52) by DNA determination in perfusion fluid from intestinal loops. We share the latter investigators' suspicion that crypt hypoplasia is a primary phenomenon in patients with refractory sprue. The flat mucosa in these patients, resembling that in coeliac sprue, is nothing but the end-result of this hypoplasia. Analogous to comparing the turnover pattern of the intestinal epithelium in coeliac patients with haemolytic anaemia (89, 186), one might compare the pattern in refractory sprue with aplastic anaemia. Although this hypothesis might explain the morphogenesis of the intestinal mucosa in these patients, it fails to explain the cause of this primary crypt hypoplasia.

CHAPTER 12

METHODS AND PROCEDURES

12.1 BIOCHEMICAL ASSAYS

12.1.1 Determinations in blood

Albumin concentration in serum was determined electrophoretically with cellulose acetate as vehicle (483). Since this method involves the use of amido-black which binds more strongly to albumin than to the globulin fractions, the values given are relatively high.
Controls (n = 32): 45.8-55.1 g/l.

Alkaline phosphatase activity in serum was determined according to Bessey et al. (65), using 2-amino-2-methylpropanolol buffer.
Controls (n = 29): 45-90 U/l
(6.5-13 KAU/l).

Amino acid analysis in serum was carried out with the aid of a Beckman Multichrom amino acid analyser. The normal range of the various essential amino acids in 23 controls is listed in table 7.8.

Calcium concentration in plasma was measured with the aid of an atom absorption spectrophotometer.
Controls (n = 24): 2.35-2.50 mmole/l
(4.70-5.00 mEq/l).

Cholesterol concentration in serum was determined in accordance with the principle of Liebermann-Burchard as modified according to Huang et al. (424).
Controls (n = 37): 4.0-7.2 mmole/l
(150-275 mg/100 ml).

Folate concentration in serum was determined by means of a biological assay with Lactobacillus casei, as described by Waters et al. (893).
Controls (n = 25): 6.8-26.2 µmole/l
(3.0-11.5 ng/ml).

Haemoglobin concentration in blood was colorimetrically determined after conversion to cyanmethaemoglobin according to Van Kampen et al. (456).
Female controls (n = 47): 7.9-9.8 mmole/l (12.7-15.8 g/100 ml).
Male controls (n = 54): 8.7-10.9 mmole/l (14.0-17.6 g/100 ml).

Iron concentration in serum was determined colorimetrically as described by Ramsay (696).
Controls (n = 102): 8.9-24.7 μmole/l
(50-138 μg/100 ml)

Iron binding capacity (total) of serum was determined as described by Ramsay (697).
Controls (n = 102): 50-85 μmole/l
(280-476 μg/100 ml)

Magnesium concentration in serum was measured with the aid of an atom absorption spectrophotometer.
Controls (n = 25): 0.80-0.95 mmole/l
(1.60-1.90 mEq/l).

Thrombotest was measured in venous blood after incubation in thrombotest reagent as described by Owren (654).
Controls (n = 22): 60-100%.

Vitamin A concentration in serum was determined according to Paterson et al. (661).
Controls (n = 54): cf Fig. 7.10.

Vitamin B_{12} concentration in serum was determined by a microbiological assay with Lactobacillus Leichmanii, as described by Matthews (565).
Controls (n = 24): 220-440 μmole/l
(300-600 pg/ml)

Vitamin E concentration in serum was spectrophotometrically determined according to Hashim et al. (368).
Controls (n = 25): 25-35 μmole/l
(1075-1500 μg/100 ml).

12.1.2 Determinations in urine

Amino acid excretion was determined in 24-hour urine with the aid of a Beckman Multichrom amino acid analyser.

Hydroxyproline excretion was measured in 24-hour urine during collagen restriction. Measurements were done colorimetrically as described by Prockop et al. (692).
Controls (n = 23): 150-400 μmole/24 hrs
(19.5-52.5 mg/24 hrs).

Indican excretion was determined in 24-hour urine according to Müting et al. (622).
Controls (n = 33): 180-480 μmole/24 hrs
(45-120 mg/24 hrs).

12.1.3 Absorption tests

Calcium absorption was determined by measuring the radioactivity in plasma after oral administration of 10 μCi [47]Ca in the form of calcium citrate together with 200 ml cow's milk, 1 hour after breakfast. Blood samples were obtained after 10, 20, 30, 45, 60, 120, 180 and 240 minutes. Radioactivity was measured in a well-type scintillation detector and expressed as per cent of the dose administered per litre of plasma. Radioactivity in the organism was determined 1 hour after administration of the [47]Ca, with the aid of a whole-body counter. Retention of [47]Ca in the organism was determined after 1, 7, 14 and 21 days, and expressed as per cent of the activity measured in the body 1 hour after administration of the dose.

Fat absorption coefficient was calculated by relating the amount of fat in the faeces to the oral intake. This was done in the course of a 5-day balance period during which a diet with a fixed amount of fat (60-100 g) was used. Faeces was marked with carmine red before and after this 5-day period. The faecal fat was determined according to Van de Kamer et al. (452). Lower limit of normal range: 95%.

Glucose tolerance test was carried out with 100 g glucose. The blood sugar concentration was measured by the potassium ferricyanide method according to Hoffman (407). Blood samples were obtained from the fasting subject and 30, 60, 90 and 120 minutes after glucose ingestion.
Controls (n = 22): cf Fig. 7.2.

Iron retention was determined by measuring [59] Fe activity with the aid of a whole-body counter after oral administration of 2 μCi ^{59}Fe in a 50 ml solution of 0.2 mmole ferroammonium sulphate and 2 mmole ascorbic acid in 0.004 n HC1 to the fasting subject. Radioactivity measured 3 weeks after administration of the ^{59}Fe was expressed as per cent of the activity present in the body 1 hour after administration of the dose.

Lactose tolerance test was carried out with 50 g lactose. The blood sugar concentration was determined according to Hoffman (407) in the fasting subject and 10, 20, 30, 45, 60 and 90 minutes after lactose ingestion.
Maximal increase in blood sugar concentration in controls (n = 22): 1.2-3.8 mmole/l (22-68 mg/100 ml).

Maltose tolerance test was carried out with 50 g maltose.

Sucrose tolerance test was carried out with 50 g sucrose.

Vitamin A tolerance test was carried out after oral administration of 600,000 IU (= 320 mg) vitamin A palmitate in aqueous solution (Arovit^R) to the fasting subject. Blood samples were obtained from the fasting subject and 3, 6 and 9 hours after administration of the dose. The serum vitamin A concentration was determined according to Paterson et al. (661).
Maximal increase in serum vitamin A concentration in controls (n = 24): 1.8-21.0 μmole/l (170-2000 μg/100 ml).

Vitamin B_{12} absorption was determined according to Schilling (758), using 0.5 μCi ^{57}Co vitamin B_{12} (1.1 μg vitamin B_{12}). Together with oral administration to the fasting patient, 1 mg vitamin B_{12} was injected i.m. Radioactivity was measured in the urine of the 48-hour period after ingestion. Patients in whom achlorhydria was not excluded in advance, were given intrinsic factor as well.
Controls (n = 28): 15-35% of dose excreted in 48 hours.

Xylose absorption was studied by measuring the excretion of D-xylose in the 5-hour urine after ingestion of 25 g D-xylose while fasting. The D-xylose was determined colorimetrically as described by Roe et al. (712).
Controls (n = 25): 33.5-62 mmole/5 hrs
             (5.0-9.3 g/5 hrs).

12.1.4 Other determinations

Albumin synthesis rate was determined after administration of ^{14}C-labelled carbonate according to McFarlane (575), as described by Hafkenscheid et al. (349).
Controls (n = 15): 22.3 ± 6.8 g/175 cm/24 hrs.

Breath test with (glyco-1-^{14}C) cholic acid, for demonstration of the presence of an abnormal intestinal flora, was carried out by determining the

amount of $^{14}CO_2$ in expiratory air after ingestion of 5 μCi ^{14}C-labelled glycocholic acid with a standard breakfast. Radioactivity was determined in the breath samples collected every hour (up to 10 hours after ingestion) with the aid of a fluid scintillation counter, and expressed as proportion of the dose administered per mmole expiratory CO_2 (295, 777).
Upper limit of normal range: 1.5×10^{-5} of dose per mmole expiratory CO_2.

Enteric plasma protein leakage was determined by measuring the radioactivity of faeces and determining the plasma disappearance curve after intravenous administration of 50 μCi $^{51}CrCl_3$ as described by Van Tongeren et al. (848).
Upper limit of normal range: 30 ml plasma/24 hrs.

Intestinal juice cultures were carried out by aspirating a sample from the first jejunal loop in the fasting subject, transporting it immediately under strictly anaerobic conditions and inoculating it on a medium previously rendered free of oxygen.
Bacteria were counted by a dilution technique and counts were checked on the basis of a Gram preparation of the original jejunal juice.
Upper limit of normal range: 10^3 micro-organisms per ml.

Phosphate reabsorption was determined by measuring the ratio between phosphate and creatinine excretion in a 2-hour urine portion as described by Bijvoet et al. (67).

12.2 STATISTICAL ANALYSES

12.2.1 Calculation of normal values

In order to ensure correct interpretation of the values found in patients, virtually every biochemical test was also done in a group of controls, consisting partly of healthy staff-members and partly of out-patients in whom no abnormalities had been found. The number of control values always exceeded 20, with a maximum of 102.

Since it was not always clear whether a normal distribution of control values existed, a distribution-free method as described by Mainland (545) and Elveback et al. (248) was used. By this method the inside limits for the 2.5 and 97.5 percentile lines with 90% confidence were calculated. The values found were interpreted as limits of the normal range, represented by the shaded area in each figure.

12.2.2 *Calculation of significances*

In an effort to establish whether the biochemical determinations and the results of the absorption tests showed differences between individuals with a flat mucosa and those with a convoluted pattern in the jejunal biopsy specimen, the Mann-Whitney test (552) was applied. This test was preferred because the samples did not impress as having been drawn from a normally distributed population, and because the variances were usually unequal. For the same reasons, Wilcoxon's signed-rank test (916) was used in comparing results before and after gluten withdrawal. In order to characterize the relation between various parameters, Pearson's correlation coefficient was calculated if necessary.

12.3 BIOPSY OF THE SMALL INTESTINE

Prior to 1970, the capsule of Crosby et al. (185) was used for taking biopsies of the small intestine. Later the multiple biopter according to Becker, as described by Haex et al (347), or that according to Quinton-Flick-Rubin (278) was used. Immediately before taking biopsies, the exact position of the capsule was determined under fluoroscopic control.

The biopsy specimens were rinsed with physiological saline, and subsequently spread on paper with the submucosal surface adherent to the paper towelling. This was immediately followed by fixation in formalin, and also in Bouin's fluid to facilitate stereomicroscopic evaluation and photography.

At stereomicroscopy, the biopsy specimens were named according to the most conspicuous type of villus: finger-shaped, leaf-shaped, convoluted or flat.

The biopsies were carefully embedded in paraffin in order to avoid tangential cutting. The histological sections were stained with haematoxylin-eosin and PAS; for better evaluation of the presence of collagen with van Gieson elastin stain, and for detection of ceroid according to Ziehl-Neelsen or with auramin-rhodamin.

Lactase activity in biopsy specimens was determined as described by Dahlqvist (190) and expressed as Units per gramme wet weight of tissue. Lower limit of normal range: 1.5 Unit.

REFERENCES

1. ABELS J: Intrinsic factor van Castle en resorptie van vitamine B_{12}. MD Thesis, Groningen, 1959.
2. ABELS J, VEEGER JJM, WOLDRING MG, et al: The physiologic mechanism of vitamin B_{12} absorption. Acta Med Scand 165: 105-113, 1959.
3. ABELS J, SCHILLING RF: Protection of intrinsic factor by vitamin B_{12} J Lab Clin Med 64: 375-384, 1964.
4. ADIBI SA: Leucine absorption rate and net movements of sodium and water in human jejunum. J Applied Physiol 28: 753-757, 1970.
5. ADIBI SA, MERCER DW: Protein digestion in human intestine as reflected in luminal, mucosal and plasma amino acid concentrations after meals. J Clin Invest 52: 1586-1594, 1973.
6. ADIBI SA, FOGEL MR, AGRAWAL RM: Comparison of free amino acid and dipeptide absorption in the jejunum of sprue patients. Gastroenterology 67: 586-591, 1974.
7. ADDISON IM, MATTHEWS DM, BURSTON D: Competition between carnosine and other peptides for transport by hamster jejunum in vitro. Clin Sci 46: 707-714, 1974.
8. ADLERSBERG D, COLCHER H, DRACHMAN SR: Studies on the effects of cortisone and pituitary adrenocorticotropic hormone (ACTH) in the sprue syndrome. Gastroenterology 19: 674-697, 1951.
9. ADMIRAND W, WAY LW: Bile formation and biliary tract function, in 'Gastrointestinal disease'. Ed by MH SLEISENGER, JS FORDTRAN; pp 352-358. Saunders, Philadelphia, 1973.
10. AGNEW JE, KEHAYOGLOU AK, HOLDSWORTH CD: Comparison of three isotopic methods for the study of calcium absorption. Gut 10: 590-597, 1969.
11. AGNEW JE, HOLDSWORTH CD: The effect of fat on calcium absorption from a mixed meal in normal subjects, patients with malabsorptive disease, and patients with a partial gastrectomy. Gut 12: 973-977, 1971.
12. ALARCON-SEGOVIA D, HERSKOVIC T, WAKIM KG, et al: Presence of circulating antibodies to gluten and milk fractions in patients with nontropical sprue. Am J Med 36: 485-499, 1964.
13. ALBERT ED, HARMS K, WANK R, et al: Segregation analysis of HL-A antigens and haplotypes in 50 families with coeliac disease. Transpl Proceed 5: 1785-1789, 1973.
14. ALBERT ED: Participation in the discussions, in 'Coeliac Disease'. Ed by WTJM HEKKENS, AS PENA; p 337. Stenfert Kroese, Leiden, 1974.
15. ALCOCK N, MACINTYRE I: Interrelation of calcium and magnesium absorption. Clin Sci 22: 185-193, 1962.
16. ALLEN A, SNARY D: The structure and function of gastric mucus. Gut 13: 666-672, 1972.
17. ALP MH, WRIGHT R: Autoantibodies to reticulin in patients with idiopathic steatorrhoea, coeliac disease, and Crohn's disease, and their relation to immunoglobulins and dietary antibodies. Lancet 2: 682-685, 1971.
18. ALVARADO F: D-xylose active transport in the hamster small intestine. Biochim Biophys Acta 112: 292-306, 1966.
19. AMENT EM, SHIMODA SS, SAUNDERS DR, RUBIN CE: Pathogenesis of steatorrhea in three cases of small intestinal stasis syndrome. Gastroenterology 63: 728-747, 1972.
20. AMMAN HV, PHILLIPS SF: Inhibition of colonic water and electrolyte absorption by fatty acids in man. Gastroenterology 65: 744-749, 1973.
21. AMMAN HV, THOMAN PJ, PHILLIPS SF: Effects of oleic and ricinoleic acids on net jejunal water and electrolyte movement. J Clin Invest 53: 374-379, 1974.

22. ANDERSON BB, PEART MB, FULFORD-JONES CE: The measurement of serum pyridoxal by a microbiological assay using Lactobacillus casei. J Clin Pathol 23: 232-242, 1970.
23. ANDERSON CM, GRACEY M, BURKE V: Coeliac disease. Arch Dis Child 47: 292-298, 1972.
24. ANDERSON CM: Participation in the discussions, in 'Coeliac Disease'. Ed by WTJM HEKKENS, AS PENA; p 337. Stenfert Kroese, Leiden, 1974.
25. ARNOLD R, EBERT R, BROWN JC, CREUTZFELDT W: Gastrin (IRG) and gastric inhibitory polypeptide (GIP) after partial duodeno-pancreatectomy and in coeliac disease. Eur J Clin Invest 6: 327, 1976.
26. ARTHUR AB, CLAYTON BE, COTTOM DG, SEAKINS JWT: Importance of disaccharide intolerance in the treatment of coeliac disease. Lancet 1: 172-174, 1966.
27. ASCHHEIM E, ZWEIFACH BW: Quantitative studies of protein and water shifts during inflammation. Am J Physiol 202: 554-558, 1962.
28. ASQUITH P, THOMPSON RA, COOKE WT: Serum-immunoglobulins in adult coeliac disease. Lancet 2: 129-131, 1969.
29. ASQUITH P: Immunology. Clinics in Gastroenterology III, 1: 213-234, 1974.
30. ASQUITH P: Participation in the discussions, in 'Coeliac Disease'. Ed by WTJM HEKKENS, AS PENA; p 24. Stenfert Kroese, Leiden, 1974.
31. ASQUITH P: Family studies in coeliac disease, in 'Coeliac Disease'. Ed by WTJM HEKKENS, AS PENA; pp 322-325. Stenfert Kroese, Leiden, 1974.
32. AUSTAD WI, CORNES JS, GOUGH KR et al: Steatorrhoea and malignant lymphoma – the relationship of malignant tumours of lymphoid tissue and coeliac disease. Am J Dig Dis 12: 475-490, 1967.
33. BADENOCH J: Steatorrhoea in the adult. Br Med J 2: 879-887, 963-974, 1960.
34. BADENOCH J, CALLENDER ST: Effect of corticosteroids and gluten-free diet on absorption of iron in idiopathic steatorrhoea and coeliac disease. Lancet 1: 192-194, 1960.
34a. BAKER H, FRANK O, SOBOTKA H: Mechanisms of folic acid deficiency in nontropical sprue. Jama 187: 119-121, 1964.
35. BAKER H, FRANK O, ZIFFER H, FEINGOLD S: Reversal of folate malabsorption in tropical and non-tropical sprue by calf jejunum. Br Med J 3: 472-474, 1968.
36. BAKER PG, BARRY RE, READ AE: Detection of continuing gluten ingestion in treated coeliac patients. Br Med J 1: 486-488, 1975.
37. BAKER PG, READ AE: Reversible infertility in male coeliac patients. Br Med J 2: 316-317, 1975.
38. BAKER PG: Facts about gluten. Lancet 2: 1307, 1975.
39. BAKER PG, READ AE: Oats and barley toxicity in coeliac patients. Postgrad Med J 52: 264-268, 1976.
40. BAKER SJ, KUMAR S, SWAMINATHAN SP: Excretion of folic acid in bile. Lancet 1: 685, 1965.
41. BAKER SJ, MATHAN VI: Syndrome of tropical sprue in South India. Am J Clin Nutr 21: 984-993, 1968.
42. BAKER SJ: Geographical variations in the morphology of the small intestinal mucosa in apparently healthy individuals. Pathologia et Microbiologia 39: 222-237, 1973.
43. BALINT JA, HIRSCHOWITZ BI: Hypomagnesemia with tetany in nontropical sprue. N Eng J Med 265: 631-633, 1961.
44. BANERJEE DK, CHATTERJEE JB: Observations on the presence of pteroyl polyglutamates in human serum. Blood 28: 913-917, 1966.
45. BANWELL JG, HUTT MRS, LEONARD PJ et al: Exocrine pancreatic disease and the malabsorption syndrome in tropical Africa. Gut 8: 388-401, 1967.
46. BARAONA E, ORREGA H, FERNANDEZ O, et al: Absorptive function of the small intestine in liver cirrhosis. Am J Dig Dis 7: 318-330, 1962.
47. BARNES BA, COPE O, HARRISON T: Magnesium conservation in human being on low magnesium diet. J Clin Invest 37: 430-440, 1958.
48. BARRETT CR, HOLT PR: Postgastrectomy blind-loop syndrome. Megaloblastic anaemia secondary to malabsorption of folic acid. Am J Med 41: 629-637, 1967.
49. BARRY RE, MORRIS JS, READ AE: A case of small-intestinal mucosal atrophy. Gut 11: 743-747, 1970.
50. BARRY RE, MORRIS JS, KENWRIGHT S, READ AE: Coeliac disease and malignancy. Scand J Gastroenterol 6: 205-207, 1971.
51. BARRY RE, READ AE: Two types of 'coeliac' disease? Gut 13: 846-847, 1972.

52. BARRY RE, READ AE: Coeliac disease and malignancy. Q J Med 42: 665-675, 1973.
53. BARRY RE, BAKER P, READ AE: The clinical presentation. Clinics in Gastroenterology III, 1: 55-69, 1974.
54. BAYLESS TM, SWANSON VL: Comparison of tropical sprue and adult celiac disease (nontropical sprue). Gastroenterology 46: 731, 1964.
55. BAYLESS TM, KAPELOWITZ RF, SHELLEY WM, et al: Intestinal ulceration – a complication of celiac disease. N Eng J Med 276: 996-1002, 1967.
56. BAYLESS TM, YARDLEY JH, HENDRIX TR: Coeliac disease and possible disease relationships, in 'Coeliac Disease'. Ed by WTJM HEKKENS, AS PENA; pp 351-359. Stenfert Kroese, Leiden, 1974.
57. BENDL BJ, WILLIAMS PB: Histopathological changes in the jejunal mucosa in dermatitis herpetiformis. Can Med Assoc J 98: 575-577, 1968.
58. BENEKE K: Ueber der Spruekrankheit. Verhandl Deutsch Pathol Ges 14: 132, 1910.
59. BENNETT RA, WHITELOCK T, KELLEY JL: Eosinophilic gastroenteritis, gluten enteropathy, and dermatitis herpetiformis. Am J Dig Dis 19: 1154-1161, 1974.
60. BENSON GD, KOWLESSAR OD, SLEISENGER MH: Adult celiac disease with emphasis upon response to the gluten-free diet. Medicine (Baltimore) 43: 1-40, 1964.
61. BERG NO, DAHLQVIST A, LINDBERG T et al; Small intestinal mucosal structure, disaccharidases and dipeptidases in different types of malabsorption in childhood. A longitudinal study, in 'Coeliac Disease'. Ed by CC BOOTH, RH DOWLING; pp 187-195. Churchill Livingstone, London, 1970.
62. BERNIER JJ, SOULE C, GALIAN A et al: Etude de l'absorption intestinale de l'eau, des électrolytes et du glucose dans la maladie coeliaque de l'adulte par la méthode de la perfusion intestinale. Arch Fr Mal App Dig 64: 495-506, 1975.
63. BERNSTEIN LH, GUTSTEIN S, WEINER S, EFRON G: The absorption and malabsorption of folic acid and its polyglutamates. Am J Med 48: 570-579, 1970.
64. BERRILL WT, FITZPATRICK PF, MACLEOD WM, et al: Bird-fancier's lung and jejunal villous atrophy. Lancet 2: 1006-1008, 1975.
65. BESSEY OA, LOWRY OH, BROCK MJ: Method for rapid determination of alkaline phosphatase with 5 cubic millimeters of serum. J Biol Chem 164, 321-329, 1946.
66. BIBER B, FARA J, LUNDGREN O: Intestinal vasodilatation in response to transmural electrical field stimulation. Acta Physiol Scand 87: 277-282, 1973.
67. BIJVOET OLM, MORGAN DB, FOURMAN P: The assessment of phosphate reabsorption. Clin Chim Acta 26, 15-24, 1969.
68. BILLICH CO, LEVITHAN RI: Effects of sodium concentration and osmolality on water and electrolyte absorption from the intact human colon. J Clin Invest 48: 1336-1347, 1969.
69. BINDER HJ, HERTING DC, HURST V, et al: Tocopherol deficiency in man. N Eng J Med 273: 1289-1297, 1965.
70. BINDER HJ, SOLITARE GB, SPIRO HM: Neuromuscular disease in patients with steatorrhoea. Gut 8: 605-611, 1967.
71. BIRGE SJ, PECK WA, BERMAN M, WHEDON GD: Study of calcium absorption in man: a kinetic analysis and physiologic model. J Clin Invest 48: 1705-1713, 1969.
72. BIRKBECK JA: Coeliac disease in a diabetic child. Lancet 2: 496, 1969.
73. BISHOP RF, ALLCOCK EA: Bacterial flora of the small intestine in acute intestinal obstruction. Br Med J 1: 766-770, 1960.
74. BLACK JA: Possible factors in the incidence of coeliac disease. Acta Paediatr Scand 53: 109-116, 1964.
75. BLANKENHORN DH, HIRSCH J, AHRENS EH: Transintestinal intubation: Technic for measurement of gut length and physiologic sampling at known loci. Proc Soc Exp Biol & Med 88, 356-362, 1955.
76. BLECHER TE, BRZECHWA-ADJUKIEWICZ A, MCCARTHY CF, READ AE: Serum immunoglobulins and lymphocyte transformation studies in coeliac disease. Gut 10: 57-62, 1969.
77. BLEUMINK E: Allergens and toxic proteins in food, in 'Coeliac Disease'. Ed by WTJM HEKKENS, AS PENA; pp 46-55. Stenfert Kroese, Leiden, 1974.
78. BLOCH R, MENGE H, LINGELBACH B, et al: The relationship between structure and function of small intestine in patients with a sprue syndrome and in healthy controls. Klin Wochenschr 51: 1151-1158, 1973.
79. BLOOM SR, BRYANT MG: Distribution of radioimmunoassayable gastrin, secretin, pan-

creozymin and enteroglucagon in rat, dog, and baboon gut. J. Endocrinol 59: XLIV, 1973.
80. BODEN G, MURPHY NS, SILVER E: 'Big' secretin. Clin Res 23: 245, 1975.
81. BOENDER CA, VERLOOP MC: Iron absorption, iron loss and iron retention in man: studies after oral administration of a tracer dose of $^{59}FeSO_4$ and $^{131}BaSO_4$. Br J Haematol 17: 45-48, 1969.
82. BOLT RJ, PARRISH JA, FRENCH AB, POLLARD HM: Adult coeliac disease. Ann Intern Med 60: 581-586, 1964.
83. BOOTH CC, MOLLIN DL: Plasma, tissue and urinary radioactivity after oral administration of ^{56} Co-labelled vitamin B_{12}. Brit J Haematol 2: 223-236, 1956.
84. BOOTH CC, MOLLIN DL: The site of absorption of vitamin B_{12} in man. Lancet 1: 18-21, 1959.
85. BOOTH CC: The metabolic effects of intestinal resection in man. Postgrad Med J 37: 725-739, 1961.
86. BOOTH CC, STEWART JS, HOLMES R, BRACKENBURY W: Dissecting microscope appearances of intestinal mucosa, in 'Intestinal biopsy'. Ed by GEW WOLSTENHOLME, MP CAMERON; pp 2-19. Churchill, London, 1962.
87. BOOTH CC, BABOURIS N, HANNA S, MACINTYRE I: Incidence of hypomagnesaemia in intestinal malabsorption. Br Med J 3: 141-144, 1963.
88. BOOTH CC: Effect of location along the small intestine on absorption of nutrients, in 'Handbook of Physiology'. Ed by CF CODE, section 6 vol 3; pp 1513-1528. American Physiological Society, Washington, 1968.
89. BOOTH CC: Enterocyte in coeliac disease. Br Med J 3: 725-731; 4: 14-17, 1970.
90. BOOTH CC: Definition of adult coeliac disease, in 'Coeliac Disease'. Ed by WTJM HEKKENS, AS PENA; pp 17-22. Stenfert Kroese, Leiden, 1974.
91. BORGSTRÖM B, DAHLQVIST A, LUNDH G, SJÖVALL J: Studies of intestinal digestion and absorption in the human. J Clin Invest 36: 1521-1536, 1957.
92. BORGSTRÖM B: Studies on intestinal cholesterol absorption in the human. J Clin Invest 39: 809-815, 1960.
93. BORGSTRÖM B: Quantification of cholesterol absorption in man by fecal analysis after the feeding of a single isotope labeled meal. J Lipid Res 10: 331-337, 1969.
94. BORGSTRÖM B: Absorption of fats, in 'Malabsorption'. Ed by RH GIRDWOOD, AN SMITH; pp 14-23. University Press, Edinburgh, 1969.
95. BOSCH W: Over de indische sprouw (aphthae orientales). Sulpke, Amsterdam, 1837.
96. BOSSART R, HENRY K, BOOTH CC, DOE WF: Subepithelial collagen in intestinal malabsorption. Gut 16: 18-22, 1975.
97. BOWEN JC, FANG W, PAWLIK W: Gastrointestinal hormones and blood flow, in 'Gastrointestinal hormones'. Ed by JC THOMPSON; pp 391-400. University of Texas Press, Austin, 1975.
98. BRAGANZA J, HOWAT HT: Gallbladder inertia in coeliac disease. Lancet 1: 1133, 1971.
99. BRAIN MC, BOOTH CC: The absorption of tritium-labelled pyridoxine HCL in control subjects and in patients with intestinal malabsorption. Gut 5: 241-247, 1964.
100. BRANDBORG LL, RUBIN CE, QUINTON WE: A multipurpose instrument for suction biopsy of the esophagus, stomach, small bowel, and colon. Gastroenterology 37, 1-16, 1959.
101. BRANDBORG LL: Pancreatic Physiology, in 'Gastrointestinal disease'. Ed by MH SLEISENGER, JS FORDTRAN; pp 359-364, Saunders, Philadelphia, 1973.
102. BRICE RS, OWEN EE, TYOR MP: Amino acid uptake and fatty acid esterification by intestinal mucosa from patients with Whipple's disease and nontropical sprue. Gastroenterology 48: 584-592, 1965.
103. BRISCOE AM, RAGAN C: Bile and endogenous calcium in man. Am J Clin Nutr 16: 281-286, 1965.
104. BROOKS FP, POWELL KC, CERDA JJ: Variable clinical course of adult celiac disease. Arch Intern Med 117: 789-794, 1966.
105. BROOKS SG, DOBBINS WO: Autoradiographic localization of I-125 labeled albumin in the intestine of guinea pigs: a light and electron microscopic study. Gastroenterology 62: 1001-1012, 1972.
106. BROW JR, PARKER F, WEINSTEIN WM, RUBIN CE: The small intestinal mucosa in dermatitis herpetiformis. Gastroenterology 60: 355-361, 1971.
107. BROWN IL, FERGUSON A, CARSWELL F, et al: Autoantibodies in children with coeliac disease. Clin Exp Immunol 13: 373-382, 1973.

108. BROWN WR, BUTTERFIELD D, SAVAGE D, TADA T: Clinical, microbiological and immunological studies in patients with immunoglobulin deficiencies and gastrointestinal disorders. Gut 13: 441-449, 1972.
109. BROWNING TH, TRIER JS: Organ culture of mucosal biopsies of human small intestine. J Clin Invest 48: 1423-1432, 1969.
110. BROZOVIC B: Absorption of iron, in 'Intestinal absorption in man'. Ed by I MCCOLL, GE SLADEN; pp 263-314. Academic Press, London, 1975.
111. BRUIN EJP DE, JANSEN CR, BERG AS VAN DEN: Iron absorption in the Bantu. J Am Diet Ass 57: 129-131, 1970.
112. BRUNT PW, SIRCUS W, MACLEAN N: Neoplasia and the coeliac syndrome in adults. Lancet 1: 180-184, 1969.
113. BUCHAN DJ, GERRARD JW: Celiac disease. Ann Intern Med 57: 85-95, 1962.
114. BURG CL VAN DER: Indische spruw (aphthae Tropicae). Geneeskundig Tijdschrift voor Nederlands Indië, N S 10, 1-127, 1881.
115. BURGER GCE, DRUMMOND JC, SANDSTEAD HR: Malnutrition and starvation in Western Netherlands, september 1944- july 1945. General State Printing Office, The Hague, 1948.
116. BURKE V, ANDERSON CM: Investigation of gastrointestinal function, in 'Paediatric gastroenterology.. Ed by CM ANDERSON, V BURKE; pp 633-670. Blackwell, Oxford, 1975.
117. BURKHOLDER PK, DUBOFF EA, FILMANOWICZ EV: Nontropical sprue with secondary hyperparathyroidism. Am J Dig Dis 10: 75-85, 1965.
118. BURROWS FGO, TOYE DKM: Barium studies. Clinics in Gastroenterology III, 1: 91-107. Saunders, London, 1974.
119. BURROWS PJ, FLEMMING JS, GARNETT ES, et al; Clinical evaluation of the ^{14}C fat absorption test. Gut 15: 147-150, 1974.
120. BUTTERWORTH CE: Participation in general discussion, in 'Intestinal biopsy'. Ed by GEW WOLSTENHOLME, MP CAMERON; pp 109-112. Churchill, London, 1962.
121. BUTTERWORTH CE, BAUGH CM, KRUMDIECK C: A study of folate absorption and metabolism in man utilizing Carbon-14-labeled polyglutamates synthesized by the solid phase method. J Clin Invest 48: 1131-1142, 1969.
122. CALLENDER ST, MARNEY SR, WARNER GT: Eggs and iron absorption. Brit J Haematol 19: 657-665, 1970.
123. CAMERON AH, ASTLEY R, HALLOWELL M, et al: Duodeno-jejunal biopsy in the investigation of children with coeliac disease. Q J Med 31: 125-140, 1962.
124. CANTLIE 1936; quoted by EK, 1970: 9.
125. CARMEL R, ROSENBERG AH, KAM-SENG LAU, et al: Vitamin B_{12} uptake by human small bowel homogenate and its enhancement by intrinsic factor. Gastroenterology 56: 548-555, 1969.
126. CARTER C, SHELDON W, WALKER C: The inheritance of coeliac disease. Ann Hum Genet 23: 266-278, 1959.
127. CERDA JJ: Celiac sprue, in 'Gastrointestinal pathophysiology'. Ed by FP BROOKS; pp 238-249. Oxford University Press, London, 1974.
128. CERF M, MARCHE C, FRÉMONT A, et al: Régime sans gluten et évolution de la maladie coeliaque de l'adulte. Arch Fr Mal App Dig 64: 483-493, 1975.
129. CHALLACOMBE DN, DAWKINS PD, BAYLIS JM, ROBERTSON K: Small-intestinal histology in coeliac disease. Lancet 1: 1345-1346, 1975.
130. CHALLACOMBE DN, ROBERTSON K: Enterochromaffin cells and coeliac disease. Lancet 1: 370-371, 1976.
131. CHANARIN I, ROTHMAN D, PERRY J, STRATFULL D: Normal dietary folate, iron and protein intake with special reference to pregnancy. Br Med J 2: 394-397, 1968.
132. CHANARIN I, PERRY J: Evidence for reduction and methylation of folate in the intestine during normal absorption. Lancet 2: 776-778, 1969.
133. CHANARIN I: Absorption of cobalamins. J Clin Pathol 24 suppl 5: 60-65, 1971.
134. CHAPMAN BL, HENRY K, PAICE F, et al: A new technique for examining intestinal biopsies. Gut 13: 846, 1972.
135. CHAPMAN BL, HENRY K, PAICE F, et al: Measuring the response of the jejunal mucosa in adult coeliac disease to treatment with a gluten-free diet. Gut 15: 870-874, 1974.
136. CHARLEY PJ, STITT C, SHORE E, SALTMAN P: Studies in the regulation of intestinal iron absorption. J Lab Clin Med 61: 397-410, 1963.

242

137. CHRISTENSEN J, CLIFTON JA, SCHEDL HP: Variations in the frequency of human duodenal basic electrical rhythm in health and disease. Gastroenterology 51: 200-206, 1966.
138. CHRISTENSEN J: Movements of the small intestine, in 'Gastrointestinal disease'. Ed by MH SLEISENGER, JS FORDTRAN; pp 216-228. Saunders, Philadelphia, 1973.
139. CHUNG ASM, PEARSON WN, DARBY WJ, et al: Folic acid, vitamin B_6, pantothenic acid and vitamin B_{12} in human dietaries. Am J Clin Nutr 9: 573-582, 1961.
140. CITRIN Y, STERLING K, HALSTED JA: The mechanism of hypoproteinemia associated with giant hypertrophy of the gastric mucosa. N Eng J Med 257: 906-912, 1957.
141. CLINICOPATHOLOGICAL CONFERENCE: A case of adult coeliac disease resistent to treatment. Br Med J 2: 678-684, 1968.
142. CLINICOPATHOLOGICAL CONFERENCE: A case of malabsorption, intestinal mucosal atrophy and ulceration, cirrhosis and emphysema. Br Med J 3: 207-212, 1970.
143. CLINICOPATHOLOGICAL CONFERENCE: Non-responsive coeliac disease. Br Med J 3: 624-631, 1972.
144. CLUYSENAER OJJ, CORSTENS FHM, HAFKENSCHEID JCM, et al: Mechanisms of hypoalbuminaemia in coeliac sprue in 'Coeliac Disease'. Ed by WIJM HEKKENS, AS PENA; pp 386-398. Stenfert Kroese, Leiden, 1974.
145. CLUYSENAER OJJ, ENGELS LGJ, TONGEREN JHM VAN: De waarde van het microscopische verteringsonderzoek van faeces. Ned Tijdschr Geneesk 121: 315-319, 1977.
146. COCCO AE, DOHRMANN MJ, HENDRIX TR: Reconstruction of normal jejunal biopsies: Three-dimensional histology. Gastroenterology 51: 24-31, 1966.
147. CODE CF: Normal rates of absorption of water, sodium and potassium in man and animal. Am J Dig Dis 7: 50-56, 1962.
148. COELIAC HANDBOOK, The Coeliac Society, London, 1972.
149. COHEN M, MORGAN RGH, HOFMANN AF: Lipolytic activity of human gastric and duodenal juice against medium and long chain triglycerides. Gastroenterology 60: 1-15, 1971.
150. COHEN MI, MCNAMARA H, BLUMENFELD O, ARIAS IM: The relationship between glutamyl transpeptidase and the syndrome of celiac-sprue, in 'Coeliac Disease'. Ed by CC BOOTH, RH DOWLING; pp 91-102. Churchill Livingstone, London, 1970.
151. COLLINS FD, SINCLAIR AJ, ROYLE JP, et al: Plasma lipids in human linoleic acid deficiency. Nutr Metabol 13, 150-167, 1971.
152. COLLINS JR, ISSELBACHER KJ: Treatment of adult celiac disease (nontropical sprue). N Eng J Med 271: 1153-1156, 1964.
153. COLLINS JR, ISSELBACHER KJ: The occurrence of severe small intestinal mucosal damage in conditions other than celiac disease (nontropical sprue). Gastroenterology 49: 425-431, 1965.
154. CONNON JJ, MCFARLAND J, KELLY A, et al: Acute abdominal complications of coeliac disease. Scand J Gastroenterol 10: 843-846, 1975.
155. CONRAD ME, CROSBY WH: Intestinal mucosal mechanisms controlling iron absorption. Blood 22: 406-415, 1963.
156. CONRAD ME. WEINTRAUB LR, SEARS DA, CROSBY WH: Absorption of hemoglobin iron. Am J Physiol 211: 1123-1130, 1966.
157. CONRAD ME, BENJAMIN BI, WILLIAMS HL, FOY AL: Human absorption of hemoglobiniron. Gastroenterology 55: 35-45, 1967.
158. COOK PB, NASSIM JR, COLLINS J: The effects of thyreotoxocosis upon the metabolism of calcium, phophorus and nitrogen. Q J Med 28: 505-529, 1959.
159. COOKE WT, PEENEY ALP, HAWKINS CF: Symptoms, signs, and diagnostic features of idiopathic steatorrhoea. Q J Med 22: 59-77, 1953.
160. COOKE WT, FONE DJ, COX EV, MEYNELL MJ, GADDIE R: Adult coeliac disease. Gut 4: 279-291, 1963.
161. COOKE WT, FONE DJ, COX EV, et al: Acute folic acid deficiency of unknown aetiology: temperate sprue. Gut 4: 292-298, 1963.
162. COOKE WT, SMITH WT: Neurological disorders associated with adult coeliac disease. Brain 89: 683-722, 1966.
163. COOKE WT: Adult celiac disease, in 'Progress in gastroenterology vol I'. Ed by GB JERZY GLASS; pp 299-338. Grune & Stratton, New York, 1968.
164. COOKE WT, ASQUITH P, Introduction and definition. Clinics in Gastroenterology III, 1: 3-10. Saunders, London, 1974.

165. CORCINO JJ, WAXMAN S, HERBERT V: Absorption and malabsorption of vitamin B_{12}. Am J Med 48: 562-569, 1970.
166. CORCINO JJ: Recent advances in tropical sprue, in 'Intestinal absorption and malabsorption'. Ed by TZ CSAKY; pp 285-299. Raven Press, New York, 1975.
167. CORMANE RH: Immunofluorescent studies of the skin in lupus erythematosus and other diseases. Pathologia Europaea 2: 170-180, 1967.
168. CORNELL HJ, TOWNLEY RRW: Investigation of possible intestinal peptidase deficiency in coeliac disease. Clin Chim Acta 43: 113-125, 1973.
169. COTTON PB: Non-dietary lipid in the intestinal lumen. Gut 13: 675-681, 1972.
170. COX EV, MEYNELL MJ, COOKE WT, GADDIE R: The folic acid excretion test in the steatorrhea syndrome. Gastroenterology 35: 390-397, 1958.
171. CRABBÉ PA, HEREMANS JF: Lack of gamma A-immunoglobulin in serum of patients with steatorrhoea. Gut 7: 119, 1966.
172. CRABBÉ PA, DOUGLAS AP, HOBBS JR: Immunopathology and coeliac disease, in 'Coeliac Disease'. Ed by CC BOOTH, RH DOWLING; pp 134-142. Churchill Livingstone, London, 1970.
173. CRAFT IL, GEDDES D, HYDE CW, et al: Absorption and malabsorption of glycine and glycine peptides in man. Gut 9: 425-437, 1968.
174. CRAMER CF: Site of calcium absorption and the calcium concentration of gut contents in the dog. Can J Physiol Pharmacol 43: 75-78, 1965.
175. CRANE RK: Na^+ dependent transport in the intestine and other animal tissues. Fed Proc 24: 1000-1006, 1965.
176. CREAMER B: Malignancy and the small intestinal mucosa. Br Med J 2: 1435-1436, 1964.
177. CREAMER B: Histology and dynamics, in 'Postgraduate gastroenterology'. Ed by TJ THOMSON, IE GILLESPIE; pp 16-21. Baillière, Tindall & Cassell, London, 1966.
178. CREAMER B: The turnover of the epithelium of the small intestine. Br Med Bull 23: 226-230, 1967.
179. CREAMER B, CROFT DN: Losses from the gut in the coeliac syndrome, in 'Coeliac Disease'. Ed by CC BOOTH, RH DOWLING; pp 21-24. Churchill Livingstone, London, 1970.
180. CREAMER B: Mainly about structure, in 'The small intestine'. Ed by B CREAMER; pp 1-23. Heinemann, London, 1974.
181. CREAMER B, HELLIER MD: Mainly about function, in 'The small intestine'. Ed by B CREAMER; pp 24-46. Heinemann, London, 1974.
182. CREAMER B: Coeliac disease, in 'The small intestine'. Ed by B CREAMER; pp 91-114. Heinemann, London, 1974.
183. CREAMER B: Intestinal permeability as a screening test for mucosal damage, in 'Coeliac disease'. Ed by WTJM HEKKENS, AS PENA; pp 348-349. Stenfert Kroese, Leiden, 1974.
184. CROFT DN, LOEHRY CA, CREAMER B: Small-bowel cell-loss and weight-loss in the coeliac syndrome. Lancet 2: 68-70, 1968.
185. CROSBY WH, KUGLER HW: Intraluminal biopsy of the small intestine. Am J Dig Dis 2: 236-241, 1957.
186. CROSBY WH: Concept of the pathogenesis of anemia applied to disorders of the intestinal mucosa. Am J Dig Dis 6: 492-498, 1961.
187. CUMMISKEY J, KEELAN P, WEIR DG: Coeliac disease and diffuse pulmonary disease. Br Med J 1, 1401, 1976.
188. DA COSTA LR, CROFT DN, CREAMER B: Protein loss and cell loss from the small-intestinal mucosa. Gut 12: 179-183, 1971.
189. DAHLQVIST A, BORGSTRÖM B: Digestion and absorption of disaccharides in man. Biochem J 81: 411-418, 1961.
190. DAHLQVIST A: Method for assay of intestinal disaccharidases. Anal Biochem 7, 18-25, 1964.
191. DAHLQVIST A, LINDBERG T, MEEUWISSE G, ÄKERMAN M: Intestinal dipeptidases and disaccharidases in children with malabsorption. Acta Paediatr Scand 59: 621-630, 1970.
192. DAVENPORT HW: 'Physiology of the digestive tract' 3rd ed. Year Book Medical Publishers, Chicago, 1971.
193. DAVID TJ, AJDUKIEWICZ AB, READ AE: Fingerprint changes in coeliac disease. Br Med J 4: 594-596, 1970.

194. DAVID TJ, AJDUKIEWICZ AB, READ AE: Dermal and epidermal ridge atrophy in celiac sprue. Gastroenterology 64: 539-544, 1973.
195. DAVIDSON AR: Recurrent benign ileal ulcer occurring with the coeliac syndrome. Br Med J 3: 341, 1969.
196. DAVIDSON S, PASSMORE R, BROCK JF: 'Human nutrition and dietetics'. Churchill Livingstone, London, 1972.
197. DAVIS PS, LUKE CG, DELLER BG: Reduction of gastric iron binding protein in haemochromatosis. Lancet 2: 1431-1433, 1966.
198. DAWSON AM, HOLDSWORTH CD, PITCHER CS: Sideroblastic anaemia in adult coeliac disease. Gut 5: 304-308, 1964.
199. DAWSON AM: The absorption of fat. J Clin Pathol 24 suppl 5: 77-84, 1971.
200. DELLER DJ, MURRELL TGC, BLOWES R: Jejunal biopsy in malignant disease. Aust Ann Med 16: 236-241, 1967.
201. DELLIPIANI AW: Observations on the bacteriology of the gastro-intestinal tract in man, in 'Malabsorption'. Ed by RH GIRDWOOD, AN SMITH; pp 193-216. University Press, Edinburgh, 1969.
202. DE LUCA HF: Vitamin D. N Eng J Med 281, 1103-1104, 1969.
203. DE LUCA HF: The kidney as an endocrine organ for the production of 1,25-dihydroxy-vitamin D_3, a calcium-mobilizing hormone. New Eng J Med 289, 359-365, 1973.
204. DE LUCA L, SCHUMACHER M, WOLF G: Biosynthesis of a fucose-containing glycopeptide from rat small intestine in normal and vitamin A deficient conditions. J Biol Chem 245: 4551, 1970.
205. DENCKER H, MEEUWISSE G, NORRYD C, et al: Intestinal transport of carbohydrates as measured by portal catheterization in man. Digestion 9: 514-524, 1973.
206. DESNUELLE P, REBOUD JP, BEN ABDELJLIL A: Diet and enzyme content of pancreas, in 'The exocrine pancreas'. Ed by AVS DE RAUCH, MP CAMERON. Little, Brown & Co, Boston, 1962.
207. DEVROEDE GJ, PHILLIPS SF: Conservation of sodium, chloride and water by the human colon. Gastroenterology 56: 101-109, 1969.
208. DICKE WK: Coeliakie. Een onderzoek naar de nadelige invloed van sommige graansoorten op de lijder aan coeliakie. MD Thesis Utrecht, 1950.
209. DICKE WK, WEYERS HA, KAMER JH VAN DE: Coeliac disease; presence in wheat of a factor having deleterious effect in cases of coeliac disease. Acta Paediatr Scand 42, 34-42, 1953.
210. DIETSCHY JM, SOLOMON HS, SIPERSTEIN MD: Bile acid metabolism. J Clin Invest 45: 832-846, 1966.
211. DIETSCHY JM, WILSON JD: Cholesterol synthesis in the squirrel monkey: relative rates of synthesis in various tissues and mechanisms of control. J Clin Invest 47: 166-174, 1968.
212. DIETSCHY JM: The role of the intestine in the control of cholesterol metabolism. Gastroenterology 57: 461-464, 1969.
213. DIETSCHY JM, SALLEE VL, WILSON FA: Unstirred water layers and absorption across the intestinal mucosa. Gastroenterology 61: 932-934, 1971.
214. DIMAGNO EP, GO VLW, SUMMERSKILL WHJ: Impaired cholecystokinin-pancreozymin secretion, intraluminal dilution, and maldigestion of fat in sprue. Gastroenterology 63: 25-32, 1972.
215. DIMAGNO EP, GO VLW, SUMMERSKILL WHJ: Gallbladder function in nontropical sprue. N Eng J Med 293: 359-360, 1975.
216. DISSANAYAKE AS: Coeliac disease, in 'Topics in Gastroenterology'. Ed by SC TRUELOVE, DP JEWELL; pp 167-183. Blackwell, Oxford, 1973.
217. DISSANAYAKE AS, TRUELOVE SC, WHITEHEAD R: Lack of harmful effect of oats on small-intestinal mucosa in coeliac disease. Br Med J 4: 189-191, 1974.
218. DISSANAYAKE AS, TRUELOVE SC, WHITEHEAD R: Jejunal mucosal recovery in coeliac disease in relation to the degree of adherence to a gluten-free diet. Q J Med 53: 161-185, 1974.
219. DOBBINS WO: Electron microscopy of intestinal fat absorption under normal conditions and in malabsorptive states, in 'Progress in gastroenterology' vol I. Ed by GB JERZY GLASS; pp 261-276. Grune & Stratton, New York, 1968.
220. DOBBINS WO: Hypo-β-lipoproteinemia and intestinal lymphangiectasia. A new syn-

drome of malabsorption and protein-losing enteropathy. Arch Intern Med 122: 31-38, 1968.

221. DOE WF, EVANS D, HOBBS JR, BOOTH CC: Coeliac disease, vasculitis and cryoglobulin-aemia. Gut 13: 112-123, 1972.

222. DOE W, HENRY K, HOLT L, BOOTH CC: An immunological study of adult coeliac disease. Gut 13: 324-325, 1972.

223. DOE WF, HENRY K, BOOTH CC: Complement in coeliac disease, in 'Coeliac Disease'. Ed by WTJM HEKKENS, AS PENA; pp 189-194. Stenfert Kroese, Leiden, 1974.

224. DOLLY JO, FOTTRELL PF: Multiple forms of dipeptidases in normal human intestinal mucosa and in mucosa from children with coeliac disease. Clin Chim Acta 26: 555-558, 1969.

225. DONALDSON RM JR, MACKENZIE IL, TRIER JS: Intrinsic factor mediated attachment of vitamin B_{12} to brush borders and microvillous membranes of hamster intestine. J Clin Invest 46: 1215-1228, 1967.

226. DONALDSON RM: The relation of enteric bacterial populations to gastrointestinal function and disease, in 'Gastrointestinal disease'. Ed by MH SLEISENGER, JS FORDTRAN; pp 70-82. Saunders, Philadelphia, 1973.

227. DONALDSON RM, GRYBOSKI JD: Carbohydrate intolerance, in 'Gastrointestinal disease'. Ed by MH SLEISENGER, JS FORDTRAN; pp 1015-1030. Saunders, Philadelphia, 1973.

228. DONIACH I, SHINER M: Duodenal and jejunal biopsies. Gastroenterology 33: 71-86, 1957.

229. DORMANDY KM, WATERS AH, MOLLIN DL: Folic-acid deficiency in coeliac disease. Lancet 1: 632-635, 1963.

230. DOUGLAS AP, BOOTH CC: Post-prandial plasma-free amino acids in adult coeliac disease after oral gluten and albumin. Clin Sci 37: 643-653, 1969.

231. DOUGLAS AP, PETERS TJ, HOFFBRAND AV, BOOTH CC: Studies of intestinal peptidases with special reference to coeliac disease, in 'Coeliac Disease'. Ed by CC BOOTH, RH DOWLING; pp 115-122. Churchill Livingstone, 1970.

232. DOUGLAS AP, CRABBÉ PA, HOBBS JR: Immunochemical studies of the serum, intestinal secretions and intestinal mucosa in patients with adult celiac disease and other forms of the celiac syndrome. Gastroenterology 59: 414-425, 1970.

233. DOUGLAS AP: Long term prognosis and relation to diets, in 'Coeliac Disease'. Ed by WTJM HEKKENS, AS PENA; pp 399-405. Stenfert Kroese, Leiden, 1974.

234. DOWD, B WALKER-SMITH J: Samuel Gee, Aretaeus, and the coeliac affection. Br Med J 2: 45-47, 1974.

235. DOWLING RH: The enterohepatic circulation. Gastroenterology 62: 122-140, 1972.

236. DRASAR BS, SHINER M: Studies on the intestinal flora. Gut 10: 812-819, 1969.

237. DRASAR BS, HILL MJ: 'Human intestinal flora'. Academic Press, London, 1974.

238. DREILING DA, JANOWITZ HD: The secretion of electrolytes by the human pancreas. Gastroenterology 30: 382-390, 1956.

239. DUNNILL MS, WHITEHEAD R: A method for the quantitation of small intestinal biopsy specimens. J Clin Path 25: 243-246, 1972.

240. DUPRÉ J: Gastroeintstinal hormones, in 'Modern trends in endocrinology 4'. Ed by FTG PRUNTY, H GARDINER-HILL; pp 278-301. Butterworths, London, 1972.

241. DYMOCK IW, MACKAY N, MILLER V, et al: Small intestinal function in neoplastic disease. Br J Cancer 21: 505-511, 1967.

242. EASTHAM RD: 'Clinical haematology' 3rd ed. Wright & Sons, Bristol, 1970.

243. EDMONDS CJ: Transport of potassium by the colon of normal and sodium-depleted rats. J Physiol (London) 193: 603-617, 1967.

244. EGGERMONT E, LOEB H, MAINGUET P: Glucose absorption in coeliac disease. Lancet 2: 1315, 1967.

245. EIDELMAN S, PARKINS RA, RUBIN CE: Abdominal lymphoma presenting as malabsorption; Medicine 45: 111-137, 1966.

246. EIDELMAN S, DAVIS SD, RUBIN CE: Immunologic studies in 'hypogamma-globulinaemic sprue.' Clin Res 16: 117, 1967.

247. EK B: Studies on idiopathic non-tropical sprue. Acta Med Scand Supp 508, 1970.

248. ELVEBACK LR, TAYLOR WF: Statistical methods of estimating percentiles. Ann N Y Acad Sci 161, 538-548, 1969.

246

249. EMONS D, BOHM ER, ROTTHAUWE HW: Ergebnisse einer Nachuntersuchung von Coeliakie-Patienten. Dtsch Med Wochenschr 99: 1847-1853, 1974.
250. EMTAGE JS, LAWSON EM, KODICEK E: The response of the small intestine to vitamin D. Biochem J 140: 239-247, 1974.
251. ERTAN A, BROOKS FP, OSTROW JD, et al: Effect of jejunal amino acid perfusion and exogenous cholecystokinin on the exocrine pancreatic and biliary secretions in man. Gastroenterology 61: 686-692, 1971.
252. ESSEN R VON, SAVILAHTI E, PELKONEN P: Reticulin antibody in children with malabsorption. Lancet 1: 1157-1159, 1972.
253. EVANS DJ, BOOTH CC: Fatal malabsorption unresponsive to gluten-free diet in the adult. Gut 12: 858, 1971.
254. EVANS DJ, PATEY AL: Chemistry of wheat proteins and the nature of the damaging substances. Clinics in Gastroenterology III, 1: 199-211, Saunders, London, 1974.
255. FABER K: Ein Fall chronischer Tropendiarrhoea ('Sprue') mit anatomischer Untersuchungen des Digestionstraktus. Arch Verdauungskrankh 9: 333, 1904.
256. FAHRLAENDER H, SEIGEL M: Die klinischer Symptome der gluteninduzierten Enteropathie. Gastroenterologia 105: 283-293, 1966.
257. FALCHUK KR, FALCHUK ZM: Selective immunoglobulin A deficiency, ulcerative colitis, and gluten-sensitive enteropathy – a unique association. Gastroenterology 69: 503-506, 1975.
258. FALCHUK ZM, ROGENTINE GN, STROBER W: Predominance of histocompatibility antigen HL-A8 in patients with gluten-sensitive enteropathy. J Clin Invest 51: 1602-1605, 1972.
259. FALCHUK ZM, STROBER W: Gluten-sensitive enteropathy: synthesis of antigliadin antibody in vitro. Gut 15: 947-952, 1974.
260. FALCHUK ZM, GEBHARD RL, STROBER W: The pathogenesis of gluten sensitive enteropathy (celiac sprue): organ culture studies, in 'Coeliac Disease'. Ed by WTJM HEKKENS, AS PENA; pp 107-117. Stenfert Kroese, Leiden, 1974.
261. FANCONI G: Die chronischen Verdauungsstörungen der alteren Kinder (Herterscher infantilismus) und ihre Behandlung mit Früchten und Gemüse. Schweiz Med Wochenschr 58: 789-893, 1928.
262. FARA J, RUBINSTEIN EH, SONNENSCHEIN RR: Intestinal hormones in mesenteric vasodilatation after intraduodenal agents. Am J Physiol 223: 1058-1067, 1972.
263. FAWWAZ RA, WINCHELL HS, POLLYCOVE M, et al: Intestinal iron absorption studies using iron-52 and Anger positron camera. J Nucl Med 7: 569-574, 1966.
264. FENNIS JFM: Absorptie van ijzer bij achylia gastrica. MD Thesis, Nijmegen, 1975.
265. FERGUSON A, MAXWELL JD, HUTTON MM, MURRAY D; Adult coeliac disease in hyposplenic patients. Lancet 1:163-164, 1970.
266. FERGUSON A, MURRAY D: Quantitation of intraepithelial lymphocytes in human jejunum. Gut 12: 988-994, 1971.
267. FERGUSON A, CARSWELL F: Precipitins to dietary proteins in serum and upper intestinal secretions of coeliac children. Br Med J 1: 75-77, 1972.
268. FERGUSON A: Lymphocytes in coeliac disease, in 'Coeliac Disease'. Ed by WTJM HEKKENS, AS PENA; pp 265-276, Stenfert Kroese, Leiden, 1974.
269. FERGUSON A: Thymus-dependence of experimental villous atrophy, in 'Coeliac Disease'. Ed by WTJM HEKKENS, AS PENA; pp 286-287. Stenfert Kroese, Leiden, 1974.
270. FERGUSON A: Celiac disease and gastrointestinal food allergy, in 'Immunological aspects of the liver and gastrointestinal tract'; pp 153-202. MTP Press, London, 1976.
271. FERGUSON R, BASU MK, ASQUITH P, COOKE WT: Jejunal mucosal abnormalities in patients with recurrent aphthous ulceration. Br Med J 1: 11-13, 1976.
272. FERNANEZ LB, PAULA A DE, PRIZONT R, et al: Exocrine pancreas insufficiency secondary to gluten-enteropathy. Am J Gastroenterol 53: 564-569, 1970.
273. FEYRTER F: 'Ueber diffuse endokrine epitheliale Organe'. Barth, Leipzig, 1938.
274. FIELD M: Intestinal secretion. Gastroenterology 66: 1063-1084, 1974.
275. FISH JC, MCNEEL L, HOLADAY WJ: Lymphatic obstruction in the pathogenesis of intestinal mucosal atrophy. Ann Surg 169: 316-325, 1969.
276. FLENDRIG JA, TONGEREN JHM VAN, HOGEWEG B. VERHOEF CW: Aspects of iron absorption and iron retention, especially in patients with idiopathic haemochromatosis, in 'Radio-aktive Isotope in Klinik und Forschung, Band VIII'. Ed by K FELLINGER, R HÖFER; pp 138-150. Urban & Schwarzenberg, München, 1968.

247

277. FLESHLER B, BUTT JH, WISMAR JD: Absorption of glycine and L-alanine by the human jejunum. J Clin Invest 45: 1433-1441, 1966.
278. FLICK AL, QUITON WE, RUBIN CE: A peroral hydraulic biopsy tube for multiple sampling at any level of the gastrointestinal tract. Gastroenterology 40: 120-127, 1961.
279. FLOREY HW: The secretion and function of intestinal mucus. Gastroenterology 43: 326-329, 1962.
280. FORDTRAN JS, SCROGGIE JB, POLTER DE: Colonic absorption of tryptophan metabolites in man. J Lab Clin Med 64: 125-132, 1964.
281. FORDTRAN JS, LOCKLEAR JW: Ionic constituents and osmolality of gastric and small intestinal fluids after eating. Am J Dig Dis 11: 503-521, 1966.
282. FORDTRAN JS, RECTOR FC, WARD LOCKLEAR T, EWTON MF: Water and solute movement in the small intestine of patients with sprue. J Clin Invest 46: 287-298, 1967.
283. FORDTRAN JS, RECTOR FC, CARTER NW: The mechanisms of sodium absorption in the human small intestine. J Clin Invest 47: 884-900, 1968.
284. FORDTRAN JS: Diarrhea, in 'Gastrointestinal Disease'. Ed by MH SLEISENGER, JS FORDTRAN; pp 291-319. Saunders, Philadelphia, 1973.
285. FOTTRELL PF, DOLLY JO, DILLON A, et al: Multiple forms of peptidases in intestinal mucosa from children with coeliac disease, in 'Coeliac Disease'. Ed by CC BOOTH, RH DOWLING; pp 124-131. Churchill Livingstone, 1970.
286. FRANK BW, KERN F: Intestinal and liver lymph and lymphatics. Gastroenterology 55: 408-422, 1968.
287. FRASER NG, MURRAY D, ALEXANDER JO'D: Structure and function of the small intestine in dermatitis herpetiformis. Br J Dermatol 79: 509-518, 1967.
288. FRAZER AC: Discussion on some problems of steatorrhoea and reduced stature. Proc Roy Soc Med 49: 1009-1013, 1956.
289. FRAZER AC: Fat absorption and its disorders. Br Med Bull 14: 212-220, 1958.
290. FRAZER AC, FLETCHER RF, ROSS CAC, et al: Gluten-induced enteropathy. The effect of partially digested gluten. Lancet 2: 252-255, 1959.
291. FRAZER AC: 'Malabsorption Syndromes'. Heinemann, London, 1968.
292. FRICK PG, RIEDLER G, BRÖGLI H: Dose response and minimal daily requirement for vitamin K in man. J Appl Physiol 23: 387-389, 1967.
293. FRIEDMAN G, WAYE JD, WOLF BS, JANOWITZ HD: Manometric and cineradiographic motility patterns in disorders of the small bowel, in 'Progress in gastroenterology vol II'. Ed by GB JERZY GLASS; pp 178-199. Grune & Stratton, New York, 1970.
294. FRIEDMAN M, HARE PJ; Gluten-sensitive enteropathy and eczema. Lancet 1: 521-524, 1965.
295. FROMM H, HOFMANN AF: Breath test for altered bile-acid metabolism. Lancet 2: 621-625, 1971.
296. FRY L, KEIR P, MCMINN RMH, et al: Small-intestinal structure and function and haematological changes in dermatitis herpetiformis. Lancet 2: 729, 1967.
297. FRY L, SEAH PP, MCMINN RMH, HOFFBRAND AV: Lymphocytic infiltration of epithelium in diagnosis of gluten-sensitive enteropathy. Br Med J 3: 371, 1972.
298. FRY L, SEAH PP: Dermatitis herpetiformis: an evaluation of diagnostic criteria. Br J Dermatol 90: 137-146, 1974a.
299. FRY L, SEAH PP, HOFFBRAND AV: Dermatitis herpetiformis, in 'Coeliac Disease'. Ed by WT COOKE, P ASQUITH; Clinics in Gastroenterology vol III, 1 pp 148-157. Saunders, London, 1974b.
300. GALJAARD H, MEER-FIEGGEN W VAN DER, GIESEN J: Feedback control by functional villus cells on cell proliferation and maturation in intestinal epithelium. Exp Cell Res 73: 197-207, 1972.
301. GALJAARD H, MEER-FIEGGEN W VAN DER, BOTH NJ DE: Cell differentiation in gut epithelium, in: 'Cell differentiation' (D Viza & H Harris eds) pp 322-328. Munksgaard, Copenhagen, 1972.
302. GANGULY J: Absorption of vitamin A. Am J Clin Nutr 22: 923-933, 1969.
303. GARABEDIAN M, TANAKA Y, HOLICK MF, DE LUCA HF: Response of intestinal calcium transport and bone calcium mobilization to 1,25 dihydroxyvitamin D_3 in thyroparathyroidectomised rats. Endocrinology 94:1022-1027, 1974.
304. GEBHARD RL, KATZ SI, MARKS J, et al: Hl-A antigen type and small-intestinal disease in dermatitis herpetiformis. Lancet 2: 760-762, 1973.
305. GEE SJ: On the coeliac affection. St Bartholomew's Hosp Rep, London 24: 17-20, 1888.

306. GENT AE, CREAMER B: Faecal fats, appetite, and weightloss in the coeliac syndrome. Lancet 1: 1063-1064, 1968.
307. GENT AE: Coeliac primary amenorrhoea. Digestion 8: 509-512, 1973.
308. GERSON CD, COHEN N, BROWN N, et al: Folic acid and hexose absorption in sprue. Am J Dig Dis 19:911-919, 1974.
309. GIANNELLA RA, BROITMAN SA, ZAMCHECK N: Vitamin B_{12} uptake by intestinal microorganisms: Mechanism and relevance to syndromes of intestinal bacterial overgrowth. J Clin Invest 50: 1100-1107, 1971.
310. GIANNELLA RA, ROUT WR, TOSKES PP: Jejunal brush border injury and impaired sugar and amino acid uptake in the blind loop syndrome. Gastroenterology 67: 965-974, 1974.
311. GIBBONS RJ, KAPSIMALIS B: Estimates of the overall rate of growth of the intestinal microflora of hamsters, guinea pigs, and mice. J Bacteriol 93, 510-512, 1967.
312. GITLER C: Protein digestion and absorption in nonruminants, in 'Mammalian protein metabolism'. Ed by HN MUNRO, JB ALLISON; pp 35-39. Academic Press, London, 1964.
313. GITLIN D, CRUSHAUD A: On the kinetics of iron absorption in mice. J Clin Invest 41: 344-350, 1962.
314. GO VLW, HOFMANN AF, SUMMERSKILL WHJ: Pancreozymin bioassay in man based on pancreatic enzyme secretion: potency of specific amino acids and other digestive products. J Clin Invest 49: 1558-1564, 1970.
315. GOLDBERG D: A psychiatric study of patients with disaeses of the small intestine. Gut 11: 459-465, 1970.
316. GOLDBERG DM, CAMPBELL R, ROY AD: Fate of trypsin and chymotrypsin in the human small intestine. Gut 10: 477-483, 1969.
317. GOLDMAN AS, FOSSAN DD VAN, BAIRD EE: Magnesium deficiency in celiac disease. Pediatrics 29: 948-952, 1962.
318. GOLDSTEIN F, KARACADAG S, WIRTS CW, KOWLESSAR OD: Intraluminal small-intestinal utilization of D-xylose by bacteria. Gastroenterology 59: 380-386, 1970.
319. GOLDSTEIN F: Mechanisms of malabsorption and malnutrition in the blind loop syndrome. Gastroenterology 61: 780-784, 1971.
320. GOODCHILD MC, NELSON R, ANDERSON CM: Cystic fibrosis and coeliac disease: coexistence in two children. Arch Dis Child 48: 684-691, 1973.
321. GORBACH SL, NAHAS L, LERNER PI: Studies of intestinal microflora. I. Effects of diet, age and periodic sampling on numbers of fecal microorganisms in man. Gastroenterology 53: 845-855, 1967.
322. GORBACH SL, PLAUT AG, NAHAS L, et al: Studies of intestinal microflora. II. Microorganisms of the small intestine and their relations to oral and fecal flora. Gastroenterology 53: 856-867, 1967.
323. GOUDIE RB, STUART-SMITH DA, BOYLE IT, FERGUSON A: Serological diagnosis of idiopathic Addison's disease in patients on prolonged prednisolone therapy for steatorrhoea. Lancet 1: 186-188, 1969.
324. GOUGH KR, READ AE, NAISH JM: Intestinal reticulosis as a complication of idio-pathic steatorrhoea. Gut 3: 232-239, 1962.
325. GRABER W, LAISSUE J, KREBS A: Bioptische und serologische Untersuchungen zur Enteropathie bei Dermatitis herpetiformis Duhring. Dermatologica (Basel) 142: 329-339, 1971.
326. GRACEY M, BURKE V, ANDERSON CM: Association of monosaccharide malabsorption with abnormal small-intestinal flora. Lancet 2: 384-385, 1969.
327. GRACEY M, BURKE V, OSHIN A: Intestinal transport of fructose. Lancet 2: 827-829, 1970.
328. GRACEY M: Intestinal absorption in the 'contaminated small-bowel syndrome'. Gut 12: 403-410, 1971.
329. GRACEY M, BURKE V, OSHIN A, et al: Bacteria, bile salts, and intestinal monosaccharide malabsorption. Gut 12: 683-692, 1971.
330. GRAHAM LA, CAESAR JJ, BURGER ASV: Gastrointestinal absorption and excretion of Mg^{28} in man. Metabolism 9: 646-659, 1960.
331. GRANGER DN, COOK BH, TAYLOR AE: Structural locus of transmucosal albumin efflux in canine ileum. A fluorescent study. Gastroenterology 71: 1023-1027, 1976.
332. GRASBECK R, NYBERG W, REIZENSTEIN P: Biliary and fecal vitamin B_{12} excretion in man. An isotope study. Proc Soc Exp Biol Med 97: 780-784, 1958.

333. GRAY GM, SANTIAGO NA: Disaccharide absorption in normal and diseased human intestine. Gastroenterology 51: 489-498, 1966.
334. GRAY GM, COOPER HL: Protein digestion and absorption. Gastroenterology 61, 535-544, 1971.
335. GRAY GM: Mechanisms of digestion and absorption of food, in 'Gastrointestinal disease'. Ed by MH SLEISENGER, JS FORDTRAN; pp 250-258, Saunders, Philadelphia, 1973.
336. GRAY TK, BIEBERDORF FA, FORDTRAN JS: Thyrocalcitonin and the jejunal absorption of calcium, water, and electrolytes in normal subjects. J Clin Invest 52, 3084-3088, 1973.
337. GREEN FHY, CARTY JE: Coeliac disease and autoimmunity. Lancet 1: 964, 1976.
338. GREEN PA, WOLLAEGER EE: The clinical behavior of sprue in the United States. Gastroenterology 38: 399-418, 1960.
339. GREENBERGER NJ, SAEGH S, RUPPERT RD: Urine indican excretion in malabsorptive disorders. Gastroenterology 55: 204-211, 1968.
340. GREENBERGER NJ, SKILLMAN TG: Medium-Chain Triglycerides. N Eng J Med 280: 1045-1058, 1969.
341. GROSSMAN MI: Gastrointestinal hormones: spectrum of actions and structure-activity relations, in 'Endocrinology of the gut'. Ed by WY CHEY, FP BROOKS; pp 65-75. Slack, Thorofare NJ, 1974.
342. GROSSMAN MI, KONTUREK SJ: Gastric acid does drive pancreatic bicarbonate secretion. Scand J Gastroenterol 9: 299-302, 1974.
343. GROSSMAN MI, et al: Candidate hormones of the gut. Gastroenterology 67: 730-755, 1974.
344. GRUETTNER R: Stellungnahme zur Arbeit von E. Rossipal: Nachweis von präcipitierenden Antikörpern gegen wässrige Mehlextrakte bei Cöliakie. Z Kinderheilk 110: 200, 1971.
345. GUTIERREZ JG, CHEY WY, DINOSO VP: Actions of cholecystokinin and secretin on the motor activity of the small intestine in man. Gastroenterology 67: 35-41, 1974.
346. HAAS SV: The value of the banana in the treatment of celiac disease. Am J Dis Child 28: 421-437, 1924.
347. HAEX AJC, SEEDER WA, WEBBFRS JPP: Ervaringen met een apparaat voor multipele zuigbiopsieën in het maagdarmkanaal. Ned Tijdsch Geneesk 107: 783-787, 1963.
348. HAEX AJC: General introduction, in 'Coeliac Disease'. Ed by WTJM HEKKENS, AS PENA; pp 3-9. Stenfert Kroese, Leiden, 1974.
349. HAFKENSCHEID JCM, YAP SH, TONGEREN JHM VAN: Measurement of the rate of synthesis of albumin with ^{14}C-carbonate: a simplified method. Z Klin Chem Klin Biochem 11: 147-151, 1973.
350. HAKAMI N, NEIMAN PE, CANELLOS GP, et al: Neonatal megaloblastic anemia due to inherited transcobalamin II deficiency in two siblings. N Eng J Med 285: 1163-1170, 1971.
351. HALL CA, FINKLER AE: The dynamics of transcobalamin II. A vitamin B_{12} binding substance in plasma. J Lab Clin Med 65: 459-468, 1965.
352. HALL RJC, CREAMER B: Hyperphagia in intestinal disease. Gut 15: 858-861, 1974.
353. HALL WH: Proximal muscle atrophy in adult celiac disease. Am J Dig Dis 13: 697-704, 1968.
354. HALSTED CH, ROWE JW: Occurrence of celiac sprue in a patient with Fabry's disease. Ann Intern Med 83: 524-525, 1975.
355. HAMBRAEUS L, HEVESY G DE: A case of coeliac disease associated with cystine-lysinuria. Acta Paediatr 53: 213-220, 1964.
356. HAMILTON JD, DYER NH, DAWSON AM, et al: Assessment and significance of bacterial overgrowth in the small bowel. Q J Med 39: 265-285, 1970.
357. HAMILTON JD, CHAMBERS RA, WYNN-WILLIAMS A: Role of gluten, prednisone, and azathioprine in non-responsive coeliac disease. Lancet 1: 1213-1216, 1976.
358. HAMILTON JR, LYNCH MJ, REILLY BJ: Active coeliac disease in childhood. Q J Med 38: 135-158, 1969.
359. HANNA S, HARRISON M, MACINTYRE I, FRASER R: Syndrome of magnesium deficiency in man. Lancet 2: 172-175, 1960.
361. HANSEN AE, STEWART RA, HUGHES G, SÖDERHJELM L: The relation of linoleic acid to infant feeding. Acta Pediatr Scand 51, suppl 137, 1962.

362. HARDWICK C: Prognosis in coeliac disease. Arch Dis Childh 14: 279-294, 1939.
363. HARMS K, GRANDITSCH G, ROSSIPAL E, et al: HL-A in patients with coeliac disease and their families, in 'Coeliac Disease'. Ed by WTJM HEKKENS, AS PENA; pp 215-226. Stenfert Kroese, Leiden, 1974.
364. HARRIS F, HOFFENBERG R, BLACK E: Calcium kinetics in vitamin D deficiency rickets. II. Intestinal handling of calcium. Metabolism 14: 1112-1121, 1965.
365. HARRIS OD, COOKE WT, THOMPSON H, WATERHOUSE JAH: Malignancy in adult celiac disease and idiopathic steatorrhea. Am J Med 42: 899-912, 1967.
366. HARRIS OD, WARNER M, COOKE WT: Serum alkaline phosphatase in adult coeliac disease. Gut 10: 655-658, 1969.
367. HARRISON JE, HITCHMAN AJW, FINLAY JM, MCNEILL KG: Calcium kinetic studies in patients with malabsorption syndrome. Gastroenterology 56: 751-757, 1969.
368. HASHIM SA, SCHUTTRINGER GR: Rapid determination of tocopherol in macro- and microquantities of plasma. Results obtained in various nutrition and metabolic studies. Am J Clin Nutr 19: 137-145, 1966.
369. HAUSMAN K, KUSE R, SONNENBERG OW, et al: Inter-relations between iron stores, general factors and intestinal iron absorption. Acta Haematol (Basel) 42: 193-207, 1969.
370. HEDNER P, PERSSON H, RORSMAN G: Effect of cholecystokinin on small intestine. Acta Physiol Scand 70: 250-254, 1967.
371. HEIDEN C VAN DER, WAUTERS EAK, KETTING D, et al: Gas chromatographic analysis of urinary tyrosine and phenylalanine metabolites in patients with gastrointestinal disorders. Clin Chim Acta 34: 289-296, 1971.
372. HEINRICH HC, BARTELS H: Bestimmungsmethoden und Normalbereiche der intestinalen Eisenresorption beim Menschen. Klin Wochenschr 45: 553-558, 1967.
373. HEINRICH HC: Gastric intrinsic factor and iron absorption. Lancet 2: 1256, 1970.
374. HEKKENS WTJM, HAEX AJC, WILLIGHAGEN RG: Some aspects of gliadin fractionation and testing by a histochemical method, in 'Coeliac Disease'. Ed by CC BOOTH, RH DOWLING; pp 11-19. Churchill Livingstone, London, 1970.
375. HEKKENS WTJM, AARSEN CJ VAN DEN, GILLIAMS JP, et al: α-Gliadin structure and degradation, in 'Coeliac Disease'. Ed by WTJM HEKKENS, AS PENA; pp 39-45. Stenfert Kroese, Leiden, 1974.
376. HELLIER MD, THIRUMALAI C, HOLDSWORTH CD: The effect of amino acids and dipeptides on sodium and water absorption in man. Gut 14: 41-45, 1973.
377. HELLIER MD, HOLDSWORTH CD: Digestion and absorption of proteins, in 'Intestinal absorption in man'. Ed by I MCCOLL, GEG SLADEN; pp 143-186, Academic Press, London, 1975.
378. HENDRIX TR, BAYLESS TM: Digestion: intestinal secretion. Ann Rev Physiol 32: 139-164, 1970.
379. HENRIKSSON KG, HALLERT C, WALAN A: Gluten-sensitive polymyositis and enteropathy. Lancet 2: 317, 1976.
380. HEPNER GW, BOOTH CC, COWAN J, et al: Absorption of crystalline folic acid in man. Lancet 2: 302-306, 1968.
381. HEPNER GW: The absorption of pteroylglutamic (folic) acid in rats. Br J Haematol 16: 241-249, 1969.
382. HERBERT V: Experimental nutritional folate deficiency in man. Trans Assoc Am Phys 75: 307-320, 1962.
383. HERBERT V: Nutritional requirements for vitamin B_{12} and folic acid. Am J Clin Nutr 21, 743-752, 1968.
384. HERSKOVIC T: The exocrine pancreas in intestinal malabsorption syndromes. Am J Clin Nutr 21: 520-522, 1968.
385. HERTER CA: On infantilism from chronic intestinal infection. McMillan, New York, 1908.
386. HERTING DC, DRURY EE: Plasma tocopherol levels in man. Am J Clin Nutr 17, 351-356, 1965.
387. HESS THAYSEN TE: Non-tropical sprue. Munksgaard, Copenhagen, 1932.
388. HEYSSEL RM, BOZIAN RC, DARBAY WJ, et al: Vitamin B_{12} turnover in man. Am J Clin Nutr 18: 176-184, 1966.
389. HIGGINS JA, LEE PR, SCHOLER JF, et al: Absorption of water and sodium from the small intestine of patients with non-tropical sprue. J Clin Invest 36: 265-269, 1957.

390. HIGHTOWER NC: Motor action of the small bowel, in 'Handbook of Physiology' section 6, vol IV, pp 2001-2024. American Physiological Society, Washington, 1968.
391. HILLARY W: Observations on the changes of the air and the concomitant epidemical diseases in the island of Barbadoes Lawes, Clarke & Collins, London, 1759.
392. HIMES HW, GABRIEL JB, ADLERSBERG D: Previously undescribed clinical and post-mortem observations in non-tropical sprue: possible role of prolonged corticosteroid therapy. Gastroenterology 32: 60-71, 1957.
393. HINDLE W, CREAMER B: Significance of a flat small-intestinal mucosa. Br Med J 2: 455-458, 1965.
394. HINES JD, ROSENBERG A, HARRIS JW: Intrinsic factor mediated radio B_{12} uptake in sequential incubation studies using everted sacs of guinea pig small intestine: evidence that IF is not absorbed into the intestinal cell. Proc Soc Exp Biol Med 129: 653-658, 1968.
395. HISTOCOMPATIBILITY TESTING. Ed by J Dausset, J Colombani. Munksgaard, Copenhagen, 1973.
396. HOBBS JR, HEPNER GW: Deficiency of γM-globulin in coeliac disease. Lancet 1: 217-220, 1968.
397. HOBBS JR, HEPNER GW, DOUGLAS AP, et al: Immunological mystery of coeliac disease. Lancet 2: 649-650, 1969.
398. HOBBS JR: Participation in the discussions, in 'Coeliac Disease'. Ed by WTJM HEKKENS, AS PENA; p 337. Stenfert Kroese, Leiden, 1974.
399. HODGSON HJF, DAVIES RJ, GENT AE, HODSON ME: Atopic disorders and adult coeliac disease. Lancet 1: 115-117, 1976.
400. HOEDEMAEKER PJ, ABELS J, WACHTERS JJ, et al: Investigations about the site of production of Castle's gastric intrinsic factor. Lab Invest 13: 1394-1399, 1964.
401. HOFFBRAND AV, PETERS TJ: The subcellular localization of pteroylpolyglutamate hydrolase and folate in guinea-pig intestinal mucosa. Biochim Biophys Acta (Amst) 192: 479-485, 1969.
402. HOFFBRAND AV, DOUGLAS AP, FRY L, STEWART JS: Malabsorption of dietary folate (pteroylpolyglutamates) in adult coeliac disease and dermatitis herpetiformis. Br Med J 4: 85-89, 1970.
403. HOFFBRAND AV: Folate absorption. J Clin Pathol 24: suppl 5, 66-76, 1971.
404. HOFFBRAND AV, TABAQCHALI S, BOOTH CC, MOLLIN DL: Small intestinal bacterial flora and folate status in gastrointestinal disease. Gut 12: 27-33, 1971.
405. HOFFBRAND AV: Anaemia in adult coeliac disease. Clin gastroent III, 1: 71-89, 1974.
406. HOFFMAN HN, WOLLAEGER EE, GREENBERG E: Discordance for nontropical sprue (adult celiac disease) in a monozygotic twin pair. Gastroenterology 51: 36-42, 1966.
407. HOFFMAN WS: A rapid photoelectric method for the determination of glucose in blood and urine. J Biol Chem 120, 51-55, 1937.
408. HOFMANN AF: A physicochemical approach to the intraluminal phase of fat absorption. Gastroenterology 50: 56-64, 1966.
409. HOLDSTOCK DJ, OLEESKY S: Successful treatment of collagenous sprue with combination of prednisolone and gluten-free diet. Postgrad Med J 49: 664-667, 1973.
410. HOLDSWORTH CD, DAWSON AM: Glucose and fructose absorption in idiopathic steatorrhoea. Gut 6: 387-391, 1965.
411. HOLDSWORTH CD: Calcium absorption in man, in 'Intestinal absorption in man'. Ed by I MCCOLL, GEG SLADEN; pp 223-262. Academic Press, London, 1975.
412. HOLMES GKT, ASQUITH P, STOKES PL, COOKE WT: Cellular infiltrate of jejunal biopsies in adult coeliac disease in relation to gluten withdrawal. Gut 15: 278-283, 1974.
413. HOLMES GKT, STOKES PL, SORAHAN TM, et al: Coeliac disease, gluten-free diet, and malignancy. Gut 17: 612-619, 1976.
414. HOLMES R: The intestinal brush border. Gut 12: 668-677, 1971.
415. HOOD J, MASON AMS: Diffuse pulmonary disease with transfer defect occurring with coeliac disease. Lancet 1: 445-447, 1970.
416. HOOFF JP VAN, PENA AS, KEUNING JJ, et al: SD and LD determinants of the HL-A complex in coeliac disease, in 'Coeliac Disease'. Ed by WTJM HEKKENS, AS PENA; pp 233-237. Stenfert Kroese, Leiden, 1974.
417. HOOFT C, DEVOS E, KRIEKEMANS J, DAMME VD: Malabsorption and diabetes mellitus in children. Helv Paediatr. Acta 23, 478-488, 1968.

252

418. HOOFT C, ROELS H, DEVOS E: Diabetes and coeliac disease. Lancet 2, 1192, 1969.
419. HOETZEL D. BARNES RH: Contributions of the intestinal microflora to the nutrition of the host. Vitam and Horm 24: 115-171, 1966.
420. HOURIHANE DO'B: The histology of intestinal biopsies. Proc Roy Soc Med 56: 1073-1077, 1963.
421. HOURIHANE DO'B, WEIR DG: Malignant celiac syndrome. Gastroenterology 59: 130-139, 1970.
422. HOWE PS: 'Basic nutrition in health and disease' 5th ed. Saunders, Philadelphia, 1971.
423. HOWLAND 1921: quoted by DOUGLAS, 1974: 399.
424. HUANG TC, CHEN CP, WEFLER V, RAFTERY A: A stable reagent for the Liebermann-Burchard reaction. Application to rapid serum cholesterol determination. Ann Chem 33, 1405, 1961.
425. HUBBLE D: Diagnosis and management of coeliac disease in childhood. Br Med J 2: 701-706, 1963.
426. HUBEL KA: Secretin: a long progress note. Gastroenterology 62: 318-341, 1972.
427. IVANOVICH P, FELLOWS H, RICH C: The absorption of calcium carbonate. Ann Int Med 66: 917-923, 1967.
428. JACOBS A: Iron absorption. J Clin Pathol 24 suppl 5: 55-59, 1971.
429. JACOBS P, BOTHWELL TH, CHARLTON RW: Role of hydrochloric acid in iron absorption. J Appl Physiol 19: 187-188, 1964.
430. JAEGERSTAD M, LINDSTRAND K, NORDEN A, et al: The folate conjugase activity of the intestinal mucosa in celiac disease. Scand J Gastroenterol 9: 255-259, 1974.
431. JARNUM S: 'Protein-losing gastroenteropathy'. Blackwell, Oxford, 1963.
432. JARNUM S, JENSEN KB, SØLTOFT J, WESTERGAARD H: Protein loss and turnover of albumin, IgG and IgM in adult coeliac disease, in 'Coeliac Disease'. Ed by CC BOOTH, RH DOWLING. Churchill Livingstone, London, 1970.
433. JAWORSKI ZF, BROWN EM, FEDORUK S, SEITZ H: A method for the study of calcium absorption by the human gut using a standard dose of calcium labelled with calcium[47]. N Eng J Med 269: 1103-1111, 1963.
434. JEANS WD: An evaluation of radiological signs in small bowel examinations in children. Clin Radiol 23: 78-86, 1972.
435. JEEJEEBHOY KN, COGHILL NF: The measurement of gastrointestinal protein loss by a new method. Gut 2: 123-130, 1961.
436. JEEJEEBHOY KN: Endogenous protein loss into the bowel as a cause of hypoproteinaemia, in 'The role of the gastrointestinal tract in protein metabolism'. Ed by HN MUNRO; pp 357-383. Blackwell, Oxford, 1964.
437. JEFFRIES GH, HOLMAN HR, SLEISENGER MH: Plasma proteins and the gastrointestinal tract. N Engl J Med 266: 652-660, 1962.
438. JEFFRIES GH, STEINBERG H, SLEISENGER MH: Chronic ulcerative (nongranulomatous) jejunitis. Am J Med 44: 47-59, 1968.
439. JOHNSON CF: Disaccharidase: localization in hamster intestine brush borders. Science 155: 1670-1672, 1967.
440. JOHNSON LR: Effect of gastric mucosal acidification on the action of pepsigogues. Am J Physiol 225: 1411-1415, 1973.
441. JOHNSON LR: Gastrointestinal hormones, in 'MTP International review of science. Physiology series one, vol 4'. Ed by ED JACOBSON, LL SHANBOUR; pp 1-43. University Park Press, Baltimore, 1974.
442. JONES EA, CRAIGIE A, TAVILL AS, et al: Protein metabolism in the intestinal stagnant loop syndrome. Gut 9: 466-469, 1968.
443. JONES JE, MANALO R, FLINK EB: Magnesium requirements in adults. Am J Clin Nutr 20: 632-635, 1967.
444. JONES PE, GLEESON MH: Mucosal ulceration and mesenteric lymphadenopathy in coeliac disease. Br Med J 3: 212-213, 1973.
445. JONES RS, GROSSMAN MI: Choleretic effects of cholecystokinin, gastrin II, and caerulein in the dog. Am J Physiol 219: 1014-1018, 1970.
446. JOS J, LENOIR G, DE RITIS G, REY J: In vitro culturing of biopsies from children, in 'Coeliac Disease'. Ed by WTJM HEKKENS, AS PENA; pp 91-105. Stenfert Kroese, Leiden, 1974.
447. JOSKE RA, MARTIN JD: Coeliac disease presenting as recurrent abortion. J Obstet Gynaecol Br Commonw 78: 754-758, 1971.

253

448. KAHAN J: The vitamin A absorption test. I. Studies on children and adults without disorders in the alimentary tract. Scand J Gastroenterol 4: 313-324, 1969.
449. KAHAN J: The vitamin A absorption test. II. Studies on children and adults with disorders in the alimentary tract. Scand J Gastroenterol 5: 5-12, 1970.
450. KALIMA TV: The structure and function of intestinal lymphatics and the influence of impaired lymph flow on the ileum of rats. Scand J Gastroenterol 6, supplements 10, 1971.
451. KAMER JH VAN DE: Vet in faeces. PhD Thesis, Utrecht, 1948.
452. KAMER JH VAN DE, BOKKEL HUININK H TEN, WEIJERS HA: Rapid method for the determination of fat in faeces. J Biol Chem 177: 347-355, 1949.
453. KAMER JH VAN DE, WEYERS HA, DICKE WK: Coeliac disease; investigation into unjurious constituents of wheat in connection with their action on patients with coeliac disease. Acta Paediatr Scand 42: 223-231, 1953.
454. KAMER JH VAN DE, WEIJERS HA, WAUTERS EAK: Some biochemical aspects of coeliac disease: past, present and future, in 'Coeliac Disease'. Ed by CC BOOTH, RH DOWLING; pp 106-113, Churchill Livingstone, London, 1970.
455. KAMER JH VAN DE: Personal communication, 1977.
456. KAMPEN EJ VAN, ZIJLSTRA WG: Standardization of hemoglobinometry II. The hemiglobincyanide method. Clin Chim Acta 6: 538-544, 1961.
457. KAPADIA CR, BHAT P, JACOB E, BAKER SJ: Vitamin B_{12} absorption – a study of intraluminal events in control subjects and patients with tropical sprue. Gut 16: 988-993, 1975.
458. KARLISH AJ: Coeliac disease and diffuse lung disease. Lancet 1: 1077, 1971.
459. KASARDA DD, NIMMO CC, BERNARDIN JE: Structural aspects and genetic relationships of gliadins, in 'Coeliac Disease'. Ed by WTJM HEKKENS, AS PENA; pp 25-36. Stenfert Kroese, Leiden, 1974.
460. KASPER H: Faecal fat excretion, diarrhea, and subjective complaints with highly dosed oral fat intake. Digestion 3: 321-330, 1970.
461. KASPER H, HOSPACH R: Der diagnostische Wert der Vitamin-A- und Carotin-Bestimmung im Serum bei Maldigestion und Malabsorption. Dtsch Med Wochenschr 99: 198-200, 1974.
462. KASPER H, HOSPACH R: Der diagnostische Wert des Vitamine-A-Toleranztests bei Maldigestion und Malabsorption. Dtsch Med Wochenschr 99: 354-357, 1974.
463. KATZ AJ, FALCHUK ZM, STROBER W, SHWACHMAN H: Glutensensitive enteropathy. Inhibition by cortisol of the effect of gluten protein in vitro. N Eng J Med 295: 131-135, 1976.
464. KATZ AJ, FALCHUK ZM, SHWACHMAN H: The coexistence of cystic fibrosis and celiac disease. Pediatrics 57, 715-721, 1976.
465. KATZ J, SPIRO HM, HERSKOVIC T: Milk-precipitating substance in the stool in gastrointestinal milk sensitivity. N Eng J Med 278: 1191-1194, 1968.
466. KAUFMANN HJ: Chylous ascites and intestinal muscular hypertrophy occurring in the course of celiac sprue. Am J Dig Dis 20: 494-497, 1975.
467. KAYDEN HJ, SENIOR JR, MATTSON FH: The monoglyceride pathway of fat absorption in man. J Clin Invest 46: 1695, 1967.
468. KAYE M, PRITCHARD JE, HALPENNY GW, LIGHT W: Bone disease in chronic renal failure with particular reference to osteosclerosis. Medicine 39: 157-190, 1960.
469. KELLEHER J, LOSOWSKY MS: The absorption of α-tocopherol in man. Br J Nutr 24: 1033-1047, 1970.
470. KELLEY ML, TERRY R: Clinical and histological observations in fatal non-tropical sprue. Am J Med 25: 460-469, 1958.
471. KENDALL MJ, NUTTER S, HAWKINS CF: Bacteria and the xylose test. Lancet 1: 1017-1018, 1972.
472. KENRICK KD, WALKER-SMITH JA: Immunoglobulins and dietary protein antibodies in childhood coeliac disease. Gut 11: 635-640, 1970.
473. KENWRIGHT S: Coeliac disease and small bowel carcinoma. Postgrad Med J 48: 673-677, 1972.
474. KETELAER V: Commentarius medicus de aphthis nostratibus, seu Belgarum sprouw. MD Thesis, Leiden, 1669.
475. KEUNING JJ, PENA AS, LEEUWEN A VAN, et al: HLA-DW3 associated with coeliac disease. Lancet 1: 506-507, 1976.

476. KEUSCH GT, KAPLAN MM, SMITH D, RAVANESI P: Persistent, fulminant watery diarrhea complicating chronic active hepatitis. Gastroenterology 62, 307-313, 1972.
476a. KEYS A, FIDANZA F, KARVONEN MJ, KIMVRA N, TAYLOR HL: Indices of relative weight and obesity. J Chron Dis 25: 329-343, 1972.
477. KHOSLA T, LOWE CR: Height and weight of British men. Lancet 1, 742-745, 1968.
478. KINNEAR DG, JOHN DG, MACINTOSH PC, et al: Intestinal absorption of tritium-labelled folic acid in idiopathic steatorrhea: Effect of a gluten-free diet. Can Med Assoc J 89: 975-979, 1963.
479. KLAEVEMAN HL, GEBHARD RL, SESSOMS C, STROBER W: In vitro studies of ulcerative ileojejunitis. Gastroenterology 68: 572-582, 1975.
480. KLIPSTEIN FA: Urinary excretion of orally administered tritium-labeled folic acid as a test of folic acid absorption. Blood 21: 626-639, 1963.
481. KLIPSTEIN FA, BAKER SJ: Regarding the definition of tropical sprue. Gastroenterology 58: 717-721, 1970.
482. KOEPKE JA, STEWART WB: Role of gastric secretion in iron absorption. Proc Soc Exp Biol (NY) 115: 927-929, 1964.
483. KOHN J: A cellulose acetate supporting medium for zone electrophoresis. Clin Chim Acta 2: 297-303, 1957.
484. KOMROWER GM: Coeliac disease in a diabetic child. Lancet 1: 1215, 1969.
485. KORMAN MG, SOVENY C, HANSKY J: Effect of food on serum gastrin evaluated by radio-immunoassay. Gut 12: 619-624, 1971.
486. KOWLESSAR OD, WILLIAMS RC, LAW DH, SLEISENGER MH: Urinary excretion of 5-hydroxy-indolacetic acid in diarrheal states, with special reference to non-tropical sprue. New Eng J Med 259: 340-341, 1958.
487. KOWLESSAR OD, HAEFFNER LJ, BENSON GD: Abnormal tryptophan metabolism in patients with adult celiac disease, with evidence for deficiency of vitamin B6. J Clin Invest 43: 894-903, 1964.
488. KOWLESSAR OD, HAEFFNER LJ, BRONSTEIN HD: Evidence for aminoaciduria and peptiduria in adult celiac disease. J Clin Invest 43: 1274, 1964.
489. KOWLESSAR OD, PHILLIPS LD: Celiac disease. Med Clin North Am 54: 647-656, 1970.
490. KRAUSE MV, HUNSCHER MA: 'Food, nutrition and diet therapy', 5th ed. Saunders, Philadelphia, 1972.
491. KRAWITT EL, BEEKEN WL: Limitations of the usefulness of the d-xylose absorption test. Am J Clin Pathol 63: 261-263, 1975.
492. KRONDL A, SKÁLA I, VULTERINOVÁ M, et al: 'Fat and Malabsorption Syndrome'. Butterworths, London, 1971.
492a. KRUSKAL WH, WALLIS WA: Use of ranks in one-criterion variance analysis. J Am Stat Ass 47, 584-618, 1952.
493. KUITUNEN P, MAENPAA J, KROHN K, VISAKORPI JK: Gastrointestinal findings in auto-immune thyroiditis and nongoitrous juvenile hypothyreoidism in children. Scand J Gastroenterol 6: 336-341, 1971.
494. KUMAR PJ, SILK DBA, CLARK ML, DAWSON AM: Jejunal function in dermatitis herpetiformis and dult coeliac disease. Gut 13: 322, 1972.
495. KUMAR PJ, SILK DBA, MARKS R, et al: Treatment of dermatitis herpetiformis with corticosteroids and a gluten-free diet: a study of jejunal morphology and function. Gut 14: 280-283, 1973.
496. LAMERS CBHW: Some aspects of the Zollinger-Ellison syndrome and serum gastrin. MD Thesis, Nijmegen, 1976.
497. LANCASTER-SMITH MJ, BENSON MK, STRICKLAND ID: Coeliac disease and diffuse interstitial lung disease. Lancet 1: 473-475, 1971.
498. LANCASTER-SMITH MJ, STRICKLAND ID: Auto-antibodies in adult coeliac disease. Lancet 1: 1244, 1971.
499. LANCASTER-SMITH MJ, PERRIN J, SWARBRICK ET, WRIGHT JT: Coeliac disease and auto-immunity. Postgrad Med J 50: 45-48, 1974.
500. LANCASTER-SMITH M, KUMAR P, MARKS R, et al: Jejunal mucosal immunoglobulin-containing cells and jejunal fluid immunoglobulins in adult coeliac disease and dermatitis herpetiformis. Gut 15: 371-376, 1974.
501. LANCASTER-SMITH M, KUMAR P, CLARK ML, et al: Antireticulin antibodies in dermatitis herpetiformis and adult coeliac disease. Br J Dermatol 92: 37-42, 1975.

255

502. LANE DJ, HAMILTON WS: Idiopathic steatorrhoea and idiopathic pulmonary haemosiderosis. Br Med J 2: 89-90, 1971.
503. LANZKOWSKY P, ERLANDSON ME, BEZAN AI: Isolated defect of folic acid absorption associated with mental retardation and cerebral calcification. Blood 34: 452-465, 1969.
504. LARSON DL, BOND TP, ROBIN AE, et al: Clinical and experimental obstruction of the thoracic duct. Surgery 60: 35-42, 1966.
505. LEADING ARTICLE: Magnesium deficiency. Lancet 1: 523-524, 1976.
506. LEBENTHAL E, ANTONOWICZ I, SHWACHMAN H: Enterokinase and trypsin activities in pancreatic insufficiency and diseases of the small intestine. Gastroenterology 70: 508-512, 1976.
507. LEBLOND CP, WALKER BE: Renewal of cell population. Physiol Rev 36: 255-276, 1956.
508. LEE FD: Nature of the mucosal changes associated with malignant neoplasms in the small intestine. Gut 7: 361-367, 1966.
509. LEPORE MJ: Longterm or maintenance adrenal steroid therapy in non-tropical sprue. Am J Med 25: 381-390, 1958.
510. LESLIE GI, ROWE PB: Folate binding by the brush border membrane proteins of small intestinal epithelial cells. Biochem (Washington) 11: 1696-1703, 1972.
511. LEV R: The histochemistry of mucus-producing cells in the normal and diseased gastrointestinal mucosa, in 'Progress in gastroenterology vol II'. Ed by GB JERZY GLASS; pp 13-41. Grune & Stratton, New York, 1970.
512. LEVINE RA, BRIGGS GW, HARDING RS, NOLTE LB: Prolonged gluten administration in normal subjects. N Eng J Med 274: 1109-1114, 1966.
513. LEVINE RA: The role of cylic AMP in hepatic and gastrointestinal function. Gastroenterology 59: 280-300, 1970.
514. LEVITHAN R: Salt and water absorption from the normal human colon: effect of 9-alpha-fluorohydrocortisone administration. J Lab Clin Med 69: 558-564, 1967.
515. LEVITT MD, DUANE WC: Floating stools – flatus versus fat. N Eng J Med 286: 973-975. 1972.
516. LINDBERG T, NORDEN A, JOSEFSSON L: Dipeptidase activities in small intestine biopsy specimens from a clinical material. Scand J Gastroenterol 3: 177-182, 1968.
517. LINDENBAUM J, RYBAK B, GERSON CD, et al: Effects of ethanol on the small intestine of man. Clin Res 18: 385, 1970.
518. LINDNER J: Zur Physiologie und Pathologie der Schleimbildung des Darmes, in 'Die Malabsorption'. Ed by G SEIFERT; pp 111-154, Fischer, Stuttgart, 1970.
519. LINDSAY MKM, NORDIN BEC, NORMAN AP: Late prognosis in coeliac disease. Br Med J 1: 14-18, 1956.
520. LOEB PM, STROBER W, FALCHUK ZM, LASTER L: Incorporation of L-leucine- ^{14}C into immunoglobulins by jejunal biopsies of patients with celiac sprue and other gastrointestinal diseases. J Clin Invest 50, 559-569, 1971.
521. LOEHRY CA, CREAMER B: Post-mortem study of small-intestinal mucosa. Br Med J 1: 827-829, 1966.
522. LOEHRY CA, CREAMER B: Three-dimensional structure of the human small intestinal mucosa in health and disease. Gut 10: 6-12, 1969.
523. LOEHRY CA, CREAMER B: Vitamin B_{12} excretion by the rat small intestine. Gut 10: 662-664, 1969.
524. LOEHRY CA, PARISH D, BAKER J: The permeability of the small intestinal mucosa: A study using iron. Gut 14: 773-777, 1973.
525. LOSOWSKY MS, WALKER BE, KELLEHER J: 'Malabsorption in clinical practice'. Churchill Livingstone, London, 1974.
526. LOVE AHG, MITCHELL TG, PHILLIPS RA: Water and sodium absorption in the human intestine. J Physiol (London) 195: 133-140, 1968.
527. LOVE AHG, MATTHEWS JGW, VEALL N: Intestinal blood flow and sodium transport. Gut 13: 853-854, 1972.
528. LOW-BEER TS, HEATON ST, HEATON KW, READ AE: Gallbladder inertia and sluggish enterohepatic circulation of bile-salts in coeliac disease. Lancet 1: 991-994, 1971.
529. LOW-BEER TS, HEATON KW, POMARE EW, READ AE: The effect of coeliac disease upon bile salts. Gut 14: 204-208, 1973.
530. LOW-BEER TS, HARVEY RF, DAVIES ER, READ AE: Abnormalities of serum cholecystokinin and gallbladder emptying in celiac disease. N Eng J Med 292: 961-963, 1975.

531. LOW-BEER TS, HARVEY RF, DAVIES ER, READ AE: Letter to the editor. N Eng J Med 293: 360, 1975.
532. LUNDGREN O: Autonomic control of gastrointestinal function, in 'Pathofysiology'. Ed by ED FROHLICH; pp 615-630. Lippincott, Philadelphia, 1972.
533. LUNDGREN O: The circulation of the small bowel mucosa. Gut 15: 1005-1013, 1974.
534. LUTHER L, SANTINI R, BREWSTER C, et al: Folate binding by insoluble components of American and Puerto Rican diets. Am J Med Sci 3: 389-393, 1965.
534a. LYONS H, PINN VW, CORTELL S, et al: Allergic interstitial nephritis causing reversible renal failure in four patients with idiopathic nephrotic syndrome. N Engl J Med 288: 124-128, 1973.
535. MACCUISH AC, MUNRO JF, LAMB WL: Reversible renal tubular defects in gluten enteropathy with osteomalacia. Br Med J 2: 343-344, 1970.
536. MACDONALD WC, TRIER JS, EVERETT NB: Cell proliferation and migration in the stomach, duodenum and rectum of man: radioautographic studies. Gastroenterology 46: 405-417, 1964.
537. MACDONALD WC, DOBBINS WO, RUBIN CE: Studies of the familial nature of celiac sprue using biopsy of the small intestine. N Eng J Med 272: 448-456, 1965.
538. MACKAY IR, VOLWILER W: The effect of cortisone upon absorption of protein, fat, and calcium in idiopathic steatorrhea. Gastroenterology 28: 972-980, 1955.
539. MACKENZIE IL, DONALDSON RM: Vitamin B_{12} absorption and the intestinal cell surface Fed Proc 28: 41-45, 1969.
540. MACKINNON AM, SHORT MD, ELIAS E, DOWLING RH: Adaptive changes in vitamin B_{12} absorption in celiac disease and after proximal small-bowel resection in man. Am J Dig Dis 20: 835-839, 1975.
541. MACLAURIN BP, MATTHEWS N, KILPATRICK JA: Coeliac disease associated with autoimmune thyroiditis, Sjogren's syndrome, and a lymphocytotoxic serum factor. Aust N Z J Med 4: 405-411, 1972.
542. MACMAHON MT, NEALE G: The absorption of α-tocopherol in control subjects and in patients with intestinal malabsorption. Clin Sci 38: 197-210, 1970.
543. MADANAGOPALAN N, SHINER M, ROWE B: Measurements of small intestinal mucosa obtained by peroral biopsy. Am J Med 38: 42-53, 1965.
544. MAGALHAES AIN, PETERS TJ, DOE WF: Studies on the nature and significance of connective tissue antibodies in adult coeliac disease and Crohn's disease. Gut 15: 284-288, 1974.
545. MAINLAND D: Normal values in medicine. Ann N Y Acad Sci 161, 527-537, 1969.
546. MAJOOR CLH, TONGEREN JHM VAN: The contribution of hypoproteinaemia, due to gastrointestinal protein loss, to the formation of oedema in patients with cardiac failure. Die Heilkunst 86: 1-4, 1973.
547. MAJOR RH: 'Classic descriptions of disease', 3rd ed, 6th printing. Blackwell, Oxford, 1958.
548. MAKHLOUF GM: The neuroendocrine design of the gut: the play of chemicals in a chemical playground. Gastroenterology 67: 159-184, 1974.
549. MALDONADO JE, GREGG JA, GREEN PA, BROWN AL: Chronic idiopathic intestinal pseudoobstruction. Am J Med 49: 203-212, 1970.
550. MANIS JG, SCHACHTER D: Active transport of iron by intestine. Am J Physiol 203: 73-80, 1962.
551. MANIS JG, SCHACHTER D: Fe^{59}-amino-acid complexes: are they intermediates in Fe^{59} absorption across the intestinal mucosa. Proc Soc Exp Biol Med 119: 1185-1187, 1965.
552. MANN HB, WHITNEY DR: On a test of whether one of two variables is stochastically larger than the other. Ann Math Stat 18: 50-60, 1947.
553. MANN JG, BROWN WR, KERN F: The subtle and variable clinical expressions of gluten-induced enteropathy (adult celiac disease, non tropical sprue). Am J Med 48: 357-366, 1970.
554. MANSON-BAHR P: The morbid anatomy and pathology of sprue, and their bearing upon aetiology. Lancet 1: 1148-1151, 1924.
555. MARCHE C, BOCQUET L, MIGNON M, PREEL JL: Syndrome de malabsorption avec cavitation ganglionnaire mésentérique et atrophie splénique. Sem Hôp Paris 50: 879-886, 1974.
556. MARCUS CS, LENGEMANN FW: Absorption of Ca^{45} and Sr^{85} from solid and liquid food

257

at various levels of the alimentary tract of the rat. J Nutr 77: 155-160, 1962.

557. MARKS J, SHUSTER S, WATSON AJ: Small-bowel changes in dermatitis herpetiformis. Lancet 2: 1280-1282, 1966.
558. MARKS J, SHUSTER S: Small-intestinal mucosal abnormalities in various skin diseases – fact or fancy? Gut 11: 281-291, 1970.
559. MARKS J, SHUSTER S: Intestinal malabsorption and the skin. Gut 12: 938-947, 1971.
560. MARKS R, WHITTLE MW, BEARD RJ, et al: Small-bowel abnormalities in dermatitis herpetiformis. Br Med J 1: 552-555, 1968.
561. MARSH GW, STEWART JS: Splenic function in adult coeliac disease. Br J Haematol 19: 445-457, 1970.
562. MARSH MN, BROWN AC, SWIFT JA: The surface ultrastructure of the small intestinal mucosa of normal control human subjects and of patients with untreated and treated coeliac disease using the scanning electron microscope, in 'Coeliac Disease'. Ed by CC BOOTH, RH DOWLING; pp 26-43, Churchill Livingstone, London, 1970.
563. MARSHAK RH, LINDNER AE: 'Radiology of the small intestine'. Saunders, Philadelphia, 1970.
564. MARTINEZ-TORRES C, LAYRISSE M: Effect of amino acids on iron absorption from a staple vegetable food. Blood 35: 669-682, 1970.
565. MATTHEWS DM: Observations on the estimation of serum vitamin B_{12} using lactobacillus Leichmannii. Clin Sci 22: 101-111, 1962.
566. MATTHEWS DM: Absorption of water-soluble vitamins. Br Med Bull 23: 258-262, 1967.
567. MATTHEWS DM: Protein absorption. J Clin Pathol 24: suppl 5, 29-40, 1971.
568. MCCARTHY CF, FRASER ID, EVANS KT, READ AE: Lymphoreticular dysfunction in idiopathic steatorrhoea. Gut 7: 140-148, 1966.
569. MCCARTHY CF: Participation in the discussions, in 'Coeliac Disease'. Ed by WTJM HEKKENS, AS PENA; p 337. Stenfert Kroese, Leiden, 1974.
570. MCCARTHY CF, MYLOTTE M, STEVENS F, et al: Family studies on coeliac disease in Ireland, in 'Coeliac Disease'. Ed by WTJM HEKKENS, AS PENA; pp 311-319. Stenfert Kroese, Leiden 1974.
571. MCCRAE WM: Inheritance of coeliac disease. J Med Genet 6: 129-131, 1969.
572. MCCRAE WM, SANDOR G, SANGANI AP: Fingerprint changes in coeliac disease. Br Med J 3: 109-110, 1971.
573. MCCRAE WM, MARTIN MR, EASTWOOD MA, SIRCUS W: Neglected coeliac disease. Lancet 1: 187-190, 1975.
574. MCDONAGH TJ, GUEFT B, KIM PYUN, ARIAS IM: Hypoproteinemia, chylous ascites, steatorrhea and protein-losing enteropathy due to chronic inflammatory obstruction of major intestinal lymph vessels. Gastroenterology 48: 642-647, 1965.
574a. MCDONALD GB, EARNEST DL, ADMIRAND WH: Hyperoxaluria correlates with steatorrhea in patients with celiac sprue. Gastroenterology 68: 949, 1975.
575. MCFARLANE AS: Measurement of synthesis rates of liver-produced plasma proteins. Biochem J 89: 277-290, 1963.
576. MCGUIGAN JE, VOLWILER W: Celiac-sprue: malabsorption of iron in the absence of steatorrhea. Gastroenterology 47: 636-641, 1964.
577. MCGUIGAN JE: Gastric mucosal intracellular localization of gastrin by immunofluorescence. Gastroenterology 55: 315-327, 1968.
578. MCLEOD GM, WIGGINS HS: Bile-salts in small intestinal contents after ileal resection and in other malabsorption syndromes. Lancet 1: 873-876, 1968.
579. MCMICHAEL HB, WEBB J, DAWSON AM: The absorption of maltose and lactose in man. Clin Sci 33: 135-145, 1967.
580. MCNEISH AS, WILLOUGHBY MLN: Whole-blood folate as a screening test for coeliac disease in childhood. Lancet 1: 442-443, 1969.
581. MCNEISH AS, ANDERSON CM: The disorder in childhood. Clinics in Gastroenterology III: 1: 127-144, 1974.
582. MCNEISH AS, ROLLES CJ, NELSON R, et al: Factors affecting the differing racial incidence of coeliac disease, in 'Coeliac Disease'. Ed by WTJM HEKKENS, AS PENA; pp 330-337. Stenfert Kroese, Leiden, 1974.
583. MCNEISH AS: Participation in the discussions, in 'Coeliac Disease'. Ed by WTJM HEKKENS, AS PENA; p 419. Stenfert Kroese, Leiden, 1974.
584. MCNICHOLL B, EGAN-MITCHELL B, FOTTRELL PF: Varying gluten susceptibility in coeliac

disease, in 'Coeliac Disease'. Ed by WTJM HEKKENS, AS PENA; pp 413-418, Stenfert Kroese, Leiden, 1974.

585. MEER JB VAN DER: Granular deposits of immunoglobulins in the skin of patients with dermatitis herpetiformis. Br J Dermatol 81: 493-503, 1969.
586. MEEUWISSE GW: Diagnostic criteria in coeliac disease. Acta Paediatr Scand 59: 461-463, 1970.
587. MEINHARD EA, WADBROOK DG, RISDON RA: Computer card morphometry of jejunal biopsies in childhood coeliac disease. J Clin Path 28: 85-93, 1975.
588. MEKHJIAN HS, PHILLIPS SF, HOFMANN AF: Colonic secretion of water and electrolytes induced by bile acids: perfusion studies in man. J Clin Invest 50: 1569-1577, 1971.
589. MELVIN KEW, HEPNER GW, BORDIER P, et al: Calcium metabolism and bone pathology in adult coeliac disease. Q J Med 39: 83-113, 1970.
590. MENZIES IS: Intestinal permeability in coeliac disease. Gut 13: 847, 1972.
591. MEYER JH, WAY LW, GROSSMAN MI: Pancreatic response to acidification of various lengths of proximal intestine in the dog. Am J Physiol 219: 971-977, 1970.
592. MIDDLETON EJ, GRICE HC: Vitamin absorption studies. IV. Site of absorption of C^{14}-riboflavin and S^{35}-thiamine in the rat. Can J Biochem 42: 353-358, 1964.
593. MIETTINEN TA: Intestinal and faecal bile-acids in malabsorption. Lancet 2: 358, 1968.
594. MIETTINEN TA, SIURALA M: Micellar solubilization of intestinal lipids and sterols in gluten enteropathy and liver cirrhosis. Scand J Gastroenterol 6: 527-535, 1971.
595. MILLER B, MITCHISON R, TABAQCHALI S, NEALE G: The effects of excessive bacterial proliferation on protein metabolism in rats with self-filling jejunal sacs. Europ J Clin Invest 2: 23-31, 1971.
596. MILLER D, CRANE RK: The digestive function of the epithelium of the small intestine. Biochim Biophys Acta 52: 281-293, 1961.
597. MILLER R: Coeliac disease: its definition and diagnosis. Lancet 1: 306, 1923.
598. MILNE MD: Disorders of intestinal amino-acid transport. J Clin Pathol 24: suppl 5, 41-44, 1971.
599. MISRA RC, KASTHURI D, CHUTTANI HK: Adult coeliac disease in tropics. Br Med J 2: 1230-1232, 1966.
600. MISTILIS SP, SKYRING AP, STEPHEN DD: Intestinal lymphangiectasia. Mechanism of enteric loss of plasma protein and fat. Lancet 1: 77-79, 1965.
601. MODIGLIANI R, MATUCHANSKY C, GALIAN A, et al: Maladie coeliaque de l'adulte (48 cas). Arch Fr Mal App Dig 64: 465-481, 1975.
602. MOHAMMED I, HOLBOROW EJ, FRY L, et al: Multiple immune complexes and hypo-complementaemia in dermatitis herpetiformis and coeliac disease. Lancet 2: 487-490, 1976.
603. MONRO J: Pantothenic acid and coeliac disease. Br Med J 4: 112-113, 1972.
604. MOORE CV: Iron and the essential trace elements, in 'Modern nutrition in health and disease'. Ed by MG WOHE, RS GOODHART. Lea & Febiger, Philadelphia, 1968.
605. MOORE WEC, CATO EP, HOLDEMAN LV: Anaerobic bacteria of the gastrointestinal flora and their occurrence in clinical infections. J Inf Dis 119: 641-649, 1969.
606. MOREHEAD RM, KESSNER DM: Effects of Mg deficiency and parathyroidectomy on gastrointestinal Ca transport in the rat. Am J Physiol 217: 1608-1613, 1969.
607. MORGAN DB: Calcium and phosphorus transport across the intestine, in 'Malabsorption'. Ed by RH GIRDWOOD, AN SMITH; pp 73-91. University Press, Edinburgh, 1969.
608. MORITZ M, MORAN JM, PATTERSON JF: Chronic ulcerative jejunitis. Gastroenterology 60: 96-102, 1971.
609. MORITZ M, FINKELSTEIN G, MESHKINPOUR H, et al: Effect of secretin and cholecysto-kinin on the transport of electrolyte and water in human jejunum. Gastroenterology 64: 76-80, 1973.
610. MORRIS JS, AJDUKIEWICZ AB, READ AE: Coeliac infertility: an indication for dietary gluten restriction? Lancet 1: 213-214, 1970.
611. MORRIS JS, AJDUKIEWICZ AB, READ AE: Neurological disorders and adult coeliac disease. Gut 11: 549-554, 1970.
612. MORRIS JS, READ AE, JONES B, et al: Coeliac disease and lung disease. Lancet 1: 754, 1971.
613. MORRISON AB, CAMPBELL JA: Vitamin absorption studies. I. Factors influencing the excretion of oral test doses of thiamine and riboflavin by human subjects. J Nutr 72: 435-440, 1960.

614. MORTIMER PE, STEWART JS, NORMAN AP, BOOTH CC: Follow-up study of coeliac disease. Br Med J 3: 7-9, 1968.
615. MOSS AJ, WATERHOUSE C, TERRY R: Gluten-sensitive enteropathy with osteomalacia but without steatorrhea. N Eng J Med 272: 825-830, 1965.
616. MOUWEN JMVM: Villous atrophy in piglets, in 'Coeliac Disease'. Ed by WTJM HEKKENS, AS PENA; pp 277-284. Stenfert Kroese, Leiden, 1974.
617. MULDOWNEY FP, FREANY R, MCGEENEY D: Renal tubular acidosis and amino-aciduria in osteomalacia of dietary or intestinal origin. Q J Med 37: 517-539, 1968.
618. MULDOWNEY FP, MCKENNA TJ, KYLE LH, et al: Parathormone-like effect of magnesium replenishment in steatorrhea. N Eng J Med 281: 61-68, 1970.
619. MÜLLER WFH: Adult celiac disease, in 'Radiological atlas of common diseases of the small bowel'. Ed by JL SELLINK; pp 311-321. Stenfert Kroese, Leiden, 1976.
620. MUNRO DR: Route of protein loss during a model protein-losing gastropathy. in dogs Gastroenterology 66: 960-972, 1974.
621. MUNRO HN: Protein secretion into the gastrointestinal tract, in 'Postgraduate Gastro-enterology'. Ed by TJ THOMSON, IE GILLESPIE; pp 58-67. Baillière, Tindall & Cassell, London, 1966.
622. MÜTING D, BURGARD HJ: Zur quantitativen Bestimmung von Indican in Urin und Serum. Z Klin Chem 3: 46-49, 1965.
623. MUTT V, JORPES JE: Structure of porcine cholecystokinin-pancreozymin. Eur J Bio-chem 6: 156-162, 1968.
624. MYLOTTE M, EGAN-MITCHELL B, FOTTRELL PF: Fingerprints in patients with coeliac disease and their relatives. Br Med J 4: 144-146, 1972.
625. MYLOTTE M, EGAN-MITCHELL B, MCCARTHY CF, MCNICHOLL B: Incidence of coeliac dis-ease in the West of Ireland. Br Med J 1: 703-705, 1973.
626. MYLOTTE M, EGAN-MITCHELL B, FOTTRELL PF, et al: Family studies in coeliac disease. Q J Med 43: 359-369, 1974.
627. NASSET ES, JU JS: Mixture of endogenous and exogenous protein in the alimentary tract. J Nutr 74: 461-465, 1961.
628. NEALE G, TABAQCHALI S: Value of measuring urinary indican excretion. Gut 7: 711, 1966.
629. NEALE G, ANTCLIFF AC, WELBOURN RB, et al: Protein malnutrition after partial gast-rectomy. Q J Med 36: 469-494, 1967.
630. NEALE G, GOMPERTZ D, SCHÖNSBY H, et al: The metabolic and nutritional conse-quences of bacterial overgrowth in the small intestine. Am J Clin Nutr 25: 1409-1417, 1972.
631. NELSON R, MCNEISH AS, ANDERSON CM: Coeliac disease in children of Asian immigrants. Lancet 1: 348-350, 1973.
632. NEWCOMER AD, MCGILL DB: Distribution of disaccharidase activity in the small bowel of normal and lactase-deficient subjects. Gastroenterology 51: 481-488, 1966.
633. NEWCOMER AD: Surface digestion of carbohydrates. Mayo Clin Proc 48: 620-623, 1973.
634. NEWEY H, SMYTH DH: The intestinal absorption of some dipeptides. J Physiol (Lond.) 145: 48-56, 1959.
635. NICHOLSON JTL, CHORNOCK FW: Intubation studies of the human small intestine. XXII. An improved technic for the study of absorption; its application to ascorbic acid. J Clin Invest 21: 505-509, 1942.
636. NIEWEG HO, VEEGER W, ABELS J: Aspecten van inheemse spruw. Folia Med Neerl 6: 39-44, 1962.
637. NILSSON G, YALOW RS, BERSON SA: Distribution of gastrin in the gastrointestinal tract of human, dog, cat and hog, in 'Frontiers in gastrointestinal hormone research'; pp 95-101. Almqvist & Wiksell, Stockholm, 1973.
638. NIXON SE, MAWER GE: The digestion and absorption of protein in man. Br J Nutr 24: 227-258, 1970.
639. NOLAN S, STEPHAN T, KHURANA RC, et al: Low profile (flat) glucose tolerances. Am J Med Sci 264: 33-39, 1972.
640. NORDIN BEC: Hormones and calcium metabolism, in 'Calcified tissues'. Ed by H. Fleish; pp 226-241. Springer, Berlin, 1966.
641. NORDIN BEC: Measurement and meaning of calcium absorption. Gastroenterology 54: 294-301, 1968.

642. NORDSTRÖM C, DAHLQVIST A: The cellular localization of enterokinase. Biochim Biophys Acta (Amst.) 198: 621-622, 1970.
643. NOVIS BH, BANK S, MARKS IN, et al: Abdominal lymphoma presenting with malabsorption. Q J Med 40:521-540, 1971.
644. NOVIS BH, BANK S, MARKS IN: Exocrine pancreatic function in intestinal malabsorption and small bowel disease. Am J Dig Dis 17: 489-494, 1972.
645. NOYES WD, JORDAN PH, Small bowel iron absorption in an unusual patient. Gastroenterology 46: 421-423, 1964.
646. NUSBAUM M, BAUM S, RAJATAPITI B, BLAKEMORE WS: Intestinal lymphangiography in vivo. J Cardiovasc Surg 8: 62-68, 1967.
647. NUSSLÉ D, FREI J, BOZIC C, GAUTIER E: Proximal and distal alterations of the intestinal mucosa in coeliac disease. Relations to the degree of malabsorption, in 'Coeliac Disease'. Ed by CC BOOTH, RH DOWLING; pp 45-53. Churchill Livingstone, London, 1970.
648. NYGAARD K, ROOTWELT K: Intestinal protein in rats with blind segments on the small bowel. Gastroenterology 54: 52-55, 1968.
649. OCKNER RK: Blood supply of the gut and pathofysiology of ischemia, in 'Gastrointestinal Disease'. Ed by MH SLEISENGER, JS FORDTRAN; pp 378-383. Saunders, Philadelphia, 1973.
650. OKUDA K, GRASBECK R, CHOW B: Bile and vitamin B_{12} absorption. L Jab Clin Med 51: 17-23, 1958.
651. OKUDA K, KITAZAKI T, TAKAMATSU M: Inactivation of vitamin B_{12} by a binder in rat intestine and the role of intrinsic factor. Digestion 4: 35-48, 1971.
652. OSBORNE TB: 'The proteins of the wheat kernel'. Carnegie Institution, Washington, 1907.
653. OTAKI AT, DALY JR, MORTON-GILL A: Observations on oral betamethasone-17-valerate in the treatment of idiopathic steatorrhoea. Gut 8: 458-462, 1967.
654. OWREN PA: Thrombotest: A new method for controlling anticoagulant therapy. Lancet 2: 754-758, 1959.
655. PADYKULA HA, STRAUSS EW, LADMAN AJ, GARDNER FH: A morphologic and histochemical analysis of the human jejunal epithelium in nontropical sprue. Gastroenterology 40: 735-765, 1961.
656. PALLIS CA, LEWIS PD: 'The neurology of gastrointestinal disease'. Saunders, London, 1974.
657. PARFITT AM: Investigation of disorders of the parathyroid glands. Clinics in Endocrinology III, 3: 451-474, 1974.
658. PARKINS RA: Protein-losing enteropathy in the sprue syndrome. Lancet 2: 1366-1368, 1960.
659. PARSONS DS: Salt transport. J Clin Pathol 24 suppl 5: 90-98, 1971.
660. PARSONS LG: Celiac disease. Am J Dis Child 43: 1293-1346, 1932.
661. PATERSON JCS, WIGGINS HS: Estimation of plasma vitamin A and vitamin A absorption test. J Clin Pathol 7: 56-60, 1954.
662. PAULK CE, FARRAR WE: Diverticulosis of the small intestine and megaloblastic anaemia. Am J Med 37: 473-480, 1964.
663. PAULLEY JW: Observations on the aetiology of idiopathic steatorrhoea. Jejunal and lymph-node biopsies. Br Med J 4: 1318-1321, 1954.
664. PAULLEY JW: The jejunal mucosa in malabsorptive states with high bacterial counts, in 'Malabsorption'. Ed by RH GIRDWOOD, AN SMITH; pp 171-176. University Press, Edinburgh, 1969.
665. PAULSRUD JR, PENSLER L, WHITTEN CF, et al: Essential fatty acid deficiency in infants induced by fat free intravenous feeding. Am J Clin Nutr 25: 897, 1972.
666. PEARSE AGE: The endocrine cells of the GI tract: origins, morphology and functional relationships in health and disease. Clinics in Gastroenterology III, 3: 491-510, 1974. Saunders, London.
667. PEMBERTON PJ: Adult celiac disease, reticulosis and carcinoma. Am J Dig Dis 17: 851-855, 1972.
668. PENA AS, TRUELOVE SC, WHITEHEAD R: Disaccharidase activity and jejunal morphology in coeliac disease. Q J Med 41: 457-476, 1972.
669. PERRY J, CHANARIN I: Intestinal absorption of reduced folate compounds in man. Br J Haematol 18: 329-339, 1970.
670. PERSONAL COMMUNICATION with Deso-Glutex milling factories.

671. PERSONAL COMMUNICATION with the Dutch Coeliac Society.
672. PERSONAL COMMUNICATION with the Dutch Foundation for Medical Registration.
673. PETERS TJ: Intestinal peptidases. Gut 11: 720-725, 1970.
674. PETERS TJ, HOFFBRAND AV: Absorption of vitamin B_{12} by the guinea pig. I. Br. J Haematol 19: 369-382, 1970.
675. PETERS TJ, QUINLAN A, HOFFBRAND AV: Absorption of vitamin B_{12} by the guinea pig II. Br J Haematol 20: 123-129, 1971.
677. PETERS TJ: Intestinal hydrolysis of oligopeptides. Gastroenterology 67: 191-192, 1974.
678. PETERSEN VP, HASTRUP J: Protein-losing enteropathy in constrictive pericarditis. Acta Med Scand 173: 401-410, 1963.
679. PHELAN JJ, MCCARTHY CF, STEVENS FM, et al: The nature of gliadin toxicity in coeliac disease: a new concept, in 'Coeliac Disease'. Ed by WTJM HEKKENS, AS PENA; pp 60-70 Stenfert Kroese, Leiden, 1974.
680. PHILLIPS SF, SUMMERSKILL WHJ: Water and electrolyte transport during maintenance of isotoxicity in human jejunum and ileum. J Lab Clin Med 70: 686-698, 1967.
681. PHILLIPS SF, GILLER J: The contribution of the colon to electrolyte and water conservation in man. J Lab Clin Med 81: 733-746, 1973.
682. PINK IJ, CREAMER B: Response to a gluten-free diet of patients with the coeliac syndrome. Lancet 1: 300-304, 1967.
683. PINK IJ, CROFT DN, CREAMER B: Cell loss drom small intestinal mucosa: a morphological study. Gut 11: 217-222, 1970.
684. PINKERTON PH, BANNERMAN RM, DOEBLIN TD, et al: Iron metabolism and absorption studies in the X-linked anaemia of mice. Br J Haematol 18: 211-228, 1970.
685. PITTMAN FE, HOLUB DA: Sjögren's syndrome and adult celiac disease. Gastroenterology 48: 869-876, 1965.
686. PLOTKIN GR, ISSELBACHER KJ: Secondary disaccharidase deficiency in adult celiac disease (nontropical sprue) and other malabsorption states. N Eng J Med 271: 1033-1037, 1964.
687. POLAK JM, PEARSE AGE, NOORDEN S VAN, et al: Secretin cells in coeliac disease. Gut 14: 870-874, 1973.
688. POLLOCK DJ, NAGLE RE, JEEJEEBHOY KN, COGHILL NF: The effect on jejunal mucosa of withdrawing and adding dietary gluten in cases of idiopathic steatorrhoea. Gut 11: 567-575, 1970.
689. POLONOVSKI C, NAVARO J, FONTAINE JL, LAPLANE R: L'intolérance au gluten chez l'enfant. Ann Med Interne (Paris) 122: 911-924, 1971.
690. PORTER HP, SAUNDERS DR, TIJTGAT G, et al: Fat absorption in bile fistula man. Gastroenterology 60: 1008-1019, 1971.
691. POTTS JT, DEFTOS LJ: Parathyroid hormone, calcitonin vitamin D, bone and bone mineral metabolism, in 'Duncan's Diseases of Metabolism'. Ed by PK BONDY, LE ROSENBERG; pp 1225-1430. Saunders, Philadelphia, 1974.
692. PROCKOP DJ, UDENFRIEND S: A specific method for the analysis of hydroxyproline in tissues and urine. Anal Biochem 1: 228-239, 1960.
693. PROST A, RAMBAUD JC, MIRAVET L, et al: Les ostéomalacies révélatrices de la maladie coeliaque de l'adulte. Nouv Presse Med 1: 1329-1335, 1972.
694. PUBLICATION (10.8.1973 TV) of Centraal Instituut voor Voedingsonderzoek TNO, Zeist.
695. RAMBAUD JC, AYMES C, ZITTOUN J, BERNIER JJ: D-xylose and folic acid tolerance tests as screening tests for adult coeliac disease, in 'Coeliac Disease'. Ed by WTJM HEKKENS, AS PENA; pp 346-347. Stenfert Kroese, Leiden, 1974.
696. RAMSAY WNM: The determination of iron in blood plasma or serum. Clin Chim Acta 2: 214-220, 1957.
697. RAMSAY WNM: The determination of the total iron-binding capacity of serum. Clin Chim Acta 2: 221-226, 1957.
698. RASMUSSEN H: The parathyroids, in 'Textbook of endocrinology'. Ed by RH WILLIAMS; pp 847-965. Saunders, Philadelphia, 1968.
699. RAYFORD PL, MILLER TA, THOMPSON JC: Secretin, cholecystokinin and newer gastrointestinal hormones. N Eng J Med 294: 1093-1101, 1157-1164, 1976.
700. RECOMMENDED DIETARY ALLOWANCES: National Academy of Sciences, Washington, 1974.
701. REIFENSTEIN EC, ALBRIGHT F, WELLS SL: The accumulation, interpretation, and presen-

tation of data pertaining to metabolic balances, notably those of calcium, phosphorus and nitrogen. J Clin Endocrinol 5: 367-395, 1945.

702. RETIEF FP: Urinary folate excretion after ingestion of pteroylmonoglutamic acid and food folate. Am J Clin Nutr 22: 352-355, 1969.

703. RHIJNE W TEN: Verhandelinge van de Asiatise melaatsheid. Van Someren, Amsterdam, 1687.

704. RICHMOND J, GIRDWOOD RH: Observations on amino acid absorption. Clin Sci 22: 301-314, 1962.

705. RIECKEN EO, STEWART JS, BOOTH CC, PEARSE AGE: A histochemical study on the role of lysosomal enzymes in idiopathic steatorrhoea before and during a glutenfree diet. Gut 7: 317-332, 1966.

706. RIECKEN EO, ROSENBAUM R, BLOCH R, et al: Tierexperimentelle Untersuchungen zur Frage der Spezifität der Dünndarmschleimhautveränderungen bei der einheimischen Sprue. Kli..i Wochenschr 47: 202-214, 1969.

707. RIECKEN EO: Histochemical findings in some intestinal dustirbances in relation to structure compared with the changes in 'Idiopathic Steatorrhoea', in 'Coeliac Disease'. Ed by CC BOOTH, RH DOWLING; pp 174-185. Churchill Livingstone, London, 1970.

708. RIECKEN EO, MENGE H: Atrophic changes in rats, in 'Coeliac Disease'. Ed by WTJM HEKKENS, AS PENA; pp 292-308. Stenfert Kroese, Leiden, 1974.

709. ROBINSON DC, WATSON AJ, WYATT EH, et al: Incidence of small-intestinal mucosal abnormalities and of clinical coeliac disease in the relatives of children with coeliac disease. Gut 12: 789-793, 1971.

710. ROBINSON JWL: Intestinal malabsorption in the experimental animal. Gut 13: 938-945, 1972.

711. ROBINSON TJ: Coeliac disease with farmers' lung. Br Med J 1: 745-746, 1976.

712. ROE JH, RICE EW: Determination of free pentoses. J Biol Chem 173: 507-512, 1948.

713. ROLLES CJ, KENDALL MJ, NUTTER S, ANDERSON CM: One-hour blood-xylose screening-test for coeliac disease. Lancet 2: 1043-1045, 1973.

714. ROLLES CJ, KYAW-MYINT TO, SIN WK: Family studies of coeliac disease, in 'Coeliac Disease'. Ed by WTJM HEKKENS, AS PENA; pp 320-321. Stenfert Kroese, Leiden, 1974.

715. ROSE GA, REED GW, SMITH AH: Isotopic method for measurement of calcium absorption from the gastro-intestinal tract. Br Med J 1: 690-692, 1965.

716. ROSENBERG IH, HARDISON WG, BULL DM: Abnormal bile-salt patterns and intestinal overgrowth associated with malabsorption. N Eng J Med 276: 1391-1397, 1967.

717. ROSENBERG IH, STREIFF RR, GODWIN HA, et al: Absorption of polyglutamatic folate: participation of deconjugating enzymes of the intestinal mucosa. N Eng J Med 280: 985-988, 1969.

718. ROSENBERG IH, GODWIN HA: The digestion and absorption of dietary folate. Gastroenterology 60: 445-463, 1971.

719. ROSENBERG IH, NEUMANN H: Multi-step mechanism in the hydrolysis of pteroylpolyglutamates by chicken intestine. J Biol Chem 249: 5126-5130, 1974.

720. ROSENBERG IH: Folate absorption and malabsorption. N Eng J Med 293: 1303-1308, 1975.

721. ROSENDAHL 1927; quoted by HESS THAYSEN, 1932: 166.

722. ROSS JR, GIBB SP, HOFFMAN DE, et al: Systemic manifestations of gluten enteropathy. Med Clin North Am 50: 515-527, 1966a.

723. ROSS JR, GIBB SP, HOFFMAN DE, et al: Gluten enteropathy and skeletal disease. JAMA 196: 180-184, 1966e.

724. ROSS JR, GARABEDIAN M: Systemic manifestations of gluten enteropathies and gluten sensitivity in some other diseases, in 'Progress in Gastroenterology vol II'. Ed by GB JERZY GLASS; pp 430-449. Grune & Stratton, New York, 1970.

725. ROSSIPAL E: Die Bedeutung präzipitierender Antikörper gegen Kleberproteine in der Pathogenese der Coeliakie. Pädiatrie und Pädologie 7: 253-258, 1972.

726. ROTEM Y. CZERNIAK P: Gastrointestinal protein leakage in celiac disease. Am J Dis Child 107: 58-66, 1964.

727. ROTHMAN MM, KATZ AB: Analysis of feces, in 'Gastroenterology vol II' 2nd ed. Ed by HL BOCKUS; pp 694-725. Saunders, Philadelphia, 1964.

728. ROTHSCHILD MA, ORATZ M, MONGELLI J, et al: Amino acid regulation of albumin synthesis. J Nutrition 98: 395-403, 1969.

729. ROTHSCHILD MA, ORATZ M, SCHREIBER SS: Albumin synthesis. N Eng J Med 286: 748-757, 816-821, 1972.
730. ROTHSCHILD MA, ORATZ M, SCHREIBER SS: Albumin metabolism. Gastroenterology 64: 324-337, 1973.
731. RUBENSTEIN R, HOWARD AV, WRONG OM: In vivo dialysis of faeces as a method of stool analysis. IV. The organic anion component. Clin Sci 37: 549-564, 1969.
732. RUBIN CE: Celiac disease and idiopathic sprue. Some reflections on reversibility, gluten and the intestine. Gastroenterology 39: 260-261, 1960.
733. RUBIN CE, BRANDBORG LL, PHELPS PC, TAYLOR HC: Studies of celiac disease. I. The apparent identical and specific nature of the duodenal and proximal jejunal lesion in celiac disease and idiopathic steatorrhea. Gastroenterology 38: 28-49, 1960.
734. RUBIN CE, BRANDBORG LL, FLICK AL, et al: Studies of celiac sprue. III. The effect of repeated wheat installation into the proximal ileum of patients on a gluten-free diet. Gastroenterology 43: 621-641, 1962.
735. RUBIN CE: Electron microscopic studies of triglyceride absorption in man. Gastroenterology 50: 65-77, 1966.
736. RUBIN CE, EIDELMAN S, WEINSTEIN WM: Sprue by any other name. Gastroenterology 58: 409-412, 1970.
737. RUBIN CE: Participation in the discussions, in 'Coeliac Disease'. Ed by WTJM HEKKENS, AS PENA; p 23. Stenfert Kroese, Leiden, 1974.
738. RUBIN W, FAUCI AS, SLEISENGER MH, JEFFRIES GH: Immunofluorescent studies in adult celiac disease. J Clin Invest 44: 475-485, 1965.
739. RUFFIN JM, KURTZ SM, BORLAND JL, et al: Gluten-free diet for nontropical sprue. JAMA 188: 42-44, 1964.
740. RUPPIN H, WEIDNER F, DOMSCHKE S, et al: Dermatitis herpetiformis and small intestinal lesion – no strict association in german patients. Acta Hepato-Gastroenterol 22: 105-111, 1975.
741. RUSSEL RI, ALLAN JG, GERSKOWITCH VP, ROBERTSON JWK: A study by perfusion techniques of the absorption abnormalities in the jejunum in adult coeliac disease. Clin Sci 42: 735-741, 1972.
742. RUSSEL RI, ALLAN JG, GERSKOWITCH VP, COCHRAN KM: The effect of conjugated and unconjugated bile acids on water and electrolyte absorption in the human jejunum. Clin Sci Mol Med 45: 301-311, 1973.
743. SADIKALI F: Dipeptidase deficiency and malabsorption of glycylglycine in disease states. Gut 12: 276-283, 1971.
744. SALEM SN, TRUELOVE SC, RICHARDS WCD: Small-intestinal and gastric changes in ulcerative colitis: a biopsy study. Br Med J 1: 827-831, 1974.
745. SAMLOFF IM, DAVIS JS, SCHENK EA: A clinical and histochemical study of celiac disease before and during a gluten-free diet. Gastroenterology 48: 155-172, 1965.
746. SAMLOFF IM: Pepsinogens, pepsins, and pepsin inhibitors. Gastroenterology 60: 586-604, 1971.
747. SANTIAGO-BORRERO PJ, SANTINI R JR, PEREZ-SANTIAGO E, et al: Congenital isolated defect of folic acid absorption. J Pediatr 82: 450-455, 1973.
748. SARNA SK: Gastrointestinal electrical activity: terminology. Gastroenterology 68: 1631-1635, 1975.
749. SAUER LW: Celiac disease (chronic intestinal indigestion). Am J Dis Child 29: 155-173, 1925.
750. SCADDING JG: Lung biopsy in the diagnosis of diffuse lung disease. Br Med J 2: 557-564, 1970.
751. SCHACHTER D: Vitamin D and the intestinal transport of calcium and phosphate, in 'L'osteomalacie'. Ed by D HIOCO; pp 199-211. Masson, Paris, 1967.
752. SCHEDL HP, CLIFTON JA: Solute and water absorption by the human small intestine. Nature (London) 199: 1264-1267, 1963.
753. SCHEDL HP, PIERCE CE, RIDER A, CLIFTON JA: Absorption of L-methionine from the human small intestine. J Clin Invest 47: 417-425, 1968.
754. SCHEIG R: Diseases of lipid metabolism, in 'Duncan's Diseases of metabolism'. Ed by PK BONDY, LE ROSENBERG; pp 341-416. Saunders, Philadelphia, 1974.
755. SCHEIN J: Syndrome of non tropical sprue with hitherto undescribed lesions of the intestine. Gastroenterology 8: 438-460, 1947.
756. SCHENK EA, SAMLOFF IM, KLIPSTEIN FA: Morphologic characteristics of jejunal biopsy

in celiac disease and tropical sprue. Am J Pathol 47: 765-781, 1965.
757. SCHENK EA, SAMLOFF IM, KLIPSTEIN FA: Pathogenesis of jejunal mucosal alterations: synechia formation. Am J Pathol 50: 523-531, 1967.
758. SCHILLING RF: Intrinsic factor studies. J Lab Clin Med 42: 860-866, 1953.
759. SCHMID WC, PHILLIPS SF, SUMMERSKILL WHJ: Jejunal secretion of electrolytes and water in nontropical sprue. J Lab Clin Med 73: 772-783, 1969.
760. SCHÖNSBY H, TABAQCHALI S: Uptake of rat gastric-juice-bound vitamin B_{12} by intestinal brush borders isolated from blind-loop rats. Scand J Gastroenterol 6: 515-521, 1971.
761. SCHÖNSBY H, HOFSTAD T: The uptake of vitamin B_{12} by the sediment of jejunal contents in patients with the blind-loop syndrome. Scand J Gastroenterol 10: 305-309, 1975.
762. SCHRAGER J: The chemical composition and function of gastrointestinal mucus. Gut 11: 450-456, 1970.
763. SCHULTZ SG, CURRAN PF: Coupled transport of sodium and organic solutes. Physiol Rev 50: 637-718, 1970.
764. SCOTT BB, LOSOWSKY MS: Coeliac disease: a cause of various associated diseases. Lancet 2: 956-957, 1975.
765. SEAH PP, FRY L, HOFFBRAND AV, HOLBOROW EJ: Tissue antibodies in dermatitis herpetiformis and adult coeliac disease. Lancet 1: 834-836, 1971.
766. SEAH PP, FRY L, ROSSITER MA, et al: Anti-reticulin antibodies in childhood coeliac disease. Lancet 2: 681-682, 1971.
767. SEAH PP, FRY L, STEWART JS, et al: Immunoglobulins in the skin in dermatitis herpetiformis and coeliac disease. Lancet 1: 611-614, 1972.
768. SEAH PP, FRY L, MAZAHERI MR, et al: Alternate pathway complement fixation by IgA in the skin in dermatitis herpetiformis. Lancet 2: 175-177, 1973.
769. SELIGER G, GOLDMAN AB, FIROOZNIA H, LAWRENCE LR: Ulceration of the small intestine complicating celiac disease. Am J Dig Dis 18: 820-824, 1973.
770. SERVELLE M, TURIAF J, ALBEAUX-FERNET M, et al: Sclérose des lymphatiques intestinaux. Sem Hôp Paris 51: 799-806, 1975.
771. SESSIONS JT, VIEGAS DE ANDRADE SR, KOKAS E: Intestinal villi: form and motility in relation to function, in 'Progress in Gastroenterology vol I'. Ed by GB JERZY GLASS; pp 248-260. Grune & Stratton, New York, 1968.
772. SHANBOUR LL, JACOBSON ED: Autoregulatory escape in the gut. Gastroenterology 60: 145-148, 1971.
773. SHEARER MJ, BARKHAN P, WEBSTER GR: Absorption and excretion of an oral dose of tritiated vitamin K_1 in man. Br J Haematol 18: 297-308, 1970.
774. SHEARER MJ, MALLINSON CN, WEBSTER GR, BARKHAN P: Absorption of tritiated vitamin K_1 in patients with fat malabsorption. Gut 11: 1063-1064, 1970.
775. SHEEHY TW, FLOCH MH: 'The small intestine'. Harper & Row, New York, 1964.
776. SHELDON W: Prognosis in early adult life of coeliac children treated with a gluten-free diet. Br Med J 2: 401-404, 1969.
777. SHERR HP, SASAKI Y, NEWMAN A, et al: Detection of bacterial deconjugation of bile salts by a convenient breath-analysis technic. N Eng J Med 285: 656-661, 1971.
778. SHIMODA SS, SAUNDERS DR, RUBIN CE: The Zollinger-Ellison syndrome with steatorrhea. Gastroenterology 55: 705-723, 1968.
779. SHINER M: Duodenal biopsy. Lancet 1: 17-19, 1956.
780. SHINER M: Effect of a gluten-free diet in 17 patients with idiopathic steatorrhea. Am J Dig Dis 8: 969-983, 1963.
781. SHINER M, SHMERLING DH: The immunopathology of coeliac disease. Digestion 5: 69-88, 1972.
782. SHINER M: Ultrastructural changes suggestive of immune reactions in the jejunal mucosa of coeliac children following gluten challenge. Gut 14: 1-12, 1973.
783. SHINER M: Electron microscopy of jejunal mucosa. Clinics in Gastroenterology III, 1: 33-53, 1974.
784. SHMERLING DH, SHINER M: The response of the intestinal mucosa to the intraduodenal instillation of gluten in patients with coeliac disease, in 'Coeliac Disease' .Ed by CC BOOTH, RH DOWLING; pp 64-74. Churchill Livingstone, London, 1970.
785. SHMERLING DH, LEISINGER P, PRADER A: On the familial occurrence of coeliac disease. Acta Paediatr Scand 61: 501, 1972.
786. SHMERLING DH: Screening tests in coeliac disease, in 'Coeliac Disease'. Ed by WTJM HEKKENS, AS PENA; pp 339-345. Stenfert Kroese, Leiden, 1974.

787. SHUSTER S: Adrenal function in chronic wasting diseases. J Clin Endocrinol 20: 675-682, 1960.
788. SHUSTER S, WATSON AJ, MARKS J: Coeliac syndrome in dermatitis herpetiformis. Lancet 1: 1101-1106, 1968.
789. SIGURDSSON G, NUNZIATA V, REINER M, et al: Calcium absorption and excretion in the gut in acromegaly. Clin Endocrinol 2: 187-192, 1973.
790. SILK DBA, KUMAR PJ, PERRETT D, et al: Amino acid and peptide absorption in patients with coeliac disease and dermatitis herpetiformis. Gut 15: 1-8, 1974.
791. SILK DBA, WEBB JPW, LANE AE, et al: Functional differentiation of human jejunum and ileum: A comparison of the handling of glucose, peptides, and amino acids. Gut 15: 444-449, 1974.
792. SILK DBA, KUMAR PJ, WEBB JPW, et al: Ileal function in patients with untreated adult coeliac disease. Gut 16: 261-267, 1975.
793. SIMMONDS WJ, HOFMANN AF, THEODOR E: Absorption of cholesterol from a micellar solution: Intestinal perfusion studies in man. J Clin Invest 46: 874-890, 1967.
794. SIURALA M, IKKALA E: Changes in the upper gastrointestinal tract in leukaemia, malignant lymphoma and multiple myeloma. Ann Med Intern Fenniae 54: 43-46, 1965.
795. SIURALA M, JULKUNEN H, TOIVONEN S, et al: Digestive tract in collagen diseases. Acta Med Scand 178: 13-25, 1965.
796. SIURALA M VARIS K, LAMBERG BA: Intestinal absorption and autoimmunity in endocrine disorders. Acta Med Scand 184: 53-64, 1968.
797. SKOU JC: Enzymatic basis for active transport of Na^+ and K^+ across cell membrane. Physiol Rev 45: 596-617, 1965.
798. SLADEN GE, DAWSON AM: Interrelationships between the absorptions of glucose, sodium and water by the normal human jejunum. Clin Sci 36: 119-132, 1969.
799. SLADEN GE: Conservation of fluid and electrolytes by the human gut. J Clin Pathol 24 Suppl 5, pp 99-107, 1971.
800. SLADEN GE: The pathogenesis of cholera and some wider implications. Gut 14: 671-680, 1973.
801. SLADEN GE, KUMAR PJ: Is the xylose test still a worth-while investigation? Br Med J 3: 223-225, 1973.
802. SLADEN GE: Absorption of fluid and electrolyte in health and disease, in 'Intestinal absorption in man'. Ed by I MCCOLL, GE SLADEN; pp 51-98. Academic Press, London, 1975.
803. SLEISENGER MH: Clinical and metabolic studies in nontropical sprue. N Eng J Med 265: 49-56, 1961.
804. SMITH B: 'The neuropathology of the alimentary tract'. Edward Arnold, London, 1972.
805. SMITH CL, KELLEHER J, LOSOWSKY MS, MORRISH N: The content of vitamin E in British diets. Br J Nutr 26: 89-96, 1971.
806. SMITSKAMP H, KUIPERS FC: Steatorrhoea and ulcerative jejuno-ileitis. Acta Med Scand 177: 37-42, 1965.
807. SMYTH DH: The economy of the columnar epithelial cell. Gut 10: 2-5, 1969.
808. SOERGEL KH, HOFMANN AF: Absorption, in 'Pathofysiology'. Ed by ED FROHLICH; pp 423-453. Lippincott, Philadelphia, 1972.
809. SOLOMONS NW, ROSENBERG IH, SANDSTEAD HH: Zinc nutrition in celiac sprue. Am J Clin Nutr 29: 371-375, 1976.
810. SÖLTOFT J: Immunoglobulin-containing cells in normal jejunal mucosa and in ulcerative colitis and regional enteritis. Scand J Gastroenterol 4: 353-360, 1969.
811. SÖNNICHSEN N, KÖLZSCH J, FRANKE U, et al: Komplexe Untersuchungen zur Pathogenese der Dermatitis herpetiformis unter besonderer Berücksichtigung des Malabsorptionssyndroms. Dermatol Monatschr 157: 631-644, 1971.
812. SPENCER H, LEWIN I, FOWLER J, SAMACHSON J: Influence of dietary calcium intake on Ca^{47} absorption in man. Am J Med 46: 197-205, 1969.
813. SPENCER RP, BOW TM: In vitro transport of radiolabeled vitamins by the small intestine. J Nucl Med 5: 251-258, 1964.
814. SPINGOLA LJ, MEYER JH, GROSSMAN MI: Potentiated pancreatic response to secretin and endogenous cholecystokinin (CCK). Clin Res 18: 175, 1970.

266

815. STENING GF, GROSSMAN MI: Gastrin-related peptides as stimulants of pancreatic and gastric secretion. Am J Physiol 217: 262-266, 1969.
816. STEWART JS, BOOTH CC: Absorbic acid absorption in malabsorption. Clin Sci 27: 15-22, 1964.
817. STEWART JS, POLLOCK DJ, HOFFBRAND AV, et al: A study of proximal and distal intestinal structure and absorptive function in idiopathic steatorrhoea. Q J Med 36: 425-444, 1967.
818. STEWART JS: Clinical and morphologic response to gluten withdrawal. Clinics in Gastroenterology III, 1: 109-126. Saunders, London, 1974.
819. STOELINGA GBA MUNSTER PJJ VAN, SLOOFF JP: Chylous effusions into the intestine in a patient with protein-losing gastroenteropathy. Pediatrics 31: 1011-1018, 1963.
820. STOKES PL, ASQUITH P, HOLMES GKT, et al: Histocompatibility antigens associated with adult coeliac disease. Lancet 2: 162-164, 1972.
821. STOKES PL, ASQUITH P, COOKE WT: Genetics of coeliac disease. Clinics in Gastroenterology II, 3: 547-556, 1973.
822. STOKES PL, HOLMES GKT: Malignancy. Clinics in Gastroenterology III, 1: 159-170, 1974.
823. STRAUSS EW, DONALDSON RM, GARDNER FH: A relationship between intestinal bacteria and the absorption of vitamin B_{12} in rats with diverticula of the small bowel. Lancet 2: 736-738, 1961.
824. STREIFF RR, ROSENBERG IH: Absorption of polyglutamic folic acid. J Clin Invest 46: 1121, 1967.
825. STROBER W: Introduction HL-A in relation to coeliac disease, in 'Coeliac Disease'. Ed by WTJM HEKKENS, AS PENA; pp 203-206. Stenfert Kroese, Leiden, 1974.
826. STROBER W, FALCHUK ZM, ROGENTINE GN, et al: The pathogenesis of gluten-sensitive enteropathy. Ann Intern Med 83: 242-256, 1975.
827. STUBER JL, WIEGMAN H, CROSBY I, GONZALEZ G: Ulcers of the colon and jejunum in celiac disease. Radiol 99: 339-340, 1971.
828. SUM PT, SCHIPPER HL, PRESHAW RM: Canine gastric and pancreatic secretion during intestinal distention and intestinal perfusion with choline derivates. Can J Physiol Pharmacol 47: 115-118, 1969.
829. SUTHERLAND EW, RALL TW: The relation of adenosine 3', 5'-phosphate and phosphorylase to the actions of catecholamines and other hormones. Pharm Rev 12: 265-299, 1960.
830. SUTTON DR, MCLEAN BAIRD I, STEWART JS, COGHILL NF: 'Free' iron loss in atrophic gastritis, post-gastrectomy states, and adult coeliac disease. Lancet 2: 387-390, 1970.
831. TABAQCHALI S, HATZIOANNOU J, BOOTH CC: Bile salt deconjugation and steatorrhoea in patients with the stagnant loop syndrome. Lancet 2: 12-16, 1968.
832. TABAQCHALI S: The pathophysiological role of small intestinal bacterial flora. Scand J Gastroenterol 5, suppl 6: 139-163, 1970.
833. TABAQCHALI S, PALLIS C: Reversible nicotinamide-deficiency encephalopathy in a patient with jejunal diverticulosis. Gut 11: 1024-1028, 1970.
834. TANDON BN, BANKS PA, GEORGE PK, et al: Recovery of exocrine pancreatic function in adult protein calorie malnutrition. Gastroenterology 58: 358-362, 1970.
835. TARLOW MJ, HADORN B, ARTHURTON MW, LLOYD JK: Intestinal enterokinase deficiency. A newly recognised disorder of protein digestion. Arch Dis Child 45: 651-655, 1970.
836. TAYLOR B, SOKOL G: Cystic fibrosis and coeliac disease: Report of two cases. Arch Dis Child 48: 692-696, 1973.
837. TAYLOR KB, THOMSON DL, TRUELOVE SC, WRIGHT R: An immunological study of coeliac disease and idiopathic steatorrhoea. Br Med J 2: 1727-1731, 1961.
838. TAYLOR WH: Water diuresis in idiopathic steatorrhoea. Clin Sci 13: 239-245, 1954.
839. TAYLOR WH: Water diuresis in idiopathic steatorrhoea. Clin Sci 14: 725-730, 1955.
840. TEXTER EC, CHOU CC, LAURETA HC, VANTRAPPEN GR: 'Physiology of the gastrointestinal tract'. Mosby, St Louis, 1968.
841. THOMPSON GR, LEWIS B, BOOTH CC: Absorption of vitamin D_3-^3H in control subjects and patients with intestinal malabsorption. J Clin Invest 45: 94-102, 1966.
842. THOMPSON GR: Absorption of fat-soluble vitamins and sterols. J Clin Pathol 24, suppl 5: 85-89, 1971.
843. THOMPSON H: The small intestine at autopsy. Clinics in Gastroenterology III, 1: 171-181, 1974.

844. THOMPSON MW: Heredity, maternal age, and birth order in the etiology of celiac disease. Am J Hum Genet 3: 159-166, 1951.
845. THOMSON AD: The absorption of radioactive sulphur-labelled thiamine hydrochloride in control subjects and in patients with intestinal malabsorption. Clin Sci 31: 167-179, 1966.
846. THYS O, MAINGUET P: Etude clinique de la maladie coeliaque de l'adulte: évolution classique et formes atypiques. Acta Gastroenterol Belg 34: 472-483, 1971.
847. TOFFLER AH, HUKILL PB, SPIRO HM: Brown bowel syndrome. Ann Intern Med 58: 872-877, 1963.
848. TONGEREN JHM VAN, REICHERT WJ, KAMPHUYS TM: The quantitative estimation of gastrointestinal protein loss, using ^{51}Cr-labelled plasma proteins. Clin Chim Acta 14: 42-48, 1966.
849. TONGEREN JHM VAN, STAAK WJBM VAN DER, SCHILLINGS PHM: Small-bowel changes in dermatitis herpetiformis. Lancet 1: 218, 1967.
850. TONGEREN JHM VAN: Eiwitverlies via de darmwand. MD Thesis, Nijmegen, 1967.
851. TONGEREN JHM VAN, BREED WPM, CORSTENS FHM, et al: Fatty liver and malabsorption. Folia Med Neerl 15: 246-258, 1972.
852. TOSKES PP, DEREN JJ: Vitamin B_{12} absorption and malabsorption. Gastroenterology 65: 662-683, 1973.
853. TOTHILL P, DELLIPIANI AW, CALVERT J: Plasma concentrations of radiocalcium after oral administration and their relationship to absorption. Clin Sci 38: 27-39, 1970.
854. TOWNLEY RRW: Celiac disease – An inborn error of metabolism. Am J Dig Dis 18: 797-800, 1973.
855. TREADWELL CR, VAHOUNY GV: Cholesterol absorption, in 'Handbook of Physiology' section 6, 3. Ed by CF CODE; pp 1407-1438. American Physiological Society, Washington, 1968.
856. TRIER JS, RUBIN CE: Electron microscopy of the small intestine: a review. Gastroenterology 49: 574-603, 1965.
857. TRIER JS: Morphology of the epithelium of the small intestine, in 'Handbook of Physiology' section 6, 3. Ed by CF CODE; pp 1125-1176. American Physiological Society, Washington, 1968.
858. TRIER JS: The surface coat of gastrointestinal epithelial cells. Gastroenterology 56: 618-622, 1969.
859. TRIER JS, BROWNING TH: Epithelial-cell renewal in cultured duodenal biopsies in celiac sprue. N Eng J Med 283: 1245-1250, 1970.
860. TRIER JS: Anatomy of the small intestine, in 'Gastrointestinal disease'. Ed by MH SLEISENGER, JS FORDTRAN; pp 840-853. Saunders, Philadelphia, 1973.
861. TRIERJS: Celiac sprue disease in ''Gastrointestinal disease'' Ed by MN SLEISENGER, JS FORDTRAN; pp 864-885. Saunders, Philadelphia, 1973.
862. TRIER JS: Organ culture of intestinal mucosa, in 'Coeliac disease'.Ed by WTJM HEKKENS, AS PENA; pp 81-88. Stenfert Kroese, Leiden, 1974.
863. TURNBERG LA, FORDTRAN JS, CARTER NW, RECTOR FC: Mechanism of bicarbonate absorption and its relationship to sodium transport in the human jejunum. J Clin Invest 49: 548-556, 1970.
864. TURNBERG LA: Potassium transport in the human small bowel. Gut 12: 811-818, 1971.
865. TYTGAT GN, RUBIN CE, SAUNDERS DR: Synthesis and transport of lipoprotein particles by intestinal absorptive cells in man. J Clin Invest 50: 2065-2078, 1971.
866. UGOLEV AM: Membrane (contact) digestion. Physiol Rev 45: 555-595, 1965.
867. UGOLEV AM: Membrane digestion. Gut 13: 735-743, 1972.
868. UNGER RH, KETTERER H, DUPRÉ J: The effects of secretin, pancreozymin and gastrin on insulin and glucagon secretion in anesthetized dogs. J Clin Invest 46: 630-645, 1967.
869. VALLEE BL, WACKER WEC, ULMER DD: Magnesiumdeficiency tetany syndrome in man. N Eng J Med 262: 155-161, 1960.
870. VEGHELYI PV, KEMENY TT: Protein metabolism and pancreatic function, in 'The exocrine pancreas'. Ed by AVS DE REUCK, MP CAMERON; pp 329-349. Churchill, London, 1962.
871. VINNIK IE, KERN F, STRUTHERS JE: Malabsorption and the diarrhea of diabetes mellitus. Gastroenterology 43: 507-520, 1962.
872. VISAKORPI JK, IMMONEN P: Intolerance to cow's milk and wheat gluten in the primary

malabsorption syndrome in infancy. Acta Paediatr Scand 56: 49-56, 1967.

873. VISAKORPI JK: Diabetes and coeliac disease. Lancet 2: 1192, 1969.
874. VISAKORPI JK, KUITUNEN P, PELKONEN P: Intestinal malabsorption: a clinical study of 22 children over 2 years of age. Acta Paediatr Scand 59: 273-280, 1970.
875. VISAKORPI JK: An international inquiry concerning the diagnostic criteria of coeliac disease. Acta Paediatr Scand 59: 463-464, 1970.
876. VISAKORPI JK: Definition of coeliac disease in children, in 'Coeliac Disease'. Ed by WTJM HEKKENS, AS PENA; pp 10-16. Stenfert Kroese, Leiden, 1974.
877. WACKER WEC, PARISI AF: Magnesium metabolism. N Eng J Med 278: 658-663, 712-717, 1968.
878. WAGONFELD JB, DUDZINSKI D, ROSENBERG IH: Analysis of rate controlling processes in polyglutamyl folate absorption. Clin Res 23: 259a, 1975.
879. WALDMANN TA: Protein-losing enteropathy. Gastroenterology 50: 422-443, 1966.
880. WALDRAM R: Mechanisms of lipid loss from the small intestinal mucosa. Gut 16: 118-124, 1975.
881. WALIA BNS, SIDHU JK, TANDON BN, et al: Coeliac disease in north indian children. Br Med J 2: 1233-1234, 1966.
882. WALKER WA, ISSELBACHER KJ: Uptake and transport of macromolecules by the intestine. Gastroenterology 67: 531-550, 1974.
883. WALKER-SMITH J: Transient gluten intolerance. Arch Dis Child 45: 523-526, 1970.
884. WALKER-SMITH J, ANDREWS J: Alpha-1-antitrypsin, autism, and coeliac disease. Lancet 2: 883-884, 1972.
885. WALKER-SMITH JA: Discordance for childhood coeliac disease in monozygotic twins. Gut 14: 374-375, 1973.
886. WALL AJ, DOUGLAS AP, BOOTH CC, PEARSE AGE: Response of the jejunal mucosa in adult coeliac disease to oral prednisolone. Gut 11: 7-14, 1970.
887. WALLING MW, ROTHMAN SS: Kinetic evidence for active carrier-mediated calcium transport across the small intestine. Fed Proc 27: 386, 1968.
888. WALSH J: Control of gastric secretion, in 'Gastrointestinal disease'. Ed by MH SLEISENGER, JS FORDTRAN; pp 144-162. Saunders, Philadelphia, 1973.
889. WALSH JH, GROSSMAN MI: Gastrin. N Eng J Med 292:1324-1334, 1377-1384, 1975.
890. WARSHAW AL, WALKER WA, CORNELL R, ISSELBACHER KJ: Small intestinal permeability to macromolecules. Lab Invest 25: 675-684, 1971.
891. WARSHAW AL, WALKER WA, ISSELBACHER KJ: Protein uptake by the intestine: evidence for absorption of intact macromolecules. Gastroenterology 66: 987-992, 1974.
892. WASSERMAN RH, CORRADINO RA, TAYLOR AN: Vitamine D-dependent calcium-binding protein: purification and some properties. J Biol Chem 243: 3978-3986, 1968.
893. WATERS AH, MOLLIN DL: Studies on the folic acid activity of human serum. J Clin Pathol 14, 335-344, 1961.
894. WATSON AJ, WRIGHT NA: Morphology and cell kinetics of the jejunal mucosa in untreated patients. Clinics in Gastroenterology III, 1: 11-31, 1974.
895. WATSON WC, PATON E, MURRAY D: Small bowel disease in rosacea. Lancet 2: 47-50, 1965.
896. WAYTE DM, HELWIG EB: Small-bowel ulceration – iatrogenic or multifactorial origin. Am J Clin Pathol 49: 26-40, 1968.
897. WEBB MGT, TAYLOR MRH, GATENBY PBB: Iron absorption in coeliac disease of childhood and adolescence. Br Med J 2: 151-152, 1967.
898. WEBLING DDA, HOLDSWORTH ES: Bile salts and calcium absorption. Biochem J 100: 652-660, 1966.
899. WEINSTEIN LD, HERSKOVIC T: Rectal seepage of oil in a patient with celiac disease and secondary pancreatic insufficiency. Am J Dig Dis 13: 762-765, 1968.
900. WEINSTEIN WM, SAUNDERS DR, TIJTGAT GN, RUBIN CE: Collagenous sprue – an unrecognized type of malabsorption. N Eng J Med 283: 1297-1301, 1970.
901. WEINSTEIN WM: Latent celiac sprue. Gastroenterology 66: 489-493, 1974.
902. WEINTRAUB LR, CONRAD ME, CROSBY WH: Regulation of the intestinal absorption of iron by the rate of erythropoiesis. Brit J Haematol 11: 432-438, 1965.
903. WEINTRAUB LR, WEINSTEIN MB, HUSER HJ, RAFAL S: Absorption of haemoglobin iron: the role of a haem-splitting substance in the intestinal mucosa. J Clin Invest 47: 531-539, 1968.

904. WEISER MM, DOUGLAS AP: An alternative mechanism for gluten toxicity in coeliac disease. Lancet 1: 567-569, 1976.
905. WELLS GC: Skin disorders in relation to malabsorption. Br Med J 2: 937-943, 1962.
906. WENSEL RH, RICH C, BROWN AC, VOLWILER W: Absorption of calcium measured by intubation and perfusion of the intact human small intestine. J Clin Invest 48: 1768-1775, 1969.
907. WESER E, SLEISENGER MH: Lactosuria and lactase deficiency in adult celiac disease. Gastroenterology 48: 571-578, 1965.
908. WEIJERS HA: De vetabsorptie van gezonde en zieke zuigelingen en kinderen in het bijzonder van coeliakie patiënten. MD Thesis, Utrecht, 1950.
909. WHEBY MS: Site of iron absorption in man. Scand J Haematol 7: 56-62, 1970.
910. WHITE AG, BARNETSON RSC, DA COSTA JAG, MCCLELLAND DBL: The incidence of HL-A antigens in dermatitis herpetiformis. Br J Dermatol 89: 133-136, 1973.
911. WHITECROSS DP, ARMSTRONG C, CLARKE AD, PIPER DW: The pepsinogens of human gastric mucosa. Gut 14: 850-855, 1973.
912. WHITEHEAD R: Primary lymphadenopathy complicating idiopathic steatorrhoea. Gut 9: 569-575, 1968.
913. WHITEHEAD R: The interpretation and significance of morphological abnormalities in jejunal biopsies. J Clin Pathol, 24 suppl 5: 108-124, 1971.
914. WHORWELL PJ, ALDERSON MR, FOSTER KJ, WRIGHT R: Death from ischaemic heart-disease and malignancy in adult patients with coeliac disease. Lancet 2: 113-114, 1976.
915. WIERINGEN JC VAN: Seculaire groeiverschuiving. PhD Thesis, Leiden, 1972.
916. WILCOXON F: Individual comparisons by ranking methods. Biometrics Bull I: 80-83, 1945.
917. WILK P, KARIPINENI R, DREILING DA, DANESE C: Studies of the effects of blockage of intestinal lymphatics. Am J Gastroenterol 63: 400-403, 1975.
918. WILLIAMS REO, HILL MJ, DRASAR BS: The influence of intestinal bacteria on the absorption and metabolism of foreign compounds. J Clin Pathol, 24 suppl 5: 125-129, 1971.
919. WILLIAMSON JM, GOLDBERG A, MOORE FML: Leucocyte ascorbic acid levels in patients with malabsorption or previous gastric surgery. Br Med J 2: 23-25, 1967.
920. WILLS MR, DAY RC, PHILLIPS JB, BATEMAN EC: Phytic acid and nutritional rickets in immigrants. Lancet 1: 771-773, 1970.
921. WILSON JP: Surface area of the small intestine in man. Gut 8: 618-621, 1967.
922. WINTROBE MM, LEE GR, BOGGS DR, et al: 'Clinical Hematology'. Lea & Febiger, Philadelphia, 1974.
923. WISEMAN G: 'Absorption from the intestine'. Academic Press, London, 1964.
924. WOLLAEGER EE, SCRIBNER BH: Delayed excretion of water with regular nocturnal diuresis in patients with nontropical sprue (idiopathic steatorrhea). Gastroenterology 19: 224-240, 1951.
925. WOODLEY JF, KEANE R: Enterokinase levels in intestinal mucosa from normal subjects and patients with coeliac disease. Gut 13: 850-851, 1972.
926. WOODLEY JF: Pyrrolidonecarboxylyl peptidase activity in normal intestinal biopsies and those from coeliac patients. Clin Chim Acta 42: 211-213, 1972.
927. WORWOOD M, EDWARDS A, JACOBS A: A non-ferritin iron compound in the rat small intestinal mucosa during iron absorption. Nature 229: 409-410, 1971.
928. WRAY D, FERGUSON MM, MASON DK, et al: Recurrent aphthae: treatment with vitamin B_{12}, folic acid, and iron. Br Med J 2: 490-493, 1975.
929. WRIGHT N, WATSON A, MORLEY A, et al: Cell kinetics in flat (avillous) mucosa of the human small intestine. Gut 14: 701-710, 1973.
930. WIJK N VAN: 'Franck's etymologisch woordenboek der Nederlandsche taal', 2nd ed; p 653. Martinus Nijhoff, 's-Gravenhage, 1971.
931. YAMAGUCHI N, ROSENTHAL WS, GLASS GBJ: Study of the intestinal absorption of ^{61}Cr-labeled intrinsic factor. Am J Clin Nutr 23: 156-164, 1970.
932. YAP SH, HAFKENSCHEID JCM, TONGEREN JHM VAN, TRIJBELS JMF: Rate of synthesis of albumin in relation to serum levels of essential amino acid in patients with bacterial overgrowth in the small bowel. Europ J Clin Invest 4: 279-284, 1974.
933. YAP SH: De synthese en afbraak van albumine bij de mens onder normale en patho-logische omstandigheden. MD Thesis, Nijmegen, 1975.
934. YAP SH, HAFKENSCHEID JCM, TONGEREN JHM VAN: Important role of tryptophan on

270

albumin synthesis in patients suffering from anorexia nervosa and hypoalbuminemia. Am J Clin Nutr 28: 1356-1363, 1975.

935. YARDLEY JH, BAYLESS TM, NORTON JH, HENDRIX TR: Celiac disease. A study of the jejunal epithelium before and after a gluten-free diet. N Eng J Med 267: 1173-1179, 1962.

936. YOUNG WF, PRINGLE EM: 110 children with coeliac disease, 1950-1969. Arch Dis Child 46: 421-436, 1971.

937. ZIEVE L. SILVIS SE, MULFORD B, BLACKWOOD WD: Secretion of pancreatic enzymes. I, Response to secretin and pancreozymin. Am J Dig Dis 11: 671-684, 1966.

SURVEY OF REFERENCES TO PATIENTS

PATIENT	YEAR OF BIRTH	SEX	CASE HISTORY	TEXT	TABLE	FIGURE
# 1	1929	m			6.3, 7.8 7.10	
# 2	1912	m	p 207	pp 202, 204, 206, 209, 219, 224	6.4, 7.10	11.3
# 3	1923	m				
# 4	1932	m				
# 5	1910	m	p 202	pp 90, 202, 204	6.3, 6.4, 7.8, 7.10, 9.4	6.3
# 6	1924	m				
# 7	1945	f			6.4	
# 8	1922	f				
# 9	1926	m			7.13	
# 10	1921	m			7.10, 7.13	
# 11	1931	m				
# 12	1934	f				
# 13	1925	f			6.3, 7.10	
# 14	1943	f				
# 15	1938	f				
# 16	1939	f				
# 17	1921	f	p 200	pp 202, 204, 219, 224	6.2	9.7, 11.3
# 18	1938	f				
# 19	1932	f				9.3
# 20	1940	f			6.2, 6.3, 7.8, 7.10	
# 21	1914	f	p 204	p 204	6.4	
# 22	1930	f			6.4	
# 23	1925	f				
# 24	1944	f				
# 25	1915	m				
# 26	1912	m			6.3, 7.8	
# 27	1914	f	p 205	pp 204, 206	6.3, 7.8, 7.16	
# 28	1904	m			6.3, 7.10	
# 29	1926	f			6.3, 7.10, 7.13	
# 30	1925	f			6.3, 7.8, 7.10	

PATIENT	YEAR OF BIRTH	SEX	CASE HISTORY	TEXT	TABLE	FIGURE
# 31	1887	m			9.1	
# 32	1949	f			6.3, 7.13	
# 33	1943	f				
# 34	1903	m	p 206	pp 90, 204, 224	7.10	6.4, 11.3
# 35	1932	f			9.1	
# 36	1934	f				9.2
# 37	1921	f				
# 38	1938	f				
# 39	1918	m				
# 40	1931	f			6.4	
# 41	1926	f				
# 42	1935	f				
# 43	1933	f				
# 44	1938	m				
# 45	1912	f			6.4	
# 46	1912	f	p 219	pp 202, 204, 223	6.2. 11.1	11.1
# 47	1925	m	p 207	p. 204		

Sympathetic (cf Autonomic nervous system)
Symptomatology (cf Coeliac sprue)

Target cells   183
Tetany   75, 88, 144, 157, 158, 184, 192
Thiamine   83, 84, 177, 181, 185, 186
Thrombotest   70, 126, 127, 135
Thyroid hormone   75
Tight junction   49, 55, 57, 102
Transcobalamin   81
Transferrin   77
Transit time   54, 61, 89-91, 107, 112, 117, 121, 158
Translocation process   54, 55, 57, 58, 60, 63, 72
Transport carriers   54, 55, 57, 63, 72, 76, 79, 82, 117, 141, 175
Treatment antibiotics   91, 92, 107, 109, 168, 170, 175, 183
- azathioprine   203
- corticosteroids   5, 8, 15, 16, 165, 201-203, 206, 218, 223, 226
- fungistatics   107
- (cf Dietary restriction, Replacement therapy)
Triglyceride absorption   53, 64, 66, 93, 133
- emulsification   64, 66
- hydrolysis   64, 66
- intake   63
- long-chain   63, 93
- medium- chain   63, 64, 66
- re-esterification   66, 133
- short-chain   63
- solubilization   64, 66
Tropical sprue   1, 2, 226
Trypsin   42, 71, 97, 140
Tuberculosis   95, 230

Unclassified sprue (cf Coeliac sprue)
Unstirred layer   33, 55, 56, 91

Vasoconstriction/-dilatation (cf Blood vessels)
Vertigo   75, 183
Villikinin   33
Villus aspect   19, 20, 28
- atrophy   5-8, 23, 25, 86, 91, 93, 197, 198, 213-215, 223
- histology   21, 25
- motility   33, 41, 91

Vitamin A absorption   133
- body stores   68
- deficiency   68, 186
- dietary sources   68
- precursors   68
- serum level   68, 124, 127, 133, 134
- synthesis   68
- tolerance test   125, 127, 134, 135
Vitamin B_1 (cf Thiamine)
Vitamin B_2 (cf Riboflavin)
Vitamin B_3 (cf Niacin)
Vitamin B_6 84, 177, 186
Vitamin B_{12} absorption   31, 80, 81, 108, 109, 170, 171, 183
- body stores   80, 171
- consumption   170
- deficiency   161, 169, 171, 183
- degradation   80, 170
- dietary sources   80
- endogenous loss   81, 100, 103
- function   80
- hydrolysis   80
- intake   80
- requirements   80
- serum level   81, 162, 166, 171, 186, 214
- synthesis   80
- transport   81
Vitamin C   83, 176, 177, 183
Vitamin D absorption   133, 153, 154, 183
- deficiency   69, 152, 154, 183, 184
- dietary sources   69
- function   69, 75, 77, 153
- metabolism   67, 69, 75
- resistance   69, 153
- serum level   153
Vitamin E absorption   133
- deficiency   69, 91, 134
- dietary sources   69
- function   69
- serum level   125, 127, 133-135
Vitamin K   70, 133, 183
Vomiting (cf Nausea)

Water absorption   43, 46, 59-61, 110-112
- intake   59
- loss   59
- requirements   59
- secretion   43, 45, 97, 111, 112
Weight loss (cf Body weight)

Xylose (cf D-xylose)